Muscle Energy Techniques

With accompanying DVD

Leon Chaitow ND DO

Registered Osteopathic Practitioner and Senior Lecturer, University of Westminster, London, UK

With contributions by
Ken Crenshaw BS ATC CSCS
Sandy Fritz BS MS
Gary Fryer BSc ND DO
Craig Liebenson DC
Ron J Porterfield BS ATC
Nathan Shaw ATC CSCS
Eric Wilson PT DSc OCS SCS CSCS

Foreword by
Donald R Murphy DC DACAN

Illustrations by
Graeme Chambers BA(Hons)
Medical Artist

THIRD EDITION

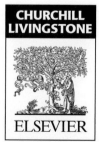

CHURCHILL
LIVINGSTONE

ELSEVIER

EDINBURGH   LONDON   NEW YORK   OXFORD   PHILADELPHIA   ST LOUIS   SYDNEY   TORONTO 2006

CHURCHILL
LIVINGSTONE
ELSEVIER

An imprint of Elsevier Limited

© Pearson Professional Limited 1996
© Elsevier Limited 1999
© 2006, Elsevier Limited. All rights reserved.

First edition 1996
Second edition 1999
Third edition 2006

ISBN 10: 0443 101140
ISBN 13: 978 0443 101144

British Library Cataloguing in Publication Data
A catalogue record for this book is available from the British Library

Library of Congress Cataloging in Publication Data
A catalog record for this book is available from the Library of Congress

---

Notice

Neither the Publisher nor the Author assume any responsibility for any loss or injury and/or damage to persons or property arising out of or related to any use of the material contained in this book. It is the responsibility of the treating practitioner, relying on independent expertise and knowledge of the patient, to determine the best treatment and method of application for the patient.

The Publisher

Printed in China

Muscle Energy Techniques

For Churchill Livingstone:

Senior Commissioning Editor: Sarena Wolfaard
Associate Editor: Claire Wilson
Project Manager: David Fleming
Design: Stewart Larking
Illustration Manager: Bruce Hogarth

Treatment table in the CD-Rom videoclips supplied
by Russell Medical Worcestershire UK.

Contents

The CD-ROM accompanying this text includes video sequences of all the techniques indicated in the text by the icon. To look at the video for a given technique, click on the relevant icon in the contents list on the CD-ROM. The CD-ROM is designed to be used in conjunction with the text and not as a stand-alone product.

Contributors vii

Foreword ix

Preface xi

Acknowledgements xiii

1. **An introduction to muscle energy techniques** 1

2. **Patterns of function and dysfunction** 23

3. **How to use MET** 77

4. **MET: efficacy and research** 107
   Gary Fryer

5. **Sequential assessment and MET treatment of main postural muscles** 131

6. **MET and the treatment of joints** 199

7. **Integrated neuromuscular inhibition technique (INIT)** 247

8. **Manual resistance techniques in rehabilitation** 257
   Craig Liebenson

9. **MET in the physical therapy setting** 273
   Eric Wilson

10. **MET in a massage therapy setting** 299
    Sandy Fritz

11. **MET in treatment of athletic injuries** 311
    Ken Crenshaw, Nathan Shaw, Ron J Porterfield

    Index 341

Contributors

Ken Crenshaw BS ATC CSCS
Head Athletic Trainer, Arizona Diamondbacks
Baseball Team, Phoenix, AZ, USA

Sandy Fritz BS MS
Director, Health Enrichment Center, School of
Therapeutic Massage, Lapeer, MI, USA

Gary Fryer BSc ND DO
Senior Lecturer, School of Health Science,
Victoria University, Melbourne, Australia;
Centre for Aging, Rehabilitation, Exercise and
Sport, Victoria University, Melbourne, Australia

Craig Liebenson DC
L.A. Sports and Spine, Los Angeles, CA, USA

Ron J Porterfield BS ATC
Head Athletic Trainer, Tampa Bay Devil Rays
Baseball Team, St Petersburg, FL, USA

Nathan Shaw ATC CSCS
Strength and Conditioning Coordinator,
Arizona Diamondbacks Baseball Team, Phoenix,
AZ, USA

Eric Wilson PT DSc OCS SCS CSCS
Chief, Physical Therapy Element, 7th MDG,
Dyess Air Force Base, TX, USA

Foreword

As the art and science of neuromusculoskeletal care evolve, it is becoming increasingly clear that manual techniques are essential in the proper management of patients with problems in this area. What is less easily measured, however, is the impact of the degree of skill with which these techniques are applied on the outcome of management. Most clinicians who use manual techniques in the treatment of dysfunction in the locomotor system would agree, however, that the level of skill with which a practitioner applies a certain technique is of the utmost importance in the success of any management strategy. Intuition would tell us that a clinician with limited skill and a limited variety of methods in his or her armamentarium would be less effective, especially for a difficult case, than one who possesses wide-ranging knowledge and ability.

It has been said that "you can't learn manual skills from a book". However, you can build upon an existing body of knowledge, skill and experience with a written source that introduces new methodology and instructs in the scientific basis and proper application of one's current methodology. In addition, a written source of high-quality, clinically applicable information can be an excellent source of support material when one is taking an undergraduate or postgraduate course in manual therapy. Dr. Chaitow has produced such a book.

One of the unique aspects of manual therapy that one discovers early on in practice is that no two patients are alike and no two locomotor systems are alike. As a result, each patient requires a highly individualized approach that addresses his or her unique circumstances. This means that one must be meticulous about identifying those specific dysfunctions, be they joint, muscle or otherwise, that are most important in producing the disorder from which the patient suffers, and choosing those specific treatment approaches that are most likely to correct the identified dysfunctions. Muscle energy techniques (METs) are among the most valuable tools that any manual clinician can have in his or her tool box. There are many reasons for this.

First, METs have a wide application. This is exemplified by the presence in this edition of chapters specific to massage therapy, physical therapy and athletic training. METs can be applied to muscle hypertonicity and muscle tightness, but can be equally effectively applied to joint dysfunction and joint capsule adhesions. They can be applied to little old ladies or high level athletes, and anyone in between. Important modifications must be made for each application and each individual, as is demonstrated in this book. But because the method is as flexible as it is, the clinician is provided with a tool that he or she can modify for a variety of types of dysfunction, and a variety of types of patients.

Second, METs can be applied in a gentle manner. In manual therapy, we always want to be as gentle as possible, in a way that still provides effective correction of dysfunction. MET, particularly when applied to muscle hypertonicity and to joint dysfunction, is both gentle and effective. For those of us who use thrust techniques, METs also represent a different method of applying joint manipulation that is well tolerated by the apprehensive patient, or the acute situation. And, MET has been shown to be equally effective as thrust techniques.

Third, METs actively involve the patient in the process. One of the essential ingredients in a successful management strategy involves empowering the patient to take charge of his or her own recovery. This means that the patient must not be a passive recipient of treatment, but rather and active participant. Unlike many manual procedures, with METs the patient must be involved in every step, contracting at the appropriate time, relaxing at the appropriate time, engaging in eye movements, breathing, etc. METs allow the clinician to apply corrective measures while at the same time beginning the process of transferring responsibility to the patient.

Finally, METs are effective. As Dr. Fryer demonstrates in his chapter, the research into the clinical efficacy of METs is in it's infancy. And he also points out the interesting challenges to effective research in this area. However, Dr. Fryer also reveals that those studies that have begun to assess whether METs have an impact on clinical outcome have suggested that, when an overall management strategy includes the use of skilled METs, patients benefit to a greater degree than when these methods are not included. In this book, not only is this research presented, but also, in Dr. Liebenson's chapter, the reader is instructed as to how these techniques can be incorporated into the overall rehabilitation strategy. I can say for myself that I could not imagine how I would attempt to manage the majority of patients that I see without METs at my disposal.

But, for all these benefits of METs to be realized, one must apply them with skill and precision. And they must be applied in the context of a management strategy that takes into consideration the entire person. This book represents an important step in this direction.

Donald R. Murphy, DC, DACAN
Clinical Director, Rhode Island Spine Center
Clinical Assistant Professor,
Brown University School of Medicine
Adjunct Associate Professor of Research,
New York Chiropractic College
Providence, RI USA

Preface

What has surprised and excited me most about the content of this third edition is the speed with which research and new methods of using MET have made the previous edition relatively out of date. It's not that the methods described in previous editions are inaccurate, but rather that the theoretical explanations as to how MET 'works' may have been over-simplistic. The diligent research, much of it from Australia, that is outlined by Gary Fryer DO in Chapter 4, reveals mechanisms previously unsuspected, and this may well change the way muscle energy methods are used clinically.

In addition, increasingly refined and focused ways of using the variety of MET methods are emerging, and excitingly many of these are from professions other than the usual osteopathic backgrounds.

MET emerged initially from osteopathic tradition, but what has become clear is just how well it has travelled into other disciplines, with chapters in this book variously describing MET usage in chiropractic rehabilitation, physical therapy, athletic training and massage contexts. For example:

In Chapter 8 a chiropractic perspective is offered by Craig Liebenson DC, in which MET is seen to offer major benefits in rehabilitation. The evolution of the methods outlined in that chapter also cross-fertilize with the pioneering manual medicine approaches as taught by Vladimir Janda MD and Karel Lewit MD, with both of whom Liebenson trained. These East European giants collaborated and worked with some of the osteopathic developers of MET.

The clinical use of MET in treating acute low-back pain in physical therapy settings, as described in detail in Chapter 9, has identified very precise MET applications in which acutely distressed spinal joints have been successfully treated and rehabilitated.

Captain Eric Wilson PT Dsc, author of that chapter, gained his MET knowledge from impeccable sources at Michigan State University's School of Osteopathic Medicine.

There are fascinating descriptions in Chapter 11 of MET as used by athletic trainers Ken Crenshaw, Nate Shaw and Ron Porterfield in the context of a professional baseball team's (Tampa Bay Devil Rays) need to help their athletes to remain functional, despite overuse patterns that would not be easily tolerated by normal mortals.

Chapter 10 provides a respite from extremes of pain and overuse and illustrates the efficiency with which MET can be incorporated into normal therapeutic massage settings. Here Sandy Fritz MS describes incorporation of these safe and effective approaches in ways that avoid breaking the natural flow of a traditional bodywork setting.

From my own perspective I am increasingly exploring the dual benefits gained by use of slow eccentric isotonic contraction/stretches (see Chapters 3 and 5), and of the remarkably efficient 'pulsed' MET methods devised by Ruddy (1962) over half a century ago and described in Chapters 3 and 6.

In short, the expanded content of this third edition highlights the growing potential of MET in multidisciplinary and integrated settings and, by offering an updated evidence base, takes us closer to understanding the mechanisms involved in its multiple variations.

Leon Chaitow ND DO
Corfu, Greece 2005

REFERENCES

Ruddy T J 1962 Osteopathic rhythmic resistive technic. Academy of Applied Osteopathy Yearbook 1962, pp 23–31

Acknowledgements

As in previous editions, my respect and appreciation go to the osteopathic and manual medicine pioneers who developed MET, and to those who continue its expanding use in different professional settings.

My profound thanks also go to the remarkable group of health care professionals who have contributed their time and efforts to the chapters they have authored in this new edition: Ken Crenshaw, Sandy Fritz, Gary Fryer, Craig Liebenson, Ron Porterfield, Nate Shaw and Eric Wilson.

Only those who have undertaken the writing of a chapter for someone else's book will know the effort it requires, and the space to accomplish this commonly has to be carved out of non-existent spare time. I truly cannot thank any of you enough!

I wish to thank the editorial staff at Elsevier in Edinburgh, in particular Sarena Wolfaard and Claire Wilson, who continue to help me to solve the inevitable problems associated with compilation of a new edition, not least those linked to the filming of new material for the CD-ROM.

And, for creating and maintaining the tranquil and supportive environment in Corfu that allowed me to work on this text, my unqualified thanks and love go to my wife Alkmini.

An introduction to muscle energy techniques

1

CHAPTER CONTENTS

Muscle energy techniques (MET)   1
The route of dysfunction   1
Revolution or evolution   3
MET by any other name   3
History   3
Early sources of MET   7
Postisometric relaxation and reciprocal inhibition:
two forms of MET   8
Key points about modern MET   9
Variations on the MET theme   12
Lewit's postisometric relaxation method
(Lewit 1999a)   13
What may be happening?   14
Why fibrosis occurs naturally   16
Putting it together   17
Why MET might be ineffective at times   18
To stretch or to strengthen   18
Tendons   18
Joints and MET   20
References   21

Muscle energy techniques (MET)

Muscle energy techniques are a class of soft tissue osteopathic (originally) manipulation methods that incorporate precisely directed and controlled, patient initiated, isometric and/or isotonic contractions, designed to improve musculoskeletal function and reduce pain.

As will be seen in later chapters, MET methods have transferred to almost all other manual therapeutic settings. Liebenson (chiropractic, Ch. 8), Wilson (physical therapy, Ch. 9), Fritz (massage therapy, Ch. 10) and Crenshaw and colleagues (athletic training, Ch. 11) have all described the usefulness, in their professional work, of incorporating MET methodology, while in Ch. 4 Fryer evaluates the evidence base for MET.

The route to dysfunction

Why and how we lose functional balance, flexibility, stability and strength differs from person to person, although the basic formula leading to altered functionality inevitably contains similar ingredients.

Ignoring for the moment psychosocial (anxiety, fear, depression, etc.) and biochemical (nutritional status, hormonal balance, etc.) issues, we might consider the decline into dysfunction from a largely biomechanical perspective. It should be possible to agree that the nature and degree of the demands of our active, or inactive, daily life, work and leisure activities, as well as our individual relationships with the close environment (shoes, chairs, cars, etc.), define the adaptive changes that are superimposed on our unique inherited and acquired characteristics. Leaving aside the effects of trauma, how our structures respond to the repetitive demands of living, and habits of use (posture, gait, breathing patterns, etc.), determines the dysfunctional configurations that emerge.

Liebenson (2000) has observed that to prevent musculoskeletal injury and dysfunction the individual needs to avoid undue mechanical stress (excessive adaptive demands), while at the same time improving flexibility and stability in order to acquire greater tolerance to strain. The lead author of this book has expressed Liebenson's observation differently, as follows (Chaitow & DeLany 2005):

> *Benefit will usually emerge if any treatment reduces the overall stress load to which the person is adapting (whether this be chemical, psychological, physical, or a combination of these), or if the person's mind-body can be helped to cope/adapt more efficiently to that load.*

Liebenson (2000) suggests that there is evidence that too little (or infrequent) tissue stress can be just as damaging as too much (or too frequent, or too prolonged) exposure to biomechanical stress. In other words, deconditioning through inactivity provokes dysfunction just as efficiently as does excessive, repetitive and inappropriate biomechanical stress.

If, over time, as a result of too little or too much in the way of adaptive demand, pathological changes occur in soft tissues and joints, the consequences are likely to include altered (commonly reduced) functional efficiency, often with painful consequences.

It was Korr (1976) who described the musculoskeletal system as 'the primary machinery of life.' It is, after all, largely through that system that we express our uniqueness, by means of which we walk, and move, dance, run, paint, lift and play, and generally interact with the world. But it was Lewit (1999a) who used the term 'locomotor system', and it is this descriptor that seems closer to reality than the phrase 'musculoskeletal system'. The word 'locomotor' embraces a sense of activity and movement, whereas musculoskeletal sounds passive and structural, rather than functional.

In truth, however, structure and function are so intertwined that one cannot be considered without the other. The structure of a unit, or area, determines what function it is capable of. Seen in reverse, it is function that imposes demands on the very structures that allow them to operate, and which, over time, can modify that structure – just think of the gross structural changes that occur in response to the functions involved in lifting weights or running marathons! Quite different changes emerge compared with those that would result from playing cards or chess.

On a cellular level this has been expressed succinctly by Hall & Brody (1999), who stated:

> The number of sarcomeres in theory determines the distance through which a muscle can shorten and the length at which it produces maximum force. Sarcomere number is not fixed and in adult muscle the number can increase or decrease. *The stimulus for sarcomere length changes may be the amount of tension along the myofibril or the myotendon (musculotendenous) junction, with high tension leading to an addition of sarcomeres and low tension causing a decrease* [italics added].

So, at its simplest, the load on tissue, which makes functional demands, leads to structural change. It is therefore essential, when considering dysfunction, to identify, as far as possible through observation, assessment, palpation, testing, imaging, and questioning, just what structural modifications coexist with the reported functional changes and/or pain, in order to construct a rational plan of therapeutic action. Conversely, in attempting to restore normal function, or to reduce the degree of dysfunction and/or pain, at least some of the focus needs to be towards modifying the identified structural changes that have evolved.

Fortunately a variety of methods exist that can encourage more normal function, modify structure, and reduce or eliminate pain, depending on the nature and chronicity of the problem. Among the most effective of such clinical tools – capable of assisting in both structural and functional change – are the range of methods that have been labelled muscle energy techniques (MET) (Mitchell 1967, Lewit & Simons 1984, Janda 1990, Lewit 1999a).

Revolution or evolution

As will become clear, as the content of this revised and expanded text unfolds, muscle energy techniques, originating as they did in osteopathic medicine, are now increasingly likely to be found in chiropractic (see Ch. 8), physiotherapy (see Ch. 9) and massage therapy (Ch. 10) and athletic training settings (Ch. 11).

A slow but steady (r)evolution is taking place in manual and manipulative therapy, involving a movement away from high-velocity/low-amplitude thrust methods (HVLT – now commonly known as 'mobilisation with impulse' – a characteristic of most chiropractic and, until recently, much osteopathic manipulation) towards gentler methods that take far more account of the soft tissue component (DiGiovanna 1991, Lewit 1999a, Travell & Simons 1992) and/or which focus on joint mobilisation methods, rather than high-velocity thrust manipulation (Maitland 1998).

Greenman (1996) states that:

'Early [osteopathic] techniques did speak of muscle relaxation with soft tissue procedures, but specific manipulative approaches to muscle appear to be 20th century phenomena.'

It is important to make clear that while muscle energy techniques (MET) target the soft tissues primarily, they can also make major contributions towards joint mobilisation. As an example see discussion of MET as a significant addition to Spencer mobilisation methods for the shoulder, in Ch. 6 (Patriquin 1992, Knebl 2002).

MET can also usefully be employed to 'prepare' joints for subsequent HVLA thrust application.

MET by any other name

There are a variety of other terms used to describe the MET approach. Some years ago chiropractor Craig Liebenson (1989, 1990) described 'muscle energy' techniques as 'active muscular relaxation techniques'. As will be seen in Ch. 8, Liebenson now uses the more generalised descriptor, manual resistance techniques.

Fryer (see Ch. 4) notes that,

'The most common forms of isometric stretching referred to in the literature are contract–relax (CR), where the muscle being stretched is contracted and then relaxed, agonist contract–relax (ACR), where contraction of the agonist (rather than the muscle being stretched) actively moves the joint into increased ROM, and contract–relax agonist contract (CRAC), a combination of these two methods. These techniques are commonly referred to as PNF [proprioceptive neuromuscular facilitation] stretching, but the similarity to MET methods for lengthening muscles is obvious'

(see Box 1.1, and further discussion of these methods later in this chapter).

While Fryer's description of variations on the theme of isometric contraction and stretching is helpful, it highlights a semantic problem relating to the words 'agonist' and 'antagonist'. Once it has been determined that a muscle requires releasing, relaxing or and/or stretching, the general usage in this book will describe that muscle as the 'agonist', irrespective of which muscle(s) are contracted in the procedure. Evaluation of the descriptions of ACR and CRAC, as outlined above by Fryer, will make clear that attribution of the word 'agonist' is not always applied in the same way in different therapeutic settings. (Fryer addresses this semantic confusion in Ch. 4.)

To be clear – from the perspective of the terminology that will be used in this book, *whenever a muscle, or muscle group, is being treated, it will be referred to as 'the agonist'.*

History

MET evolved out of osteopathic procedures developed by pioneer practitioners such as T. J. Ruddy (1961), who termed his approach 'resistive duction', and Fred Mitchell Snr (1967).

As will become clear in this chapter, there also exists a commonality between MET and various procedures used in orthopaedic and physiotherapy methodology, such as proprioceptive neuromuscular facilitation (PNF). Largely due to the work of

Box 1.1 Stretching variations

Facilitated stretching

This active stretching approach represents a refinement of PNF (see below), and is largely the work of Robert McAtee (McAtee & Charland 1999). This approach uses strong isometric contractions of the muscle to be treated, followed by active stretching by the patient. An acronym, CRAC, is used to describe what is done (contract–relax, antagonist contract). The main difference between this and MET lies in the strength of the contraction and the use of spiral, diagonal patterns, although these concepts (spiral activities) have also been used in MET in recent years (consider scalene MET treatment in Ch. 5 for example).

The reader is reminded to regard use of the words 'agonist' and 'antagonist' in decriptors such as CRAC as commonly being at odds with the general use of 'agonist' and 'antagonist' in the descripton of MET methods. Reminders will be made throughout the text to help avoid confusion.

The debate as to how much strength should be used in PNF-like methods is unresolved and is discussed in relation to research in Ch. 4.

In general the MET usage advocated in this text prefers lighter contractions than both facilitated stretching and PNF because:

- It is considered that once a greater degree of strength than 25–35% of available force is used, recruitment is occurring of phasic muscle fibres, rather than the postural fibres that will have shortened and require stretching (Liebenson 1996). (The importance of variations in response between phasic and postural muscles is discussed in more detail in Ch. 2.)
- It is far easier for the practitioner to control light contractions than it is strong ones, making MET a less arduous experience for practitioner and patient.
- There is far less likelihood of provoking cramp, tissue damage or pain, when light contractions rather than strong ones are used, making MET safer and gentler.
- Physicians and researchers such as Karel Lewit (1999) have demonstrated that *extremely* light isometric contractions, utilising breathing and eye movements alone, are often sufficient to produce a degree of tissue relaxation that allows greater movement, as well as facilitating subsequent stretching.

What little research there has been into the relative benefits of different degrees of contraction effort is discussed in Ch. 4.

Proprioceptive neuromuscular facilitation (PNF) variations (including hold–relax and contract–relax) (Voss et al 1985, Surburg 1981)

Most PNF variations involve stretching that is either passive or passive-assisted, following a strong (frequently all available strength) contraction. Some variations attempt incremental degrees of strength with subsequent contractions. (Schmitt et al 1999). The same reservations listed above (in the facilitated stretching discussion) apply to these methods. There are excellent aspects to the use of PNF; however, the author considers MET, as detailed in this text, to have distinct advantages, with no drawbacks.

Active isolated stretching (AIS) (Mattes 1995)

Flexibility is encouraged in AIS, which uses active stretching by the patient and reciprocal inhibition (RI) mechanisms. AIS, unlike MET (which combines RI and PIR, as well as active patient participation), does not utilise the assumed benefits of postisometric relaxation (PIR).

In AIS:

1. The muscle that needs stretching is identified.
2. Precise localisation is used to ensure that the muscle receives specific stretching.
3. Use is made of a contractile effort to produce relaxation of the muscles involved.
4. Repetitive, fairly short duration, isotonic muscle contractions are used to increase local blood flow and oxygenation.
5. A synchronised breathing rhythm is established, using inhalation as the part returns to the starting position (the 'rest' phase) and exhalation as the muscle is taken to, and through, its resistance barrier (the 'work' phase).
6. The muscle to be lengthened/released is taken into stretch just beyond a point of light irritation – with the patient's assistance – and held for 1–2 seconds before being returned to the starting position.
7. Repetitions continue (sometimes for minutes) until adequate gain has been achieved.

Mattes uses patient participation in moving the part through the barrier of resistance in order to prevent activation of the myotatic stretch reflex, and this component of his specialised stretching approach has been incorporated into MET methodology by many practitioners.

Box 1.1 Continued

As noted, a key feature of AIS is the rapid rate of stretching, and the deliberately induced irritation of the stretched tissues. The undoubted ability of AIS to lengthen muscles rapidly is therefore achieved at the expense of some degree of microtrauma, which is not always an acceptable exchange – particularly in elderly and/or already pain-ridden patients. AIS may be more suited to athletic settings than to use on more vulnerable individuals.

There is an additional concern associated with AIS that provokes a degree of anxiety. Hodges & Gandavia (2000) studied coordination between respiratory and postural functions of the diaphragm: 'The results indicate that activity of human phrenic motoneurones is organised such that it contributes to both posture and respiration during a task which repetitively challenges trunk posture.'

Put simply, active limb movement creates an entrainment pattern with respiration. Additionally the AIS protocol actually calls for active control of the breathing rate during the different phases of movement leading to a rate of one limb movement approximately every 3 seconds leading to a distinct possibility of frank hyperventilation, together with a host of symptoms.

This rate of breathing would be acceptable during running, for example, as the alkalisation caused by rapid breathing (due to CO_2 loss) would balance the acidification caused by activity (lactic acid, etc.) (Pryor & Prasad 2002). However, in a relatively static setting, respiratory alkalosis would probably emerge, at which time muscles become prone to fatigue, dysfunction (e.g. cramp), and trigger point evolution (Nixon & Andrews 1996).

Loss of intracellular magnesium occurs as part of the renal compensation mechanism for correcting alkalosis.

Supplementary magnesium can correct a tendency to hyperventilation (Pereira 1988).

Another result, identified by Hodges et al (2001), shows that after a mere 60 seconds of over-breathing, the normal stabilising functions of both transversus abdominis, and the diaphragm, are reduced or absent.

It is therefore suggested that AIS, effective though it is in achieving lengthening and increased range, should be employed cautiously.

Yoga stretching (and static stretching)
Adopting specific postures based on traditional yoga and maintaining these for some minutes at a time (combined, as a rule, with deep relaxation breathing) allows a slow release of contracted and tense tissues to take place. A form of self-induced viscoelastic myofascial release seems to be taking place as tissues are held, unforced, at their resistance barrier (see discussion of 'creep' in Ch. 2). Yoga stretching, applied carefully, after appropriate instruction, represents an excellent means of home care (Galantino et al 2004). There are superficial similarities between yoga stretching and static stretching as described by Anderson (1984). Anderson, however, maintains the stretch, at the barrier, for short periods (usually no more than 30 seconds) before moving to a new barrier. In some settings the stretching aspect of this method is assisted by the practitioner.

Ballistic stretching (Beaulieu 1981)
A series of rapid, 'bouncing', stretching movements are the key feature of ballistic stretching. Despite claims that it is an effective means of lengthening short musculature rapidly, in the view of the author the risk of irritation, or frank injury, makes this method undesirable.

---

experts in physical medicine such as Karel Lewit (1999a), MET has evolved and been refined, and now crosses all interdisciplinary boundaries.

MET has as one of its objectives the induced relaxation of hypertonic musculature and, where appropriate (see below), the subsequent stretching of the muscle. This objective is shared with a number of 'stretching' systems, and it is necessary to examine and to compare the potential benefits and drawbacks of these various methods (see Box 1.1).

MET, as presented in this book, owes most of its development to osteopathic clinicians such as T. J. Ruddy (1961) and Fred Mitchell Snr (1967), with

more recent refinements deriving from the work of researchers and clinicians such as Karel Lewit (1986, 1999) and the late Vladimir Janda (1989) of the former Czech Republic, both of whose work will be referred to many times in this text. Some of the pioneers of MET (and other methods) are briefly introduced below.

T. J. Ruddy

In the 1940s and 1950s, osteopathic physician T. J. Ruddy (1961) developed a treatment method involving patient-induced, rapid, pulsating contractions against resistance, which he termed 'rapid resistive duction'. It was in part this work which Fred Mitchell Snr used as the basis for the evolution of MET (along with PNF methodology, see Box 1.1).

Ruddy's method called for a series of rapid, low-amplitude muscle contractions against resistance, usually at a rate of 20 pulsations in 10 seconds. This approach is now known as pulsed MET, rather than the tongue-twisting 'Ruddy's rapid resistive duction'.

As a rule, at least initially, these patient-directed pulsating contractions involve an effort towards the barrier, using antagonists to shortened structures. This approach can be applied in all areas where sustained contraction MET procedures are appropriate, and is particularly useful for self-treatment, following instruction from a skilled practitioner. Ruddy (1961) suggested that the effects include improved local oxygenation, enhanced venous and lymphatic circulation, as well as having a positive influence on both static and kinetic posture, because of the effects on proprioceptive and interoceptive afferent pathways.

Ruddy's work formed part of the base on which Mitchell Snr and others constructed MET, and aspects of its clinical application are described in Ch. 3.

Ruddy's original work using pulsing isometric efforts involved treatment of the intrinsic eye muscles. See Ch. 5 (Box 5.11) for examples of this approach.

Fred Mitchell Snr

No single individual was alone responsible for MET, but its inception into osteopathic work must be credited to F. L. Mitchell Snr, in 1958. Since then his son F. Mitchell Jnr (Mitchell et al 1979) and many others have evolved a highly sophisticated system of manipulative methods (Mitchell Jnr 1976) in which the patient 'uses his/her muscles, on request, from a precisely controlled position in a specific direction, against a distinctly executed counterforce', the accepted definition of MET.

Philip Greenman

Professor of biomechanics Philip Greenman (1996) accurately and succinctly summarises most of the potential benefits of correctly applied MET:

The function of any articulation of the body, which can be moved by voluntary muscle action, either directly or indirectly, can be influenced by muscle energy procedures ... . Muscle energy techniques can be used to lengthen a shortened, contractured or spastic muscle; to strengthen a physiologically weakened muscle or group of muscles; to reduce localized edema, to relieve passive congestion, and to mobilize an articulation with restricted mobility.

Sandra Yale

Osteopathic physician Sandra Yale (in DiGiovanna 1991) extols MET's potential in even fragile and severely ill patients:

Muscle energy techniques are particularly effective in patients who have severe pain from acute somatic dysfunction, such as those with a whiplash injury from a car accident, or a patient with severe muscle spasm from a fall. MET methods are also an excellent treatment modality for hospitalized or bedridden patients. They can be used in older patients who may have severely restricted motion from arthritis, or who have brittle osteoporotic bones.

Edward Stiles

Among the key MET clinicians who have helped develop MET is Edward Stiles, who elaborates on the theme of the wide range of its application (Stiles 1984a, 1984b). He states (Stiles 1984a) that:

Basic science data suggests the musculoskeletal system plays an important role in the function of other systems. Research indicates that segmentally related somatic and visceral structures may affect one another directly, via viscerosomatic and somaticovisceral reflex pathways. Somatic dysfunction may increase energy demands, and it can affect a wide variety of bodily processes; vasomotor control, nerve impulse patterns (in facilitation), axionic flow of neurotrophic proteins, venous and lymphatic circulation and ventilation. The impact of somatic dysfunction on various combinations of these functions may be associated with myriad symptoms and signs. A possibility which could account for some of the observed clinical effects of manipulation.

As to the methods of manipulation Stiles now uses clinically, he states that he employs MET methods when treating about 80% of his patients, and functional techniques (such as strain/counterstrain) on 15–20%. He uses high-velocity thrusts in very few cases. The most useful manipulative tool available is, Stiles maintains, muscle energy technique.

J. Goodridge and W. Kuchera

Modern osteopathic refinements of MET – for example the emphasis on very light contractions, which has strongly influenced this text – owe much to osteopathic physicians such as John Goodridge and William Kuchera, who consider that (Goodridge & Kuchera 1997):

> *Localisation of force is more important than intensity. Localisation depends on palpatory proprioceptive perception of movement (or resistance to movement) at or about a specific articulation ... . Monitoring and confining forces to the muscle group or level of somatic dysfunction involved are important for achieving desirable changes. Poor results are most often due to improperly localized forces, often with excessive patient effort* [italics added].

Early sources of MET

MET emerged squarely out of osteopathic tradition, although a synchronous evolution of treatment methods, involving isometric contraction and stretching, was taking place independently in physical therapy, called proprioceptive neuromuscular facilitation (PNF) (see Box 1.1).

Fred Mitchell Snr (1958) quoted the words of the developer of osteopathy, Andrew Taylor Still: 'The attempt to restore joint integrity before soothingly restoring muscle and ligamentous normality was putting the cart before the horse.'

As stated earlier, Mitchell's work drew on the methods developed by Ruddy; however, it is unclear whether Mitchell Snr, when he was refining MET methodology in the early 1950s, had any awareness of PNF, a method which had been developed a few years earlier, in the late 1940s, in a physical therapy context (Knott & Voss 1968).

PNF methodology tended to stress the importance of rotational components in the function of joints and muscles, and employed these using resisted (isometric) forces, usually involving extremely strong contractions. Initially, the focus of PNF related to the strengthening of neurologically weakened muscles, with attention to the release of muscle spasticity following on from this, as well as to improving range of motion at intervertebral levels (Kabat 1959, Levine et al 1954) (see Box 1.1).

Box 1.2 Defining the terms used in MET

The terms used in MET require clear definition and emphasis:

1. An isometric contraction is one in which a muscle, or group of muscles, or a joint, or region of the body, is called upon to contract, or move in a specified direction, and in which that effort is matched by the practitioner/therapist's effort, so that no movement is allowed to take place.

2. An isotonic contraction is one in which movement does take place, in that the counterforce offered by the practitioner/therapist is either less than that of the patient, or is greater. In the first isotonic example there would be an approximation of the origin and insertion of the muscle(s) involved, as the effort exerted by the patient more than matches that of the practitioner/therapist. This has a tonic effect on the muscle(s) and is called a concentric isotonic contraction. This method is useful in toning weakened musculature.

3. The other form of isotonic contraction involves an eccentric movement in which the muscle, while contracting, is stretched. The effect of the practitioner/therapist offering greater counterforce than the patient's muscular effort is to lengthen a muscle which is trying to shorten. This is called an isolytic contraction when performed rapidly. This manoeuvre is useful in cases where there exists a marked degree of fibrotic change. The effect is to stretch and alter these tissues – inducing controlled microtrauma – thus allowing an improvement in elasticity and circulation. When the eccentric isotonic stretch is performed slowly the effect is to tone the muscle being stretched, while simultaneously inhibiting the antagonists, which can subsequently be stretched (Norris 1999, Lewit 1999b).

Postisometric relaxation and reciprocal inhibition: two forms of MET (Box 1.2)

A term much used in more recent developments of muscle energy techniques is *postisometric relaxation* (PIR), especially in relation to the work of Karel Lewit (1999). PIR refers to the assumed effect of reduced tone experienced by a muscle, or group of muscles, after brief periods following an isometric contraction. As will be seen in Ch. 4, the degree to which this neurological effect is indeed part of the MET process is under review, and has been disputed.

A further MET variation involves the physiological response of the antagonists of a muscle which has been isometrically contracted – reciprocal inhibition (RI). When a muscle is isometrically contracted, its antagonist will be inhibited, and will demonstrate reduced tone immediately following this. Thus, as part of an MET procedure, the antagonist of a shortened muscle, or group of muscles, may be isometrically contracted in order to achieve a degree of ease and additional movement potential in the shortened tissues. The relative importance of this process, based on research evidence, is also discussed further in Ch. 4.

Sandra Yale (in DiGiovanna 1991) acknowledges that, apart from the well-understood processes of reciprocal inhibition, the precise reasons for the effectiveness of MET remain unclear, despite the commonly (but not universally) held view that an isometric contraction seems to set the muscle to a new length by inhibiting it via the influence of the golgi tendon organ (Moritan 1987). Other methods that appear to utilise this concept include 'hold–relax' and 'contract–relax' techniques (see Box 1.1 and Ch. 4).

Lewit & Simons (1984) agree that while reciprocal inhibition is a factor in some forms of therapy related to postisometric relaxation techniques, it is not a factor in PIR itself, which they believed to involve a phenomenon resulting from a neurological loop associated with the Golgi tendon organs (see Figs 1.1 and 1.2).

Liebenson (1996) discusses both the benefits of, and the mechanisms involved in, the use of MET, which he terms 'manual resistance techniques' (MRT):

Two aspects to MRT [i.e. MET by another name] are their ability to relax an overactive muscle ... and their ability to enhance stretch of a shortened muscle or its associated fascia when connective tissue or viscoelastic changes have occurred.

As referred to above, two fundamental neurophysiological principles have long been thought to account for the neuromuscular inhibition that occurs during application of MET. These concepts are explored by Fryer in Ch. 4, where he describes current research that throws doubt on the validity of these previously widely held concepts.

One basic premise has been that post-contraction inhibition (also known as PIR) is operating. This states that after a muscle is contracted, it is automatically in a relaxed state for a brief, latent, period. The second premise relates to reciprocal inhibition (RI), which states that when one muscle is contracted, its antagonist is automatically inhibited. While neither of these hypotheses has been discredited, there do now exist doubts as to whether they are the primary, or even major, physiological reasons for the benefits noted when MET is used. In Ch. 4 Fryer shows the reasoning that leads current opinion to believe that the effect of MET is simply to increase tolerance to stretch.

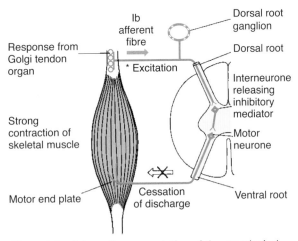

Figure 1.1 Schematic representation of the neurological effects of the loading of the Golgi tendon organs of a skeletal muscle by means of an isometric contraction, which produces a postisometric relaxation effect in that muscle. This effect occurs (Carter et al 2000), but may not be the primary reason for the benefits of MET (see Ch. 4).

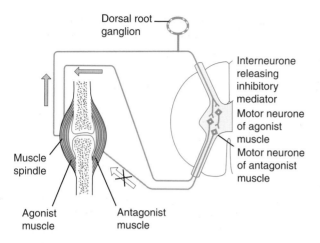

Dorsal root ganglion

Interneurone releasing inhibitory mediator

Motor neurone of agonist muscle

Motor neurone of antagonist muscle

Muscle spindle

Agonist muscle

Antagonist muscle

Figure 1.2 Schematic representation of the reciprocal effect of an isometric contraction of a skeletal muscle, resulting in an inhibitory influence on its antagonist. This effect occurs but may not be the primary reason for the benefits of MET (see Ch. 4).

A number of researchers, including Karel Lewit of Prague (Lewit 1999a), have reported on the usefulness of aspects of MET in the treatment of trigger points, and MET is indeed seen by many to be an excellent method of treating these myofascial phenomena, and of achieving the restoration of a situation where the muscle in which the trigger lies is once more capable of achieving its full resting length, with no evidence of shortening.

Travell & Simons (1983) mistakenly credited Lewit with developing MET, stating that 'The concept of applying postisometric relaxation in the treatment of myofascial pain was presented for the first time in a North American journal in 1984 [by Lewit]'. In fact Mitchell Snr had described the method some 25 years previously, a fact acknowledged by Lewit (Lewit & Simons 1984).

Key points about modern MET

MET methods all employ the use of the patient's own muscular efforts in one of a number of ways, usually in association with the restraining or assisting efforts of the therapist:

1 The practitioner/therapist's force may exactly match the effort of the patient (so producing an isometric contraction) allowing no movement to occur – and possibly producing as a result a physiological neurological response (via the Golgi tendon organs) involving a combination of:
   – reciprocal inhibition of the antagonist(s) of the muscle(s) being contracted, as well as
   – postisometric relaxation of the muscle(s) which are being contracted.

Other mechanisms are almost certainly involved in the subsequent ability to stretch the tissues more comfortably and efficiently, including a possible viscoelastic change in the connective tissues, and more probably an increased tolerance to stretching. These issues, and supporting research, are explored fully in Ch. 4.

2 The practitioner/therapist's force may overcome the effort of the patient, thus moving the area or joint in the direction opposite to that in which the patient is attempting to move it (this is an isotonic eccentric contraction, known, when performed rapidly, as an isolytic contraction). A slowly performed isotonic eccentric stretch has the effect of toning the muscle being stretched in this way, while inhibiting its antagonist(s), allowing it/them to be more easily stretched subsequently (Kolár 1999, Norris 1999). See Ch. 5 for examples of this method.

3 The practitioner/therapist may partially match the effort of the patient, thus allowing, whilst slightly retarding, the patient's effort (and so producing a toning effect by means of the isotonic concentric, isokinetic, contraction).

Other variables may be also introduced, for example involving:

- Whether the contraction should commence with the muscle or joint held at the resistance barrier or short of it – a factor decided largely on the basis of the degree of chronicity or acuteness of the tissues involved

- How much effort the patient uses – say, 20% of strength, or more, or less. Research evidence is inconclusive on this topic, and is detailed in Ch. 4.

- The length of time the effort is held – 7–10 seconds, or more, or less (Lewit (1999) favours 7–10 seconds; Greenman (1989) and Goodridge & Kuchera (1997) favour 3–5 seconds). See Ch. 4.

- Whether, instead of a single maintained contraction, to use a series of rapid, low-amplitude contractions (Ruddy's rhythmic resisted duction method, also known as pulsed muscle energy technique)

- The number of times the isometric contraction (or its variant) is repeated – three repetitions are thought to be optimal (Goodridge & Kuchera 1997). See Ch. 4.

- The direction in which the effort is made – towards the resistance barrier or away from it, thus involving either the antagonists to the muscles or the actual muscles (agonists) which require 'release' and subsequent stretching (these variations are also known as 'direct' and 'indirect' approaches. See Box 1.3)

- Whether to incorporate a held breath and/or specific eye movements (respiratory or visual synkinesis) to enhance the effects of the contraction. These tactics are desirable if possible, it is suggested – see Ch. 5 (Goodridge & Kuchera 1997, Lewit 1999a)

- What sort of resistance is offered to the patient's effort (for example by the practitioner/therapist, by gravity, by the patient, or by an immovable object)

- Whether the patient's effort is matched, overcome or not quite matched – a decision

based on the precise needs of the tissues – to achieve relaxation, reduction in fibrosis or tonifying/re-education

- Whether to take the muscle or joint to its new barrier following the contraction, or whether or not to stretch the area/muscle(s) beyond the barrier – this decision is based on the nature of the problem being addressed (does it involve shortening? fibrosis?) and its degree of acuteness or chronicity

- Whether any subsequent (to a contraction) stretch is totally passive, or whether the patient should participate in the movement, the latter being thought by many to be desirable in order to reduce danger of stretch reflex activation (Mattes 1995)

- Whether to utilise MET alone, or in a sequence with other modalities such as the positional release methods of strain/counterstrain, or the ischaemic compression/inhibitory pressure techniques of neuromuscular technique (NMT) – such decisions will depend upon the type of problem being addressed, with myofascial trigger point treatment frequently benefiting from such combinations (see description of integrated neuromuscular inhibition (INIT), in Ch. 7 (Chaitow 1993))

- Greenman summarises the requirements for the successful use of MET in osteopathic situations as 'control, balance and localisation'. His suggested basic elements of MET include the following:

- A patient/active muscle contraction, which
  - commences from a controlled position
  - is in a specific direction (towards or away from a restriction barrier)

- The practitioner/therapist applies distinct counterforce (to meet, not meet, or to overcome the patient's force)

- The degree of effort is controlled (sufficient to obtain an effect but not great enough to induce trauma or difficulty in controlling the effort)

- What is done subsequent to the contraction may involve any of a number of variables, as will be outlined in later chapters

- New chapters in this revised text outline the use of MET in a variety of settings ranging from chiropractic to physical (physio) therapy, athletic training and massage therapy.

The essence of MET then is that it uses the energy of the patient, and that it may be employed in one or other of the manners described above with any combination of variables, depending upon the particular needs of the case. Goodridge (one of the first osteopaths to train with Mitchell Snr in 1970) sum-marises as follows: 'Good results [with MET] depend on accurate diagnosis, appropriate levels of force, and sufficient localisation. Poor results are most often caused by inaccurate diagnosis, improperly localized forces, or forces that are too strong' (Goodridge & Kuchera 1997) (see also Box 1.4).

Using agonist or antagonist? (see also Box 1.3)

As mentioned, a critical consideration in MET, apart from degree of effort, duration and frequency

---

Box 1.3 Direct and indirect action

It is sometimes easier to describe the variations used in MET in terms of whether the practitioner/therapist's force is the same as, less than, or greater than that of the patient. In any given case there is going to exist a degree of limitation in movement towards end of range, in one direction or another, which may involve purely soft tissue components of the area, or actual joint restriction (and even in such cases there is bound to be some involvement of soft tissues).

The practitioner/therapist establishes, by palpation and by mobility assessments (such as motion palpation, ideally involving 'end-feel'), the direction of maximum 'bind', or restriction. This is felt as a definite point of limitation in one or more directions. In many instances the muscle(s) will be shortened and currently incapable of stretching and relaxing.

Should the isometric, or isotonic, contraction which the patient is asked to perform, be one in which the contraction of the muscles or movement of the joint is *away from the barrier* or point of bind, while the practitioner/therapist is using force in the direction which goes towards, or through that barrier, then this form of treatment involves what is called a *direct* action.

Should the opposite apply, with the patient attempting to take the area/joint/muscle towards the barrier, while the practitioner/therapist is resisting, then this is an *indirect* manoeuvre.

Experts differ
As with so much in manipulative terminology, there is disagreement even in this apparently simple matter of which method should be termed 'direct' and which 'indirect'. Grieve (1985) describes the variations thus: 'Direct action techniques [are those] in which the patient attempts to produce movement towards, into or across a motion barrier; and indirect techniques, [are those] in which the patient attempts to produce motion away from the motion barrier, i.e. the movement limitation is attacked indirectly.'

On the other hand, Goodridge (1981), having previously illustrated and described a technique where the patient's effort was directed away from the barrier of restriction, states: 'The aforementioned illustration used the direct method. With the indirect method the component is moved by the practitioner/therapist away from the restrictive barrier.'

Thus:

- If the practitioner/therapist is moving away from the barrier, then the patient is moving towards it, and in Goodridge's terminology (i.e. osteopathic) this is an indirect approach.
- In Grieve's terminology (physiotherapy) this is a direct approach.

Plainly these views are contradictory.

Since MET always involves two opposing forces (the patient's and the practitioner/therapist's/or gravity/or a fixed object), it is more logical to indicate which force is being used in order to characterise a given technique. Thus a practitioner/therapist-direct method can also equally accurately be described as a patient-indirect method.

Practitioner/therapist-direct methods (in which the patient is utilising muscles – the agonists – already in a shortened state) may be more appropriate to managing chronic conditions, rather than acute ones, for example during rehabilitation, where muscle shortening has occurred. When acute, shortened muscles could involve existing sustained fibre damage, or may be oedematous, and could be painful, and/or go into spasm, were they asked to contract. It would therefore seem both more logical, and safer, to contract their antagonists – using patient-direct methods.

Box 1.4 Muscle energy sources (Jacobs & Walls 1997, Lederman 1998, Liebenson 1996, Schafer 1987)

- Muscles are the body's force generators. In order to achieve this function, they require a source of power, which they derive from their ability to produce mechanical energy from chemically bound energy (in the form of adenosine triphosphate – ATP).
- Some of the energy so produced is stored in contractile tissues for subsequent use when activity occurs. The force which skeletal muscles generate is used to either produce or prevent movement, to induce motion or to ensure stability.
- Muscular contractions can be described in relation to what has been termed a *strength continuum*, varying from a small degree of force, capable of lengthy maintenance, to a full-strength contraction, which can be sustained for very short periods only.
- When a contraction involves more than 70% of available strength, blood flow is reduced and oxygen availability diminishes.

of use, involves the direction in which the effort is made. This may be varied, so that the practitioner/therapist's force is directed towards overcoming the restrictive barrier (created by a shortened muscle, restricted joint, etc.); or indeed opposite forces may be used, in which the practitioner/therapist's counter-effort is directed away from the barrier.

There is general consensus among the various osteopathic experts already quoted that the use of postisometric relaxation (i.e. a contraction involving the muscle that requires releasing or lengthening) is more useful than reciprocal inhibition in attempting to normalise hypertonic musculature. This, however, is not generally held to be the case by experts such as Lewit (1999) and Janda (1990), who see specific roles for the reciprocal inhibition variation.

Osteopathic clinicians such as Stiles (1984b) and Greenman (1996) believe that the muscle which requires stretching (the agonist) should be the main source of 'energy' for the isometric contraction, and suggest that this achieves a more significant degree of relaxation, and so a more useful ability to subsequently stretch the muscle,

than would be the case were the relaxation effect being achieved via use of the antagonist (i.e. using reciprocal inhibition).

Following on from an isometric contraction – whether agonist or antagonist is being used – there appears to be a refractory, or latency, period of approximately 15 seconds during which there can be an easier (due to reduced tone, or to increased tolerance to stretch) movement towards the new position (new resistance barrier) of a joint or muscle. In Ch. 4 this latency period is discussed further in relation to research evidence. A study by Moore & Kukulka (1991), for example, suggests only about 10 seconds of reduced EMG activity following an isometric contraction. However, whether this relates to the increased ease of stretching is queried by other research findings (Magnusson et al 1996).

Variations on the MET theme

As with most manual therapy approaches, the MET methods employed will vary with the objectives.

- Relaxation of soft tissues has the objective of inducing a reduction of tension in contractile structures such as muscle. Relaxation may be all that can usefully be done using MET (or other methods) during the acute and remodelling phases of soft tissue distress. An 'acute' model of MET usage will be outlined in Ch. 5.

- 'Release' of soft tissue shortening is directed towards the non-dynamic connective tissue component of soft tissues. Because such tissue is slow to shorten, it generally requires a lengthy period of applied load (minutes rather than seconds), such as is used in myofascial release. The benefit of initially using MET components (isometric contractions) will be explained. There is an undoubted increase in stretch tolerance following use of MET, which enhances 'release' techniques (Magnusson et al 1996). Release, in this context, differs from 'stretch' (see below) in that tissues tend to be held against their end of range barrier(s), rather than being forced through those barriers as they are when being stretched.

- Stretch commonly requires a relatively greater load to the tissue than relaxation or release method, as – following one or other version of MET contraction – tissues are taken to, and beyond, their end of range barriers in an attempt to increase length. Stretch methods target the non-contractile portion of muscle, the ground substance, although it also affects contractile tissues by overcoming any resistance. Stretching carries an increased risk of pain and injury that seldom applies when relaxation or release objectives are sought.

- Liebenson (1989, 1990) has described three basic variations of MET, as used by Lewit and Janda, as well as by himself in a chiropractic rehabilitation setting to achieve one or a combination of these objectives.

- Lewit's (1999a) modification of MET, which he called postisometric relaxation, is directed towards relaxation of hypertonic muscle, especially if this relates to reflex contraction, or the involvement of myofascial trigger points. Liebenson (1996) notes that 'this is also a suitable method for joint mobilisation when a thrust is not desirable'.

Lewit's postisometric relaxation method (Lewit 1999a)

1. The hypertonic muscle is taken, without force or 'bounce', to a length just short of pain, or to the point where resistance to movement is first noted (Fig. 1.3).

2. The patient gently contracts the affected hypertonic muscle away from the barrier (i.e. the agonist is contracted) for between 5 and 10 seconds, while the effort is resisted with an exactly equal counterforce. Lewit usually has the patient inhale during this effort.

3. This resistance involves the practitioner/therapist holding the contracting muscle in a direction which would stretch it, were resistance not being offered.

4. The degree of effort, in Lewit's method, is minimal. The patient may be instructed to think in terms of using only 10 or 20% of his available strength, so that the manoeuvre is never allowed to develop into a contest of strength between the practitioner/therapist and the patient.

5. After the effort, the patient is asked to exhale and to 'let go' completely, and only when this is achieved is the muscle taken to a new barrier with all slack removed – but no stretch – to the extent that the relaxation of the hypertonic muscles will now allow.

6. Starting from this new barrier, the procedure is repeated two or three times.

7. In order to facilitate the process, especially where trunk and spinal muscles are involved, Lewit usually asks the patient to assist by looking in the direction of the contraction during the contracting phase, and in the direction of stretch during the stretching phase of the procedure.

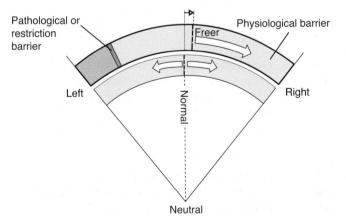

Figure 1.3 A schematic representation of the directions in which a muscle or joint can move – towards a restriction barrier (at which point MET could be usefully applied) or towards a position of relative ease.

The key elements in this approach, as in most MET methods, involve precise positioning, as well as taking out slack and using the barrier as the starting and ending points of each contraction.

What may be happening?

Karel Lewit, discussing MET methods (Lewit 1999a), states that medullary inhibition is not capable of explaining their effectiveness. He considers that the predictable results obtained may relate to the following:

- During resistance using minimal force (isometric contraction) only a very few fibres are active, the others being inhibited

- During relaxation (in which the shortened musculature is taken gently to its new limit without stretching) the stretch reflex is avoided – a reflex which may be brought about even by passive and non-painful stretch.

- He concludes that this method demonstrates the close connection between tension and pain, and between relaxation and analgesia.

- The use of eye movements (visual synkinesis) as part of the methodology is based on research by Gaymans (1980) which indicates, for example, that flexion is enhanced by the patient looking downwards, and extension by the patient looking upwards. Similarly, side-bending and rotation are facilitated by looking towards the side involved.

- The potential value of this method is easily proved by self-experiment: an attempt to flex the spine while maintaining the eyes in an upwards (towards the forehead) looking direction, will be found to be less successful than an attempt made to flex while looking downwards. These eye-direction aids are also useful in manipulation of the joints and will be mentioned in various technique descriptions in later chapters.

Effects of MET

Lewit (1999) in discussion of the element of passive muscular stretch in MET maintains that this factor does not always seem to be essential. In some areas, self-treatment, using gravity as the resistance factor, is effective, and such cases sometimes involve no actual stretch of the muscles.

Stretching of muscles during MET, according to Lewit (1999), is only required when contracture due to fibrotic change has occurred, and is not necessary if there is simply a disturbance in function. He quotes results in one series of patients (Lewit 1985, p 257), in which 351 painful muscle groups, or muscle attachments, were treated by MET (using postisometric relaxation as described above) in 244 patients. Analgesia was immediately achieved in 330 cases, and there was no effect in only 21 cases. These are remarkable results by any standards.

Lewit suggests that trigger points and 'fibrositic' changes in muscle will often disappear after MET contraction methods. He further suggests that referred local pain points, resulting from problems elsewhere, will also disappear more effectively than where local anaesthesia or needling (acupuncture) methods are employed.

Janda's postfacilitation stretch method

Janda's variation on this approach (Janda 1993), known as 'postfacilitation stretch', uses a different starting position for the contraction, and also a far stronger isometric contraction than that suggested by Lewit, and by most osteopathic users of MET:

1. The shortened muscle is placed in a mid-range position about halfway between a fully stretched and a fully relaxed state.

2. The patient contracts the muscle isometrically, using a maximum degree of effort for 5–10 seconds while the effort is resisted completely.

3. On release of the effort, a rapid stretch is made to a new barrier, without any 'bounce', and this is held for at least 10 seconds.

4. The patient relaxes for approximately 20 seconds and the procedure is repeated between three and five times more.

Some sensations of warmth and weakness may be anticipated for a short while following this more vigorous approach.

Reciprocal inhibition variation

This method, which forms a component of PNF methodology (see Box 1.1) and MET, is mainly used in acute settings, where tissue damage or pain precludes the use of the more usual agonist contraction, and also commonly as an addition to such methods, often to conclude a series of stretches whatever other forms of MET have been used (Evjenth & Hamberg 1984):

1. The affected muscle is placed in a mid-range position.

2. The patient is asked to push firmly towards the restriction barrier and the practitioner/ therapist either completely resists this effort (isometric) or allows a movement towards it (isotonic). Some degree of rotational or diagonal movement may be incorporated into the procedure.

3. On ceasing the effort, the patient inhales and exhales fully, at which time the muscle is passively lengthened.

   Liebenson notes that 'a resisted isotonic effort towards the barrier is an excellent way in which to facilitate afferent pathways at the conclusion of treatment with active muscular relaxation techniques or an adjustment (joint). This can help reprogram muscle and joint proprioceptors and thus re-educate movement patterns.' (See Box 1.2.)

Strengthening variation

Another major MET variation is to use what has been called isokinetic contraction (also known as progressive resisted exercise).

In this the patient starts with a weak effort but rapidly progresses to a maximal contraction of the affected muscle(s), introducing a degree of resistance to the practitioner/therapist's effort to put the joint, or area, through a full range of motion.

The use of isokinetic contraction is reported to be a most effective method of building strength, and to be superior to high repetition, lower resistance exercises (Blood 1980). It is also felt that a limited range of motion, with good muscle tone, is preferable (to the patient) to having a normal range with limited power. Thus the strengthening

of weak musculature in areas of permanent limitation of mobility is seen as an important contribution in which isokinetic contractions may assist.

Isokinetic contractions not only strengthen the fibres involved, but also have a training effect which enables them to operate in a more coordinated manner. There is often a very rapid increase in strength. Because of neuromuscular recruitment, there is a progressively stronger muscular effort as this method is repeated. Isokinetic contractions, and accompanying mobilisation of the region, commonly take no more than 4 seconds at each contraction, in order to achieve maximum benefit with as little fatiguing as possible, either of the patient or the practitioner/therapist. The simplest, safest, and easiest-to-handle use of isokinetic methods involves small joints, such as those in the extremities. Spinal joints may be more difficult to mobilise while muscular resistance is being fully applied.

The options available in achieving increased strength via these methods therefore involve a choice between either a partially resisted isotonic contraction, or the overcoming of such a contraction, at the same time as the full range of movement is being introduced (note that both isotonic concentric and eccentric contractions will take place during the isokinetic movement of a joint). Both of these options should involve maximum contraction of the muscles by the patient. Home treatment of such conditions is possible, via self-treatment, as in other MET methods.

Isotonic eccentric MET

Another application of the use of isotonic contraction occurs when a direct contraction is resisted and overcome by the practitioner/therapist (see Fig. 1.4). When performed rapidly this has been termed isolytic contraction, in that it involves the stretching, and sometimes the breaking down, of fibrotic tissue present in the affected muscles. Adhesions of this type are reduced by the application of force by the practitioner/therapist which is just greater than that being exerted by the patient. This procedure can be uncomfortable, and the patient should be advised of this. Limited degrees of effort are therefore called for at the outset of isolytic contractions.

An isotonic eccentric contraction involves the origins and insertions of the muscles involved becoming further separated as they contract, despite the patient's effort to approximate them.

In order to achieve the greatest degree of stretch (in the condition of myofascial fibrosis, for example), it is necessary for the largest number of fibres possible to be involved in the isotonic contraction. Thus there is a contradiction in that, in order to achieve this large involvement, the degree of contraction should be a maximal one, and yet this is likely to produce pain, which is contraindicated. The muscle force may also, in many instances, be impossible for the practitioner/therapist to overcome.

To achieve an isolytic contraction the patient should be instructed to use about 20% of possible strength on the first contraction, which is resisted and overcome by the practitioner/therapist, in a contraction lasting 3–4 seconds. This is then repeated, but with an increased degree of effort on the part of the patient (assuming the first effort was relatively painless). This continuing increase in the amount of force employed in the contracting musculature may be continued until, hopefully, a maximum contraction effort is possible, again to be overcome by the practitioner/therapist.

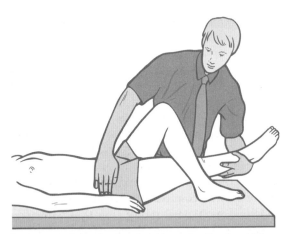

Figure 1.4   Example of an isolytic contraction in which the patient is attempting to move the right leg into abduction towards the right at exactly the same time as the practitioner/therapist is overriding this effort. This stretches the muscles which are contracting (TFL shown in example) thereby inducing a degree of controlled microtrauma, with the aim of increasing the elastic potential of shortened or fibrosed tissues.

In some muscles, of course, this may require a heroic degree of effort on the part of the practitioner/therapist, and alternative methods are therefore desirable. Deep tissue techniques, such as neuromuscular technique, would seem to offer such an alternative. The isolytic manoeuvre should have as its ultimate aim a fully relaxed muscle, although this will not always be possible.

Issues relating to the optimal degree of patient effort, and the ideal number of repetitions of such effort, based on current research evidence, will be discussed fully in Ch. 4.

When performed slowly an istonic eccentric stretch has the effect of toning the muscles involved, and of inhibiting the antagonist(s) to those muscles, with minimal or no tissue damage such as would occur if performed rapidly. The clinical use of slow eccentric isotonic stretching (SEIS) is described further in Chs 3 and 5.

Why fibrosis occurs naturally

An article in the Journal of the Royal Society of Medicine (Royal Society of Medicine 1983) discusses connective tissue changes:

> Aging affects the function of connective tissue more obviously than almost any organ system. Collagen fibrils thicken, and the amounts of soluble polymer decrease. The connective tissue cells tend to decline in number, and die off. Cartilages become less elastic, and their complement of proteoglycans changes both quantitatively and qualitatively. The interesting question is how many of these processes are normal, that contribute blindly and automatically, beyond the point at which they are useful? Does prevention of aging, in connective tissues, simply imply inhibition of crosslinking in collagen fibrils, and a slight stimulation of the production of chondroitin sulphate proteoglycan?

The effects of various soft tissue approaches such as NMT and MET will impact directly on these tissues, as well as on the circulation and drainage of the affected structures, which suggests that at least some of the effects of the ageing process can be influenced. Research has identified a feature of stiffness that may relate directly to the water content of connective tissue (see Box 1.5).

Destruction of collagen fibrils, however, is a serious matter (for example when using isolytic stretches, as described above), and although the fibrous tissue may be replaced in the process of healing, scar-tissue formation is possible, and this makes repair inferior to the original tissues, both in functional and structural terms. An isolytic contraction has the ability to break down tight, shortened tissues and the replacement of these with superior material will depend, to a large extent, on the subsequent use of the area (exercise, etc.), as well as the nutritive status of the individual. Collagen formation is dependent on adequate vitamin C, and a plentiful supply of amino acids such as proline, hydroxyproline and arginine. Manipulation, aimed at the restoration of a degree of normality in connective tissues, should therefore take careful account of nutritional requirements.

The range of choices of methods of stretching, irrespective of the form of prelude to this – strong or mild isometric contraction, starting at or short of the barrier – therefore covers the spectrum from all-passive to all-active, with many variables in between.

Box 1.5 Fascial stiffness and water

Klingler et al (2004) measured the wet, and final dry weight of fresh human fascia, and found that during an isometric stretch, water is extruded, refilling during a subsequent rest period, making the tissues stiffer.

- Using a 6% tissue elongation over 15 minutes, followed by rest, they noted the following average weight changes ($n = 21$): at end of stretch, −11.8%; after 30 min rest, −0.3%; after 1 hr, 0%; after 2 hrs, +2.1%; after 3 hrs, +3.6%.
- As water extrudes from ground substance during stretching, temporary relaxation occurs in the longitudinal arrangement of the collagen fibres and the tissue becomes more supple.
- If the strain is moderate, and there are no microinjuries, water soaks back into the tissue until it swells, becoming stiffer than before.
- The researchers question whether much manual therapy, and the tissue responses experienced, may relate to sponge-like squeezing and refilling effects in the semi-liquid ground substance, with its water binding glycosaminoglycans and proteoglycans.

Putting it together

The recommendation of this text is that the MET methods outlined above should be 'mixed and matched', so that elements of all of them may be used in any given setting, as appropriate. Lewit's (1999) approach seems ideal for more acute and less chronic conditions, while Janda's (1989) more vigorous methods seem ideal for hardy patients with chronic muscle shortening. There is a time to relax, to release and to stretch tissues, and sometimes to do all three.

MET offers a spectrum of approaches which range from those involving hardly any active contraction at all, relying on the extreme gentleness of mild isometric contractions induced by breathholding and eye movements only, all the way to the other extreme of full-blooded, total-strength contractions. Subsequent to isometric contractions – whether strong or mild – there is an equally sensitive range of choices, involving either energetic stretching or very gentle movement to a new restriction barrier.

We can see why Sandra Yale (in DiGiovanna 1991) speaks of the usefulness of MET in treating extremely ill patients. As will be reported in subsequent chapters, when used appropriately, MET, a major element in osteopathic care, fits well as an integrative tool in physical therapy, chiropractic, athletic training and massage therapy settings.

Many patients present with a combination of recent dysfunction (acute in terms of time, if not in degree of pain or dysfunction) overlaid on chronic changes that have set the scene for acute problems. It seems perfectly appropriate to use methods that deal gently with hypertonicity, and to employ more vigorous methods to help to resolve fibrotic change, in the same patient, at the same time, using different variations on the theme of MET. Other variables can be used which focus on joint restriction, or which utilise RI, pulsed MET or visual synkinesis, should conditions be too sensitive to allow PIR methods, or variations on Janda's more vigorous stretch methods (see Box 1.1).

Discussion of common errors in application of MET will help to clarify these thoughts.

Why MET might be ineffective at times

Poor results from use of MET may relate to an inability to localise muscular effort sufficiently, since unless local muscle tension is produced in the precise region of the soft tissue dysfunction, the method may fail to achieve its objectives. Also, of course, underlying pathological changes may have taken place, in joints or elsewhere, which make any soft tissue relaxation/release or stretching procedure of short-term value only, since pathology may well ensure recurrence of muscular spasms, sometimes almost immediately.

MET will be ineffective, or may cause irritation and pain, if excessive force is used in either the contraction phase or the stretching phase.

The keys to successful application of MET therefore lie in a precise focusing of muscular activity, with an appropriate degree of effort used in the isometric contraction, for an adequate length of time, followed by a safe movement to, or through, the previous restriction barrier, usually with patient assistance.

Use of variations such as stretching chronic fibrotic conditions following an isometric contraction and use of the integrated approach (INIT – see Ch. 7), mentioned earlier in this chapter, represent two examples of further adaptations of Lewit's basic approach which, as described above, is ideal for acute situations of spasm and pain.

To stretch or to strengthen?

There exists a tendency in some schools of therapy to encourage the strengthening of weakened muscle groups in order to normalise postural and functional problems as a priority, before attention is given to short/tight antagonists of the inhibited, weak muscles.

Janda (1978) has offered reasons why this approach is 'putting the cart before the horse': 'In pathogenesis, as well as in treatment of muscle imbalance and back problems, tight muscles play a more important, and perhaps even primary, role in comparison to weak muscles' (see Fig. 1.5).

He continues with the following observation:

Clinical experience, and especially therapeutic results, support the assumption that (according to Sherrington's law of reciprocal innervation)

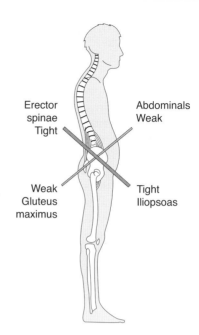

Figure 1.5 Lower crossed syndrome. An example of a common postural imbalance pattern, involving a chain reaction of hypertonia and hypotonia in which excessively tight and short muscles are inhibiting their antagonists.

Erector spinae Tight

Abdominals Weak

Weak Gluteus maximus

Tight Iliopsoas

tight muscles act in an inhibitory way on their antagonists. Therefore, it does not seem reasonable to start with strengthening of the weakened muscles, as most exercise programmes do. It has been clinically proved that it is better to stretch tight muscles first. It is not exceptional that, after stretching of the tight muscles, the strength of the weakened antagonists improves spontaneously, sometimes immediately, sometimes within a few days, without any additional treatment.

This well-reasoned, clinical observation, which directs our attention and efforts towards the stretching and normalising of those tissues which have shortened and tightened, seems irrefutable, and this theme will be pursued further in Ch. 2.

MET is designed to assist in this endeavour and, as discussed above, also provides an excellent method for assisting in the toning of weak musculature, should this still be required, after the stretching of the shortened antagonists, by means of isotonic methods.

Tendons

Aspects of the physiology of muscles and tendons are worthy of a degree of review, in so far as MET and its effects are concerned (see also Box 1.6). The

Box 1.6 Muscle tone and contraction

- Muscles display excitability – the ability to respond to stimuli, and, by means of a stimulus, to be able to *actively contract, extend* (lengthen), or to *elastically recoil* from a distended position, as well as to be able to *passively relax* when stimulus ceases.
- Lederman (1998) suggests that *muscle tone* in a resting muscle relates to biomechanical elements – a mix of fascial and connective tissue tension together with intramuscular fluid pressure, with no neurological input (therefore, not measurable by electromyogram (EMG)).
- If a muscle has altered morphologically (due to chronic shortening, for example, or compartment syndrome), then muscle tone, even at rest, will be altered and palpable.
- Lederman (1998) differentiates this from *motor tone* which is measurable by means of EMG, and which is present in a resting muscle only under abnormal circumstances – for example when psychological stress or protective activity is involved.
- Motor tone is either *phasic* or *tonic*, depending upon the nature of the activity being demanded of the muscle – to move something (phasic) or to stabilise it (tonic). In normal muscles, both activities vanish when gravitational, and activity, demands are absent.
- Contraction occurs in response to a motor nerve impulse acting on muscle fibres.
- A motor nerve fibre will always activate more than one muscle fibre, and the collection of fibres it innervates is the *motor unit.*
- The greater the degree of fine control a muscle is required to produce, the fewer the number of muscle fibres a nerve fibre will innervate, in that muscle. This can range from between 6 and 12 muscle fibres being innervated by a single motor neuron in the extrinsic eye muscles, to one motor neuron innervating 2000 fibres in major limb muscles (Gray's Anatomy 1973).
- Because there is a diffuse spread of influence from a single motor neuron throughout a muscle (i.e. neural influence does not necessarily correspond to fascicular divisions), only a few need to be active to influence the entire muscle.
- The functional contractile unit of a muscle fibre is its sarcomere, which contains filaments of actin and myosin. These myofilaments (actin and myosin) interact in order to shorten the muscle fibre.
- When a muscle is idle some of its extrafusal fibres (innervated by motor neurons) will contract to maintain normal tone while others rest.
- The muscle spindles (intrafusal fibres innervated by gamma fibres) monitor both the tone and length of the muscle. When the spindles are stretched they report to the cord both the fact of changing length and also the rate at which this is taking place.
- The Golgi tendon organs report on muscle tension so that, as this increases, fine tuning of tone occurs via the cord. As Greenman (1996) reports: 'The control of muscle tone is highly complex and includes afferent information coming from mechanoreceptors of the articulations, periarticular structures, and from the muscle spindle and Golgi tendon apparatus. This information is processed at the cord level with many muscle functions being preprogrammed … through local reflexes and propriospinal tracts. *The cord has the capacity to learn both normal and abnormal programs*' [italics added].

---

tone of muscle is largely the job of the Golgi tendon organs. These detect the load applied to the tendon, via muscular contraction. Reflex effects, in the appropriate muscles, are the result of this information being passed from the Golgi tendon organ back along the cord. The reflex is an inhibitory one, and thus differs from the muscle spindle stretch reflex. Sandler (1983) describes some of the processes involved:

When the tension on the muscles, and hence the tendon, becomes extreme, the inhibitory effect from the tendon organ can be so great that there is sudden relaxation of the entire muscle under

stretch. This effect is called the lengthening reaction, and is probably a protective reaction to the force which, if unprotected, can tear the tendon from its bony attachments. Since the Golgi tendon organs, unlike the [muscle] spindles, are in series with the muscle fibres, they are stimulated by both passive and active contractions of the muscles.

Pointing out that muscles can either contract with constant length and varied tone (isometrically), or with constant tone and varied length (isotonically), he continues:

'In the same way as the gamma efferent system operates as a feedback to control the length of

muscle fibres, the tendon reflex serves as a reflex to control the muscle tone'.

The relevance of this to soft tissue techniques is explained as follows:

In terms of longitudinal soft tissue massage, these organs are very interesting indeed, and it is perhaps the reason why articulation of a joint, passively, to stretch the tendons that pass over the joint, is often as effective in relaxing the soft tissues as direct massage of the muscles themselves. Indeed, in some cases, where the muscle is actively in spasm, and is likely to object to being pummelled directly, articulation, muscle energy technique, or functional balance techniques, that make use of the tendon organ reflexes, can be most effective.

The use of this knowledge in therapy is obvious and Sandler explains part of the effect of massage on muscle:

The [muscle] spindle and its reflex connections constitute a feedback device which can operate to maintain constant muscle length, as in posture; if the muscle is stretched the spindle discharges increase, but if the muscle is shortened, without a change in the rate of gamma discharge, then the spindle discharge will decrease, and the muscle will relax.

Sandler believes that massage techniques cause a decrease in the sensitivity of the gamma efferent, and thus increase the length of the muscle fibres rather than a further shortening of them; this produces the desired relaxation of the muscle. MET offers the clinician the ability to influence both the muscle spindles and also the Golgi tendon organs.

Joints and MET

Bourdillon (1982) tells us that shortening of muscle seems to be a self-perpetuating phenomenon which results from an over-reaction of the gamma-neuron system. It seems that the muscle is incapable of returning to a normal resting length as long as this continues. While the effective length of the muscle is thus shortened, it is nevertheless capable of shortening further. The pain factor seems related to the muscle's inability to then be restored to its anatomically desirable length. The conclusion is that much joint restriction is a result of muscular tightness and shortening.

The opposite situation may also apply, where damage to the soft or hard tissues of a joint is a key factor. In such cases the periarticular and osteophytic changes, all too apparent in degenerative conditions, are the major limiting factor in joint restrictions. In both situations, however, MET may be useful, although more useful where muscle shortening is the primary feature of restriction.

Restriction that takes place as a result of tight, shortened muscles is usually accompanied by some degree of lengthening and weakening (inhibition) of the antagonists (Lewit 1999a). A wide variety of possible permutations exists, in any given condition involving muscular shortening that may be initiating, or be secondary to, joint dysfunction combined with weakness of antagonists. A combination of isometric and isotonic MET methods can effectively be employed to lengthen and stretch the shortened groups, and to strengthen and tone the weak, overlong muscles.

Paul Williams (1965) stated a basic truth that is often neglected by the professions that deal with musculoskeletal dysfunction:

The health of any joint is dependent upon a balance in the strength of its opposing muscles. If for any reason a flexor group loses part, or all of its function, its opposing tensor group will draw the joint into a hyperextended position, with abnormal stress on the joint margins. This situation exists in the lumbar spine of modern man.

Lack of attention to the muscular component of joints in general, and spinal joints in particular, results in frequent inappropriate treatment of the joints so affected. Correct understanding of the role of the supporting musculature would frequently lead to normalisation of these tissues, without the need for heroic manipulative efforts. MET and other soft tissue approaches focus attention on these structures and offer the opportunity to correct both the weakened musculature and the shortened, often fibrotic, antagonists (Schlenk et al 1994).

More recently, Norris (1999) has pointed out that:

The mixture of tightness and weakness seen in the muscle imbalance process alters body segment alignment and changes the equilibrium point of a joint. Normally the equal resting tone of the agonist and antagonist muscles allows the joint to take up a balanced position where the joint surfaces are evenly loaded and the inert tissues of the joint are not excessively stressed. However if the muscles on one side of a joint are tight and the opposing muscles relax, the joint will be pulled out of alignment towards the tight muscle(s).

Such alignment changes produce weight-bearing stresses on joint surfaces, and result also in shortened soft tissues chronically contracting over time. Additionally such imbalances result in reduced segmental control with chain reactions of compensation emerging (see Ch. 2).

Several studies will be detailed (see Chs 5 and 8) showing the effectiveness of MET application in diverse population groups, including a Polish study on the benefits of MET in joints damaged by haemophilia, and a Swedish study on the effects of MET in treating lumbar spine dysfunction, as well as an American/Czech study involving myofascial pain problems. In the main, the results indicate a universal role in providing resolution or relief of such problems by means of the application of safe and effective muscle energy techniques.

References

Anderson B 1984 Stretching. Shelter Publishing, Nolinas, California

Beaulieu J 1981 Developing a stretching program. Physician and Sports Medicine 9(11): 59–69

Blood S 1980 Treatment of the sprained ankle. Journal of the American Osteopathic Association 79(11): 689

Bourdillon J 1982 Spinal manipulation, 3rd edn. Heinemann, London

Carter A M, Kinzey S J, Chitwood L F 2000 Proprioceptive neuromuscular facilitation decreases muscle activity during the stretch reflex in selected posterior thigh muscles. Journal of Sport Rehabilitation 9: 269–278

Chaitow L 1993 Integrated neuromuscular inhibition technique (INIT) in treatment of pain and trigger points. British Journal of Osteopathy 13: 17–21

Chaitow L, DeLany J 2005 Clinical applications of neuromuscular techniques: Practical case study exercises. Churchill Livingstone, Edinburgh

DiGiovanna E 1991 Osteopathic approach to diagnosis and treatment. Lippincott, Philadelphia

Evjenth O, Hamberg J 1984 Muscle stretching in manual therapy. Alfta, Sweden

Galantino ML, Bzdewka TM, Eissler-Russo JL et al 2004 The impact of modified hatha yoga on chronic low back pain: a pilot study. Alternative Therapies in Health and Medicine 10(2): 56–59

Gaymans F 1980 Die Bedeuting der atemtypen fur mobilisation der werbelsaule maanuelle. Medizin 18: 96

Goodridge J P 1981 Muscle energy technique: definition, explanation, methods of procedure. Journal of the American Osteopathic Association 81(4): 249–254

Goodridge J, Kuchera W 1997 Muscle energy treatment techniques. In: Ward R (ed) Foundations of osteopathic medicine. Williams and Wilkins, Baltimore

Gray's Anatomy 1973 Churchill Livingstone, Edinburgh

Greenman P 1989 Manual therapy. Williams and Wilkins, Baltimore

Greenman P 1996 Principles of manual medicine, 2nd edn. Williams and Wilkins, Baltimore

Grieve G P 1985 Mobilisation of the spine. Churchill Livingstone, Edinburgh, p 190

Hall CM, Brody LT, 1999 Therapeutic exercise moving toward function. Lippincott, Williams & Wilkins, New York, pp 48–49

Hodges P, Gandavia S 2000 Activation of the human diaphragm during a repetitive postural task. Journal of Physiology 522(1): 165–175

Hodges P et al 2001 Postural activity of the diaphragm is reduced in humans when respiratory demand increases. Journal of Physiology 537(3): 999–1008

Jacobs A, Walls W 1997 Anatomy. In: Ward R (ed) Foundations of osteopathic medicine. Williams and Wilkins, Baltimore

Janda V 1978 Muscles, central nervous regulation and back problems. In: Korr I (ed) Neurobiological mechanisms in manipulative therapy. Plenum Press, New York

Janda V 1989 Muscle function testing. Butterworths, London

Janda V 1990 Differential diagnosis of muscle tone in respect of inhibitory techniques. In: Paterson J K, Burn L (eds) Back pain, an international review. Kluwer, New York, pp 196–199

Janda V 1993 Presentation to Physical Medicine Research Foundation, Montreal, Oct 9–11

Kabat H 1959 Studies of neuromuscular dysfunction. Kaiser Permanente Foundation Medical Bulletin 8: 121–143

Klingler W, Schleip R, Zorn A 2004 European Fascia Research Project Report. 5th World Congress Low Back and Pelvic Pain, Melbourne, November 2004

Knebl J 2002 The Spencer sequence. Journal of the American Osteopathic Association 102(7): 387–400

Knott M, Voss D 1968 Proprioceptive neuromuscular facilitation, 2nd edn. Harper and Row, New York

Kolár P 1999 Sensomotor nature of postural functions. Journal of Orthopaedic Medicine 212: 40–45

Korr I M 1976 Spinal cord as organiser of disease process. In: Academy of Applied Osteopathy Yearbook. Newark, Ohio

Lederman E 1998 Fundamentals of manual therapy. Churchill Livingstone, Edinburgh

Levine M et al 1954 Relaxation of spasticity by physiological techniques. Archives of Physical Medicine 35: 214–223

Lewit K 1986 Muscular patterns in thoraco-lumbar lesions. Manual Medicine 2: 105

Lewit K 1985 Manipulative therapy in rehabilitation of the motor system. Butterworths, London

Lewit K 1999a Manipulative therapy in rehabilitation of the motor system, 3rd edn. Butterworths, London

Lewit K 1999b Chain reactions in the locomotor system in the light of coactivation patterns based on developmental neurology. Journal of Orthopaedic Medicine 21(2): 52–58

Lewit K, Simons D 1984 Myofascial pain: relief by post isometric relaxation. Archives of Physical Medical Rehabilitation 65: 452–456

Liebenson C 1989 Active muscular relaxation techniques (part 1). Journal of Manipulative and Physiological Therapeutics 12(6): 446–451

Liebenson C 1990 Active muscular relaxation techniques (part 2). Journal of Manipulative and Physiological Therapeutics 13(1): 2–6

Liebenson C (ed) 1996 Rehabilitation of the spine. Williams and Wilkins, Baltimore

Liebenson C 2000 The quadratus lumborum and spinal stability. Journal of Bodywork and Movement Therapies 4 (1): 49–54

McAtee R, Charland J 1999 Facilitated stretching, 2nd edn. Human Kinetics, Champaign, Illinois

Magnusson S P, Simonsen E B, Aagaard P et al 1996 Mechanical and physiological responses to stretching with and without preisometric contraction in human skeletal muscle. Archives of Physical Medicine and Rehabilitation 77: 373–377

Maitland G D 1998 Vertebral manipulation, 5th edn. Butterworth-Heinemann, Oxford

Mattes A 1995 Flexibility – active and assisted stretching. Mattes, Sarasota

Mitchell F L Snr 1958 Structural pelvic function. Yearbook of the Academy of Osteopathy 1958, Carmel, p 71 (expanded in references in 1967 yearbook)

Mitchell F L Snr 1967 Motion discordance. Yearbook of the Academy of Applied Osteopathy 1967, Carmel, pp 1–5

Mitchell F Jnr, 1976 Tutorial on biomechanical procedures, Yearbook American Academy of Osteopathy, Carmel

Mitchell F Jnr, Moran P S, Pruzzo N 1979 An evaluation and treatment manual of osteopathic muscle energy procedures. Valley Park, Illinois

Moore M, Kukulka C 1991 Depression of Hoffman reflexes following voluntary contraction and implications for proprioceptive neuromuscular facilitation therapy. Physical Therapy 71(4): 321–329

Moritan T 1987 Activity of the motor unit during concentric and eccentric contractions. American Journal of Physiology 66: 338–350

Nixon P, Andrews J 1996 A study of anaerobic threshold in chronic fatigue syndrome (CFS). Biological Psychology 43(3): 264

Norris C 1999 Functional load abdominal training (part 1). Journal of Bodywork and Movement Therapies 3(3): 150–158

Patriquin D 1992 Evolution of osteopathic manipulative technique: the Spencer technique. Journal of the American Osteopathic Association 92: 1134–1146

Pereira O 1988 The hazards of heavy breathing. New Scientist, Dec: 46–48

Pryor J, Prasad S 2002 Physiotherapy for respiratory and cardiac problems, 3rd edn. Churchill Livingstone, Edinburgh, p 81

Royal Society of Medicine 1983 Connective tissues: the natural fibre reinforced composite material. Journal of the Royal Society of Medicine 76

Ruddy T 1961 Osteopathic rhythmic resistive duction therapy. Yearbook of Academy of Applied Osteopathy 1961, Indianapolis, p 58

Sandler S 1983 Physiology of soft tissue massage. British Osteopathic Journal 15: 1–6

Schafer R 1987 Clinical biomechanics, 2nd edn. Williams and Wilkins, Baltimore

Schlenk R, Adelman K, Rousselle 1994 The effects of muscle energy technique on cervical range of motion. Journal of Manual and Manipulative Therapy 2(4): 149–155

Schmitt G D, Pelham T W, Holt L E 1999 From the field. A comparison of selected protocols during proprioceptive neuromuscular facilitation stretching. Clinical Kinesiology 53(1): 16–21

Stiles E 1984a Manipulation – a tool for your practice? Patient Care May 15: 16–97

Stiles E 1984b Manipulation – a tool for your practice? Patient Care August 15: 117–164

Surburg P 1981 Neuromuscular facilitation techniques in sports medicine. Physician and Sports Medicine 9(9): 115–127

Travell J, Simons D 1983 Myofascial pain and dysfunction, vol 1. Williams and Wilkins, Baltimore

Voss D, Ionta M, Myers B 1985 Proprioceptive neuromuscular facilitation, 3rd edn. Harper and Row, Philadelphia

Williams P 1965 The lumbo-sacral spine. McGraw Hill, New York

Patterns of function and dysfunction

2

CHAPTER CONTENTS

Cellular adaptation – including gene expression	25
Constructing a credible story	25
Maps and grids	26
Questions	26
Viewing symptoms in context	31
Fascial considerations	39
Postural (fascial) patterns	42
Functional evaluation of common compensatory (fascial) patterns	43
Observed CCP signs	43
Assessment of tissue preference	43
The evolution of musculoskeletal dysfunction	46
Fitness, weakness, strength and hypermobility influences	48
Characteristics of altered movement patterns	49
Different stress response of muscles	50
Postural and phasic muscles	50
Characteristics of postural and phasic muscles	52
Rehabilitation implications	53
Stabilisers and mobilisers	54
Global and local muscles	55
Patterns of dysfunction	59
Upper crossed syndrome	59
Lower crossed syndrome	60
Identification and normalisation of patterns of dysfunction	64
Trigger points	65
Fibromyalgia and trigger points	68
Summary	69
Integrated neuromuscular inhibition technique (INIT)	72
References	73

Why do soft tissues change from their normal elastic, pliable, adequately toned functional status to become shortened, contracted, fibrosed, weakened, lengthened and/or painful? The reasons may be many and varied, and are usually compound. The causes of somatic dysfunction may be summarised under broad headings, such as biomechanical, biochemical and psychosocial – or under more pointed headings such as 'overuse, abuse, misuse, disuse', and usually with some sort of status distinction (acute, subacute or chronic) which is commonly time-related.

Much musculoskeletal dysfunction can be shown to emerge out of adaptive processes, as the body – or part of it – compensates for what is being demanded of it – suddenly or gradually – in its daily activities. As a rule these adaptive demands relate to a combination of processes including repetitive use patterns, effects of past trauma, postural habits, emotional turmoil, chronic degenerative changes (e.g. arthritic) and so on. Onto such evolving patterns, sudden blows and strains are all too often superimposed, adding new adaptive demands of, and compensation responses by, the body.

Our bodies compensate (often without obvious symptoms) until the adaptive capacities of tissues are exhausted, at which time *decompensation* begins, and symptoms become apparent: pain, restriction, limitation of range of movement, etc. (Grieve 1986, Lewit 1999). The processes of decompensation then progress towards chronic dysfunction and possibly disability. Schamberger (2002) for example describes how back dysfunction can emerge from a background of 'minor insults (e.g. repetitive lifting, bending and squatting) superimposed on tissue already tender from chronic compression, distraction and/or torsional forces'.

Grieve (1986) explains how a patient presenting with pain, loss of functional movement or altered patterns of strength, power or endurance, will probably either have suffered a major trauma which has overwhelmed the physiological tolerances of relatively healthy tissues, or will be displaying 'gradual decompensation, demonstrating slow exhaustion of the tissue's adaptive potential, with or without trauma'. As this process continues, progressive postural adaptation, influenced by time factors, and possibly by trauma, leads to exhaustion of the body's adaptive potential and results in dysfunction and, ultimately, symptoms.

Grieve reminds us of Hooke's law (see Box 2.1), which states that within the elastic limits of any substance, the ratio of the stress applied to the strain produced is constant. Hooke's law is expressed as follows: 'The stress applied to stretch or compress a body is proportional to the strain, or change in length thus produced, so long as the limit of elasticity of the body is not exceeded' (Bennet 1952, Stedman 1998).

In simple terms, this means that tissue capable of deformation will absorb or adapt to forces applied to it, within its elastic limits, beyond which it will break down or fail to compensate (leading to decompensation). Grieve rightly reminds us that while attention to those tissues incriminated in producing symptoms often gives excellent short-term results, 'unless treatment is also focused towards restoring function in asymptomatic tissues responsible for the original postural adaptation and subsequent decompensation, the symptoms will recur'.

Examples of gradual structural and functional adaptation include:

- Tendon remodels in response to different forms of exercise, although it remains unclear whether this has the effect of decreasing the likelihood of damage, increasing strength, or enhancing elastic energy storage (Buchanan & Marsh 2002).

- Muscle responds to aerobic exercise with increased mitochondrial content and respiratory capacity of muscle fibres, while resistance exercise (strength training) results in muscle hypertrophy and higher contractile force (Booth & Thomason 1991).

- Depending on the type and level of exercise, there will be either beneficial or detrimental effects on bone remodelling (Wohl et al 2000).

Examples of adaptation responses include:

- Research shows that damage to any muscle results in the patient either (1) compensating for the damaged muscle by retraining other muscles to perform the same motion, or (2) changing the motion drastically in order to reduce the work required of the damaged muscle (Lieber 1992).

- Change in the maximal muscle force of a damaged iliopsoas affects not only the hip joint, but also all of the joints of the leg. For example when iliopsoas is injured this

---

Box 2.1 Laws affecting tissues

The following summary of terms and basic laws affecting tissues has direct implications in relation to the application of stretching forces as used in MET:

Mechanical terms
- *Stress:* force normalised over the area on which it acts.
- *Strain:* change in shape as a result of stress.
- *Creep:* continued deformation (increasing strain) of a viscoelastic material over time under constant load (traction, compression, twist).
  All tissues exhibit stress/strain responses.
  Tissues comprise water-absorbing collagen and ground substance (glycosaminoglycans, glycoproteins, etc.).

Biomechanical laws
- Wolff's law states that biological systems (including soft and hard tissues) deform in relation to the lines of force imposed on them.
- Hooke's law states that deformation (resulting from strain) imposed on an elastic body is in proportion to the stress (force/load) placed on it.
- Newton's third law states that when two bodies interact, the force exerted by the first on the second is equal in magnitude and opposite in direction to the force exerted by the second on the first.

leads to a large reduction in force in the ipsilateral soleus (Komura et al 2004).

Cellular adaptation – including gene expression

In rehabilitation the phrase 'specific adaptation to imposed demands' (SAID) is commonly used to describe what happens as tissues adapt to imposed tasks and loads, when particular responses are called for (Norris 2000a).

Clearly if gross and global tissue changes occur, cellular modification is also occurring. But how?

Cells have been shown to generate, transmit and sense mechanical tension, and to use these forces to control their shape and behaviour (including genetic expression). A mechanism has been discovered in which, on a cellular level, mechanical stress is communicated from stressed to unstressed cells, in order to elicit a specific remodelling response (Swartz et al 2001).

Much of this process involves integrins, a family of cell surface receptors that attach cells to the matrix, and mediate mechanical and chemical signals from it. Many integrin signals converge on cell cycle regulation, directing cells to live or die, to proliferate, or to exit the cell cycle and differentiate (Chicural et al 1998).

A dramatic example is offered by Chen & Ingber (1999) who have shown that the 'tensegrity'-designed cytoskeletons (fascia) of cells become distorted in a gravity-free environment, such as occurs when astronauts and cosmonauts spend time in space. This altered shape modifies cellular genetic behaviour, and also the way the cells process nutrients. It seems that a distorted cell cannot absorb and metabolise nutrients (including calcium) normally, and that this is a primary cause of one of the major health risks of space travel, loss of bone density.

This has enormous implications for general health. We do not need to indulge in space travel to create changes in soft tissue structure, since the processes of general and local adaptation, compensation, ageing and disease, which affect us all, create global and localised fascial warping, crowding, compression and distortion – right

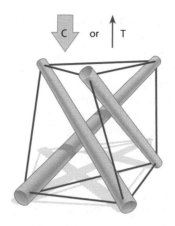

Figure 2.1 A tensegrity model showing the compressive (C) and tension (T) forces that maintain its structural stability.

down to the cellular level – and this, over time, may be as harmful to normal cellular function, and therefore gross tissue function, and ultimately general health, as would be changes caused by spending time in zero gravity (Bhatia 1999, Ruwhof 2000).

Constructing a credible story

In order to make sense of what is happening when a patient presents with symptoms, it is necessary to be able to extract information, to construct a story – or possibly several stories – based on what the patient says, what the history suggests, and what can be palpated and tested. These 'stories' should ideally tally, supporting each other to offer direction as to where therapeutic efforts should be concentrated.

Out of this should emerge a rationale for treatment, involving objectives that might reasonably be reached. Achievable objectives might sometimes involve complete recovery, or, in other circumstances, no more may be possible than a partial degree of improvement in the present condition. In other settings, ensuring that, for the time being, matters do not worsen may be the best possible scenario. Whatever the plan of action involves, it should be discussed and agreed with the patient, and should ideally involve active patient participation in the process.

Maps and grids

In order to make sense of the patient's history and of the many pieces of information made available via case history taking, observation, palpation and examination, to form a perspective on what is happening, a series of maps and grids may usefully be created. These might, for example, include (in no particular order of importance):

- A postural (structural) evaluation grid: including an anteroposterior perspective showing the relative positions of the major landmarks (ankles, knees, pelvis, spinal curves, head) as well as a bilateral comparison of the relative heights of ears, shoulders, scapulae, pelvic crest, hips and knees. The patterns observed in this way defines the structural framework to which the soft tissues are attached.

- A motion (functional) restriction grid: in which the major joints are evaluated for their functional ranges of motion, compared side with side, and with established norms. This would include spinal joints. 'End-feel', the quality of the end of range of tissues, is an important aspect of the evaluation of restriction barriers (Kaltenborn 1985).

- An individual characteristics map: demonstrating restrictions, asymmetries, or dysfunctional patterns specific to the patient, possibly including loss of range of movement, or hypermobility and/or inappropriate firing patterns in muscles when activated, and/or neurological signs.

- A postural muscle grid: including evidence of relative shortness of the postural muscles of the body. (See later in this chapter for discussion of different ways of catagorising muscles.)

- A muscular weakness grid: including evaluation of relative strength/weakness as well as endurance (stamina), of muscles associated with the patient's problem.

- Fascial patterns (for example those described by Zink & Lawson (1979) and Myers (1998 – see Box 2.2)). The Zink & Lawson description

is associated with what has been termed a 'common compensatory pattern', involving 'loose–tight' (or ease–bind) evaluations, which allows comparison of the freedom of movement of tissues on one side compared with the other (see below).

- Equilibrium/balance grid: this contains information as to stability in the upright position, for example standing on one leg, with eyes open and closed, and provides information relative to proprioceptive, visual and vestibular information delivery and processing.

- Local dysfunction maps: including detailed evidence of, for example, the presence of latent and active myofascial trigger points.

- Breathing function (and dysfunction) grid: in which aspects of breathing function are evaluated.

Space does not allow for a full discussion of all these possibilities; however, some will be explored and described.

Questions

It is useful to examine the viewpoints of different experts if we are to come to an understanding of soft tissue dysfunction in particular, and of its place in the larger scheme of things in relation to musculoskeletal and general dysfunction. A commonality will be noted in many of the views presented in this chapter. Also apparent will be distinctive differences in emphasis.

Most models include recognition of a progression, a sequence of events, chain reactions, and a process of adaptation, compensation, modification, attempted homeostatic accommodations, etc., to whatever is taking place.

In order to adequately deal with soft tissue or joint dysfunction, it is axiomatic that what is dysfunctional should first be accurately assessed and identified. Based on such verifiable data as may be available, a treatment plan with a realistic prognosis can then be formulated. The assessment findings are then capable of being used as a yardstick against which results can be assessed

Box 2.2 Myers' fascial trains (Myers 1997, 2001) (Figs 2.2–2.7)

Tom Myers, a distinguished Rolfer, has described a number of clinically useful sets of myofascial chains. The connections between different structures ('long functional continuities') which these insights allow should be kept in mind when consideration is given to the possibility of symptoms arising from distant causal sites. They are of particular importance in helping draw attention to (for example) dysfunctional patterns in the lower limb which impact directly (via these chains) on structures in the upper body.

The superficial back line (Fig. 2.2) involves a chain which starts with:

- The plantar fascia, linking the plantar surface of the toes to the calcaneus
- Gastrocnemius, linking calcaneus to the femoral condyles
- Hamstrings, linking the femoral condyles to the ischial tuberosities
- Subcutaneous ligament, linking the ischial tuberosities to sacrum
- Lumbosacral fascia, erector spinae and nuchal ligament, linking the sacrum to the occiput
- Scalp fascia, linking the occiput to the brow ridge.

The superficial front line (Fig. 2.3) involves a chain which starts with:

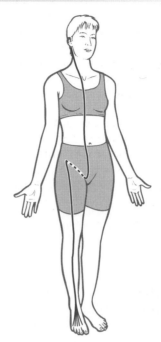

Figure 2.3 The superficial front line (SFL).

- The anterior compartment and the periosteum of the tibia, linking the dorsal surface of the toes to the tibial tuberosity

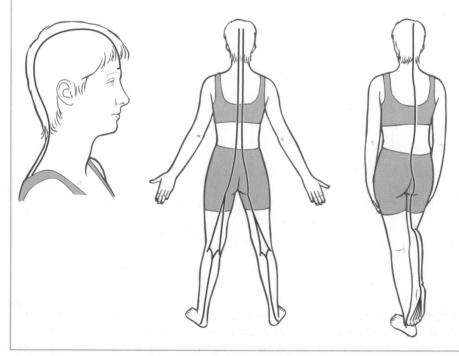

Figure 2.2 The superficial back line (SBL).

Box 2.2 Continued

- Rectus femoris, linking the tibial tuberosity to the anterior inferior iliac spine and pubic tubercle
- Rectus abdominis as well as pectoralis and sternalis fascia, linking the pubic tubercle and the anterior inferior iliac spine with the manubrium
- Sternocleidomastoid, linking the manubrium with the mastoid process of the temporal bone.

The lateral line (Fig. 2.4) involves a chain which starts with:

- Peroneal muscles, linking the 1st and 5th metatarsal bases with the fibular head
- Iliotibial tract, tensor fascia lata and gluteus maximus, linking the fibular head with the iliac crest
- External obliques, internal obliques and (deeper) quadratus lumborum, linking the iliac crest with the lower ribs
- External intercostals and internal intercostals, linking the lower ribs with the remaining ribs
- Splenius cervicis, iliocostalis cervicis, sternocleidomastoid and (deeper) scalenes, linking the ribs with the mastoid process of the temporal bone.

The spiral lines (Fig. 2.5) involve a chain which starts with:

- Splenius capitis, which wraps across from one side to the other, linking the occipital ridge (say on the right) with the spinous processes of the lower cervical and upper thoracic spine on the left

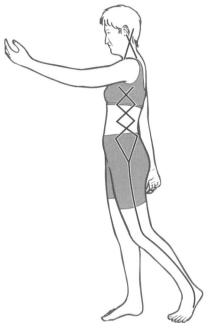

Figure 2.4
The lateral line.

- Continuing in this direction (see Fig. 2.5), the rhomboids (on the left) link via the medial border of the scapula with serratus anterior and the ribs (still on

Figure 2.5   The spiral lines.

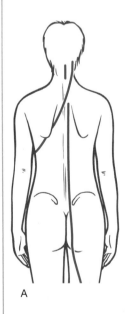

A

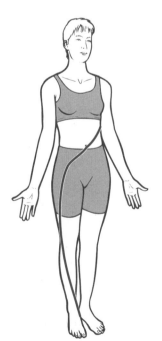

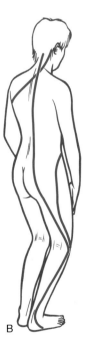

B

Box 2.2 Continued

the left), wrapping around the trunk via the external obliques and the abdominal aponeurosis on the left, to connect with the internal obliques on the right and then to a strong anchor point on the anterior superior iliac spine (right side)
- From the ASIS, the tensor fascia lata and the iliotibial tract link to the lateral tibial condyle
- Tibialis anterior links the lateral tibial condyle with the 1st metatarsal and cuneiform
- From this apparent end point of the chain (1st metatarsal and cuneiform), peroneus longus rises to link with the fibular head
- Biceps femoris connects the fibular head to the ischial tuberosity
- The sacrotuberous ligament links the ischial tuberosity to the sacrum
- The sacral fascia and the erector spinae link the sacrum to the occipital ridge.

  The deep front line describes several alternative chains involving the structures anterior to the spine (internally, for example):
- The anterior longitudinal ligament, diaphragm, pericardium, mediastinum, parietal pleura, fascia prevertebralis and the scalene fascia, which connect the lumbar spine (bodies and transverse processes) to the cervical transverse processes, and via longus capitis to the basilar portion of the occiput
- Other links in this chain might involve a connection between the posterior manubrium and the hyoid bone via the subhyoid muscles and
- The fascia pretrachealis between the hyoid and the cranium/mandible, involving suprahyoid muscles
- The muscles of the jaw linking the mandible to the face and cranium.

  Myers includes in his chain description structures of the lower limbs which connect the tarsum of the foot to the lower lumbar spine, making the linkage complete. Additional smaller chains involving the arms are described as follows:

Back of the arm lines (Fig. 2.6)
- The broad sweep of trapezius links the occipital ridge and the cervical spinous processes to the spine of the scapula and the clavicle
- The deltoid, together with the lateral intermuscular septum, connects the scapula and clavicle with the lateral epicondyle
- The lateral epicondyle is joined to the hand and fingers by the common extensor tendon

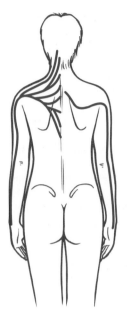

Figure 2.6 Back of arm lines.

- Another track on the back of the arm can arise from the rhomboids, which link the thoracic transverse processes to the medial border of the scapula
- The scapula in turn is linked to the olecranon of the ulna by infraspinatus and the triceps
- The olecranon of the ulna connects to the small finger via the periosteum of the ulna
- A 'stabilisation' feature in the back of the arm involves latissimus dorsi and the thoracolumbar fascia, which connects the arm with the spinous processes, the contralateral sacral fascia and gluteus maximus, which in turn attaches to the shaft of the femur
- Vastus lateralis connects the femur shaft to the tibial tuberosity and (via this) to the periosteum of the tibia.

Front of the arm lines (Fig. 2.7)
- Latissimus dorsi, teres major and pectoralis major attach to the humerus close to the medial intramuscular septum, connecting it to the back of the trunk
- The medial intramuscular septum connects the humerus to the medial epicondyle which connects with the palmar hand and fingers by means of the common flexor tendon

Box 2.2 Continued

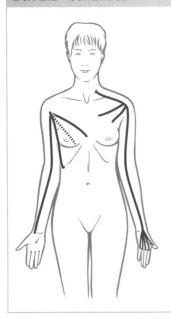

Figure 2.7   Front of arm lines.

- An additional line on the front of the arm involves pectoralis minor, the costocoracoid ligament, the brachial neurovascular bundle and the fascia clavipectoralis, which attach to the coracoid process
- The coracoid process also provides the attachment for biceps brachii (or brachialis) linking this to the radius and the thumb via the flexor compartment of the forearm
- A 'stabilisation' line on the front of the arm involves pectoralis major attaching to the ribs, as do the external obliques, which then run to the pubic tubercle, where a connection is made to the contralateral adductor longus, gracilis, pes anserinus, and the tibial periosteum.

and evaluated over time. If progress is not forthcoming, reassessment is required.

Among the many pertinent questions which need answering are:

1. Which muscle groups have shortened and contracted, and why?

2. Is identified soft tissue restriction related to neuromuscular influences (which could be recorded on an EMG reading of the muscle), or to connective tissue changes/fibrosis (which would not show on an EMG reading), or both?

3. Which muscles have become significantly weaker, and is this through inhibition or through atrophy – and why?

4. What 'chain reactions' of functional imbalance have occurred, as one muscle group (possibly because of excessive hypertonicity) has inhibited and weakened its antagonists?

5. What joint restrictions – spinal and other – are associated with identifiable soft tissue changes – either as a result, or as a cause, of these?

6. Is a restriction primarily of soft tissue or of joint origin, or a mixture of both?

7. How does the obvious dysfunction relate to neurological features and function, and to the rest of the musculoskeletal system of this patient?

8. What patterns of compensating postural stress have such changes produced (or have produced them) and how is this further stressing the body as a whole, affecting its energy levels and function?

9. Within particular muscle areas that are stressed, what local soft tissue changes (myofascial, etc.) have occurred, leading, for example, to trigger point development?

10. What symptoms, whether of pain or other forms of dysfunction, are the result of superficial, or peripheral reflexogenic activity, such as trigger points, or to central sensitisation?

In other words:

- What palpable, measurable, identifiable evidence is there which connects what we can observe, assess, test and palpate to the symptoms (pain, restriction, fatigue, etc.) of this patient?

- What's loose, what's tight, what asymmetries are there, and to what extent is malalignment a feature?

And further:

11. What, if anything, can be done to remedy or modify the situation, safely and effectively?

12. Is this a self-limiting condition which treatment can make it more tolerable as it normalises itself?

13. Is this a condition which can be helped towards normalisation by therapeutic intervention?

14. Is this a condition which cannot normalise, but which can be modified to some extent, thus making function easier or reducing pain?

15. What mobilisation, relaxation and/or toning/strengthening strategies are most likely to be of assistance, and can this individual be taught to use herself less stressfully?

16. To what degree can the patient participate in the process of recovery, normalisation, rehabilitation?

   Fortunately, as part of such therapeutic interventions, a range of MET methods exist that can be taught as self-treatment, thus involving and empowering the patient.

Viewing symptoms in context

Clearly the answers to this range of questions will vary enormously from person to person, even if symptoms appear similar at the outset. The context within which symptoms appear and exist will largely determine the opportunities available for successful therapeutic interventions.

Pain is probably the single most common symptom experienced by humans and, along with fatigue, is the most frequent reason for anyone consulting a doctor in industrialised societies – indeed the World Health Organization (1981) has suggested that pain is 'the primary problem' for developed countries.

Within that vast area of pain, musculoskeletal dysfunction in general, and back pain in particular, feature large; indeed, low-back pain is known to be the second most common reason for individuals consulting a physician in the USA (Deyo & Weinstein 2001).

If symptoms of pain and restriction are viewed in isolation, with inadequate attention being paid to the degree of acuteness or chronicity, their relationship with the rest of the body and its systems (including the musculoskeletal and nervous systems) – as well as, for example, the emotional and nutritional status of the individual, and the multiple environmental, occupational, social and other factors which impinge upon them – then it is quite possible that the presenting problem will be treated inappropriately.

A patient with major social, economic and emotional stressors current in her life, who presents with muscular pain and backache, is unlikely to respond – other than in the short term – to manual approaches that fail to take account of the enormous and multiple coping strains she is handling.

In many instances, the provision of a job, a new home, a new spouse (or removal of the present one) would be the most appropriate 'treatment' in terms of addressing the real causes of such pain or backache. However, the practitioner must utilise those skills available so that suitable treatment will, if nothing else, minimise the patient's mechanical and functional strains – even if they cannot deal with what is really wrong!

Ideal treatment of pain and dysfunction that has evolved out of the somatisation by the patient of profound emotional distress might well be helped more through counseling and/or psychotherapy, application of deep relaxation methods, and non-specific 'wellness' bodywork methods, along with enhancement of stress-coping abilities, rather than by means of specific musculoskeletal interventions which might impose even more adaptation demands on an already overextended system, and which fail to address underlying and possibly ongoing psychological features. The art of successfully applied manual approaches to healing lies, at least in part, in recognising when intervention should be specific, and when it needs to be more general, and when it needs to integrate with other approaches.

The role of the emotions in musculoskeletal dysfunction

Waersted et al (1993) have shown that a small number of motor units in particular muscles may display almost constant, or repeated, activity when influenced psychogenically. Low-amplitude levels of activity (using surface EMG) were evident even when the muscle was not being employed:

> *A small pool of low-threshold motor units may be under considerable load for prolonged periods of time ... motor units with Type 1 [postural] fibres are predominant among these. If the subject repeatedly recruits the same motor units, the overload may result in a metabolic crisis.*

This description has strong parallels with the evolution of myofascial trigger points, as suggested by Travell & Simons (1992).

Sandman (1984) has analysed the interaction between mind influences on those neurological and metabolic functions which regulate physiological responses, and concludes that there is a synergistic relationship which results in a need to address both the psychological and the physiological aspects of stress which have emerged from the effects of (among others) traumatic, social familial, relationship, career, health and financial stressors (Selye 1976, Sandman 1984). Unless mind and body are addressed, 'no permanent reduction of the negative feedback loop is possible'.

Sandman reviews the process by means of which stress and secondary stress influence muscles:

1. Stress causes biochemical changes in the brain – partly involving neurotransmitter production which increases neural excitability.

2. Postural changes follow in muscles, commonly involving increased tone, which retards circulatory efficiency and increases calcium, lactic acid and hyaluronic acid accumulation.

3. Local contractile activity in muscle is increased because of the interaction between calcium and adenosine triphosphate (ATP), leading to physiological contractions, which shorten and tense muscle bundles.

4. Sustained metabolic activity in such muscles increases neural hyper-reactivity, which may stimulate reflex vasoconstriction, leading to local tenderness and referred pain.

5. Relative oxygen lack and reduced energy supply result from decreased blood flow, leading to an energy-deficient muscle contraction in which the sarcoplasmic reticulum becomes damaged.

6. The energy-sensitive calcium pump responds by increasing muscle contraction due to the lack of energy supply, leading to ever greater depletion.

7. Pain is a feature of this process, possibly due to accumulation locally of chemicals, which might include bradykinin, substance P, inflammatory exudates, histamine and others.

8. Local pressure build-up involving these chemicals and local metabolic wastes, and/or local ischaemia, are sufficient causes to produce local spasm, which might involve local and/or referred pain.

9. If at this time the muscle is stretched, the locked actin and myosin filaments will release the contraction and sufficient ATP can then accumulate to allow a more normal sarcoplasmic reticulum, which would allow for removal of the build-up of metabolites.

10. The degree of damage which the muscle sustains due to this sequence depends entirely upon the length of time during which these conditions are allowed to continue: 'At this point physiological aspects as well as psychological should be addressed ... to stop the debilitating cycle'.

Sandman's method of relieving the physical aspects of the condition involves active and passive stretching alongside pressure and vibratory techniques.

Latey's perspective

Australian-based British osteopath Philip Latey (1996) has found a useful metaphor for describing observable and palpable patterns of distortion that coincide with particular clinical problems. He uses the analogy of 'clenched fists' (Fig. 2.8) because, he says, the unclenching of a fist correlates with physiological relaxation, while the clenched fist indicates fixity, rigidity, overcontracted muscles, emotional turmoil, withdrawal from communication and so on. Failure to express emotion results in suppression of activity and, ultimately, chronic contraction of the muscles that would have been used were these emotions (e.g. rage, fear, anger, joy, frustration, sorrow) expressed. Latey points out that all areas of the body producing sensations, which arouse emotional excitement, may have their blood supply reduced by muscular contraction.

When considering the causes of hypertonicity and muscle shortening, emotional factors should be one of the areas investigated. Failure to do so will almost certainly lead to unsatisfactory results.

Clinical question Something all practitioners and therapists facing patients with musculoskeletal pain and dysfunction should ask of themselves relates to the extent to which psychological and emotional considerations are being taken into account.

Korr's 'orchestrated movement' concept

It is necessary to conceptualise muscular function and dysfunction as being something other than a local event. Irwin Korr (1976) stated the position elegantly and eloquently:

> *The spinal cord is the keyboard on which the brain plays when it calls for activity. But each 'key' in the console sounds not an individual 'tone' such as the contraction of a particular group of muscle fibres, but a whole 'symphony' of motion. In other words, built into the cord is a large repertoire of patterns of activity, each involving the complex, harmonious, delicately balanced orchestration of the contractions and relaxation of many muscles. The brain thinks in terms of whole motions, not individual muscles. It calls, selectively, for the preprogrammed patterns in the cord and brain stem, modifying them in countless ways and combining them in an infinite variety in still more complex patterns. Each activity is subject to further modulation refinement, and adjustment by the feedback continually streaming in from the participating muscles, tendons and joints.*

We must never forget the complex interrelationships between the soft tissues, the muscles, fascia and tendons and their armies of neural reporting stations, as we attempt to understand the nature of dysfunction and of what is required to achieve normalisation.

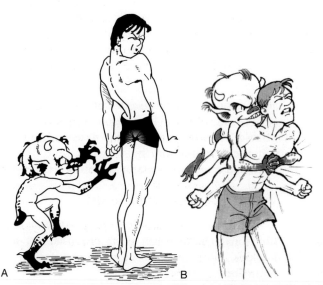

Figure 2.8 **A** Latey's lower fist concept (reproduced from Journal of Bodywork and Movement Therapies 1996 1(1): 50). **B** Latey's middle fist concept (reproduced from Journal of Bodywork and Movement Therapies 1996 1(1): 50).

A   B

A proprioceptive model of dysfunction

Let us visualise an area at relative ease, in which there is some degree of difference between antagonist muscles, one group comfortably stretched, the other short of their normal resting length and equally comfortable, such as might exist in someone comfortably bending forwards to lift something. Imagine a sudden demand for stability in this setting (the person or whatever they are lifting unaccountably slips for example). As this happened, the annulospiral receptors in the shortened (flexor) muscles would respond to the sudden demand by contracting even more (Mathews 1981).

The neural reporting stations in these shortened muscles (which would be rapidly changing length to provide stability) would be firing impulses as if the muscles were being stretched, even when the muscle remained well short of its normal resting length.

At the same time the stretched extensor muscles would rapidly shorten in order to stabilise the situation. Once stability has been achieved, they would probably still be somewhat longer than their normal resting length.

Korr (1947, 1975) has described what happens in the abdominal muscles (flexors) in such a situation. He says that because of their relaxed status, short of their resting length, there occurs a silencing of the spindles. However, due to the demand for information from the higher centres, gamma gain is increased reflexively, and as the muscle contracts rapidly to stabilise the alarm demands, the central nervous system would receive information that the muscle, which is actually short of its neutral resting length, was being stretched. In effect, the muscles would have adopted a position of *somatic dysfunction* as a result of 'garbled', or inappropriate, proprioceptive reporting.

As DiGiovanna (1991) explains:

With trauma or muscle effort against a sudden change in resistance, or with muscle strain incurred by resisting the effects of gravity for a period of time, one muscle at a joint is strained and its antagonist is hyper-shortened. When the shortened muscle is suddenly stretched the annulospiral receptors in that muscle are stimulated causing a reflex contraction of the already shortened muscle. The proprioceptors in the short muscle now fire impulses as if the shortened muscle were being stretched. Since this inappropriate proprioceptor response can be maintained indefinitely a somatic dysfunction has been created.

In effect, the two opposing sets of muscles would have adopted a stabilising posture to protect the threatened structures, and in doing so would have become locked into positions of imbalance in relation to their normal function. One set of muscles would be shorter, and one longer, than its normal resting length. In this example any attempt to extend the area/joint(s) would be strongly resisted by the tonically shortened flexor group. The individual would be locked into a forward-bending distortion. The joint(s) involved would not have been taken beyond their normal physiological range, and yet the normal range would be unavailable due to the shortened status of the flexor group. Going further into flexion, however, would present no problems or pain.

Walther (1988) summarises the situation as follows (see Fig. 2.9A–C):

When proprioceptors send conflicting information there may be simultaneous contraction of the antagonists ... without antagonist muscle inhibition, joint and other strain results ... a reflex pattern develops which causes muscle or other tissue to maintain this continuing strain. It [strain dysfunction] often relates to the inappropriate signaling from muscle proprioceptors that have been strained from rapid change that does not allow proper adaptation.

We can recognise this 'strain' situation in an acute setting such as torticollis following whiplash, as well as in acute 'lumbago'. It is also recognisable as a feature of many types of chronic somatic dysfunction in which joints remain restricted due to muscular imbalances of this type.

Van Buskirk's nociceptive model

A variation on the theme of a progression of dysfunctional changes has been proposed by Van Buskirk (1990), who suggests the following sequence:

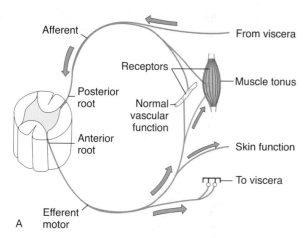

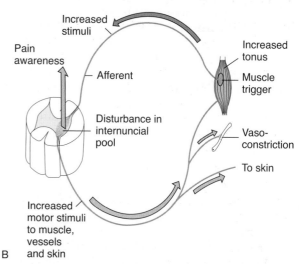

Figure 2.9A Schematic representation of normal afferent influences deriving from visceral, muscular and venous sources, on the efferent supply to those same structures.

Figure 2.9B Schematic representation of normal afferent influences deriving from a muscle which displays excessively increased tonus and/or trigger point activity, both in pain awareness and on the efferent motor supply to associated muscular, venous and skin areas.

Figure 2.9C Schematic representation of the secondary spread of neurologically induced influences deriving from acute or chronic soft tissue dysfunction, and involving trigger point activity and/or spasm.

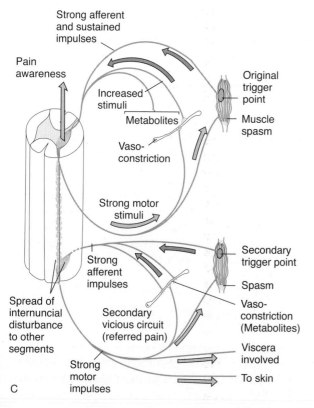

1. Nociceptors (peripheral pain receptors) in a muscle are activated by minor trauma from chemical, mechanical, or thermal stimuli, or sources such as disease or trauma, involving somatic or visceral structures producing nociceptive activation.

2. Nociceptive activation transmits impulses to other axons in the same nociceptor, as well as to the spinal cord.

3. Various peptide transmitters in the axon branches are released, resulting in vasodilatation and the gathering of immune cells around, and in, the trauma site.

4. These in turn release chemicals, which enhance the vasodilatation and extravasation while also lowering the nociceptive threshold.

5. Organs at a distance may display axon reflex effects; for example, skeletal muscles and the heart may be simultaneously affected.

6. Spinal neurons will be stimulated by impulses entering the cord synaptically, which influences aspects of the higher CNS that register pain; or the impulses might stimulate preganglionic autonomic neurons or even the spinal skeletal muscle motor pool, producing nocifensive reflexes.

7. There may be poor localisation of pain at this stage, if it is perceived at all, due to the many sources influencing the same spinal neurons, as well as the divergence of signals along neighbouring spinal segments. Pain will, however, be most noticeable in the originating segment.

8. Any sympathetic response to this chain of events will depend upon the effects of sympathetic stimuli to the target organ, and could (among others) involve cardiopressor, gastrointestinal stasis, bronchodilatation, vasopressor or vasodilator or negative immune function effects.

9. Muscular responses could involve local or multisegmental changes, including shortening of the injured muscle itself via synergistic or self-generated action from non-injured fibres; or overlying muscle might attempt to guard underlying tissues, or some other defensive action might ensue.

10. Direct mechanical restriction of the affected muscles derives from vasodilatation which, along with chemicals associated with tissue injury (bradykinin, histamine, serotonin, etc.) causes stimulation of local nociceptors in the muscle associated with the original trauma, or those reflexively influenced.

11. A new defensive muscular arrangement will develop which will cause imbalance and a shortening of the muscles involved. These will not be held at their maximal degree of shortening nor in their previously neutral position.

12. This continued contraction results in additional nociceptive action as well as fatigue, which tends to cause recruitment of additional muscular tissues to maintain the abnormal situation.

13. After a matter of hours or days the abnormal joint positions which result from this defensive muscular activity become chronic as connective tissue reorganisation involving tissue fibrocytes commences.

14. Connective tissues will be randomly orientated in the shortened muscles and less capable of handling stress along normal lines of force.

Van Buskirk (1990) describes the progression as follows:

'In the lengthened muscles, creep will elongate the connective tissue, producing slack without stressing the lengthened muscles. Now maintenance of the joint in the non-neutral position dictated by both the nocifensive reflexes and the connective tissue changes no longer requires continuous muscle activity.'

Now:

- Active contraction only occurs when the area is stressed, which would reactivate the nociceptors.

- At the same time the joint is neither 'gravitationally, posturally, nor functionally balanced', making it far more likely to be stressed and to produce yet more nociceptive activation.

- There would exist a situation of restricted motion deriving from the original shortening, chronic nociceptive activation, and autonomic activation.

- In effect, there would now be a neurologically derived restriction, as well as structural modifications and fibrotic connective tissue changes, both of which require normalising in order to restore normal function. Both the original tissues which were stressed, as well as others which have modified in a protective manner, would be influencing the unbalanced, unphysiological situation.

An example of nociceptively modulated dysfunction   Let us consider someone in a car whose neck is injured as it comes to an unexpected halt. The neck would be thrown backwards into hyperextension, stressing the flexor group of muscles. The extensor group would be rapidly shortened and various proprioceptive changes would operate (as described above in relation to a bending strain), leading to strain and reflexive shortening, inducing them to remain in a shortened state. At the time of the sudden hyperextension, the flexors of the neck would be violently stretched, inducing actual tissue damage (Nordhoff 2000).

Nociceptive responses (which are more powerful than proprioceptive influences) would occur, and these multisegmental reflexes would produce a flexor withdrawal – increasing tone in the flexor muscles.

The neck would display hypertonicity of both the extensors and the flexors – pain, guarding and stiffness would be apparent, and the role of the clinician would be to remove these restricting influences layer by layer.

Where pain is a factor in strain this has to be considered as producing an overriding influence over whatever other more 'normal' (proprioceptive) reflexes might be operating. In the example of neck strain described, it is obvious that in real-life matters are likely to be even more complicated, since a true whiplash would introduce both rapid hyperextension and hyperflexion, so producing a multitude of conflicting layers of dysfunction.

The proprioceptive and nociceptive reflexes which might be involved in the production of strain are likely to also involve other factors. As

Bailey (Bailey & Dick 1992) explains: 'Probably few dysfunctional states result from a purely proprioceptive or nociceptive response. Additional factors such as autonomic responses, other reflexive activities, joint receptor responses, or emotional states must also be accounted for.'

However, it is at the level of our basic neurological awareness that understanding of the complexity of these problems commences, and we need to be aware of the choices which are available for resolving such dysfunction.

How would MET be able to influence this situation?   Various approaches are likely to be helpful, including a variety of techniques derived from positional release methods, such as strain/counterstrain (SCS) (Jones 1964), facilitated positional release (DiGiovanna 1991) and functional technique (Greenman 1989), as well as various modifications of MET.

Van Buskirk (1990) states it thus:

In [patient] indirect 'muscle energy' the skeletal muscles in the shortened area are initially stretched to the maximum extent allowed by the somatic dysfunction [to the barrier]. With the tissues held in this position the patient is instructed to contract the affected muscle voluntarily. This isometric activation of the muscle will stretch the internal connective tissues. Voluntary activation of the motor neurons to the same muscles also blocks transmission in spinal nociceptive pathways. Immediately following the isometric phase, passive extrinsic stretch is imposed, further lengthening the tissues towards the normal easy neutral position.

It is as well to emphasise that these models of the possible chain reaction of events taking place in acute and chronic musculoskeletal dysfunction are included in order to help us to understand what might be happening in the complex series of events which surround, and which flow from, such problems. These elegant attempts at interpreting our understanding of stress and strain are not definitive; there are other models, and some of them will be touched on as we progress through our exploration of the patterns of dysfunction which confront us clinically. A reading of Ch. 4 will confirm that van Buskirk's model is not fully in tune with more recent research, and that we have much to learn about the actual effects of isometric contractions in an MET or PNF setting.

Janda's 'primary and secondary' responses

It has become a truism to say that we need to consider the body as a whole. However, all too often local focus seems to be the dominant clinical approach. Janda (1988) gives examples of why this is short-sighted in the extreme.

He discusses the events which follow on from the presence of a short leg – which might well include an altered pelvic position, scoliosis, altered head position, changes at the cervicocranial junction, compensatory activity of the small cervico-occipital muscles, later compensation of neck musculature, increased muscle tone, muscle spasm, probable joint dysfunction, particularly at cervicocranial junction ... and a sequence of events which would then include compensation and adaptation responses in many muscles, followed by the evolution of a variety of possible syndromes involving head/neck, TMJ, shoulder/arm or others (see discussion of upper and lower 'crossed' syndromes later in this chapter).

Janda's point is that at such a time, after all the adaptation that has taken place, treatment of the most obvious cervical restrictions, where the patient might complain of pain and restriction, would be of limited benefit.

He points to the existence of oculopelvic and pelviocular reflexes, which determine that any change in pelvic orientation alters the position of the eyes, and vice versa. He further notes the synkinetic effect that ensures that eye position modifies muscle tone. As an example, when the individual looks upwards, suboccipital (and other) extensors tighten, while looking down tones the flexors as they prepare for activity (Komendatov 1945). 'These examples', Janda says, 'serve to emphasise that one should not limit consideration to local clinical symptomatology ... but [that we] should always maintain a general view'.

Prior's 'foot dysfunction' example

Consultant podiatrist Trevor Prior (1999) reminds us of the ways in which body-wide dysfunctional patterns can evolve from a very simple foot dysfunction. He points out that normal flexibility of the first metatarsophalangeal joints (MTPJ) is essential to normal gait. Dysfunction of this joint might occur in a condition known as functional halux limitus ('stiff big toe').

He observes:

1st MPTJ dorsiflexion is essential to allow the metatarsal rocker phase to occur ... . 1st MTPJ dorsiflexion is accompanied by ankle plantarflexion. A failure of this to occur results in early knee joint flexion (prior to heel strike of the [other] swing limb) and thus reduced hip joint extension. Insufficient hip joint extension prevents the hip flexors gaining mechanical advantage and thus removes their ability to initiate motion via a swing of the limb. As a result, the gluteals and quadratus lumborum on the contralateral side become active in order to help pull the weight-bearing leg into swing.

This will destabilize the contralateral lower back and sacroiliac joint and may predispose to piriformis overactivity. Furthermore the position of the hip at the time of hip flexor activity means that the leg effectively acts as a dead weight. As the hip flexors are unable to accelerate the leg forwards, they effectively pull the leg downwards, exacerbating the effect of the dead weight. This results in lateral rotation on the spine and trauma to the intervertebral disks. Whilst this abnormal function is of low magnitude, it is its repetitive nature that causes the problem over a sustained period of time. The average person takes 5000 steps per day, or 2500 per foot, thus subtle imbalances are repeated thousands of times per day.

It is easy to relocate the picture drawn by Prior, and to move the dysfunctional stresses upwards towards the upper back, neck and shoulders. The lesson that we can learn from this excellent example of 'chain reactions of dysfunction' is that, whatever else is done, efforts to normalise postural stresses should always involve attention to the foundations of the body – the feet.

Isaacson's 'functional unit'

Isaacson (1980) helps us to understand the interaction of associated parts in terms of spinal motion.

He describes spinal muscles as being divided into two groups, with one set being prime movers (extrinsic) and the others stabilisers (intrinsic), including the erector spinae muscle mass. Although the component parts of the erector spinae muscle group are often referred to individually as discrete entities (multifidus, intertransverse, interspinal, etc.), this is basically inaccurate.

He states that: 'Various functions have been assigned to these intrinsic muscles, on the assumption that they actually move vertebrae; however, the arrangement and position of the muscle bundles making up this group would seem to make it improbable that they have much to do in this regard.' They are, instead, stabilisers and proprioceptive sensory receptors which facilitate the coordinated activity of the vertebral complex (as in Korr's 'whole motions').

The force required to move the vertebral column comes from the large, extrinsic, muscles. Analysis of the multifidus group, which is particularly thick in the lumbar region, indicates that its component fascicles could not be prime movers, and that they serve effectively as maintainers of the position, normal or abnormal, in which the prime movers place the vertebrae.

The same finding is made in relation to the semi-spinal group of muscles. These are responsible for compensatory dysfunction, derived from the vertebra above and below, by virtue of the arrangement of groups of pairs of stabilising fascicles. These groups of muscles are, Isaacson maintains, responsible in large part for the coordinated, synchronous, function of the spinal column, which is a complex of the two functions of the different types of muscles in the region; those that stabilise, and those that move.

Isaacson goes so far as to suggest that the evidence points to the spinal region being a vast network of information gathering tissues: 'Arranged as they are in a variety of positions some of the individual muscle bundles are placed on a stretch by any change of position in the vertebral column, and the tension so produced is translated into terms of proprioceptive sensation and reported to the CNS.'

Thus the vertebral column and the body may need to be viewed as a functional unit, and not as a collection of parts and organs which function independently of each other. This is a concept which, while obvious, is often neglected in practice.

As we will discover later in this chapter, extrinsic prime movers and intrinsic stabilisers behave differently, not only in their normal function but also, most importantly, in their dysfunction (see notes on *stabilisers* and *mobilisers*, as well as *postural* and *phasic* muscles, later in this chapter).

Fascial considerations

If we are to have anything like a clear overview of soft tissue dysfunction it is necessary to add into the equation the influence of fascia, which invests, supports, divides, enwraps, gives cohesion to and is an integral part of every aspect of soft tissue structure and function throughout the body and which represents a single structural entity, from the inside of the skull to the soles of the feet.

Rolf (1962) put fascia and its importance into perspective when she discussed its properties:

Our ignorance of the role of fascia is profound. Therefore even in theory it is easy to overlook the possibility that far-reaching changes may be made not only in structural contour, but also in functional manifestation, through better organisation of the layer of superficial fascia which enwraps the body. Experiment demonstrates that drastic changes may be made in the body, solely by stretching, separating and relaxing superficial fascia in an appropriate manner. Osteopathic practitioners have observed and recorded the extent to which all degenerative changes in the body, be they muscular, nervous, circulatory or organic, reflect in superficial fascia. Any degree of degeneration, however minor, changes the bulk of the fascia, modifies its thickness and draws it into ridges in areas overlying deeper tensions and rigidities. Conversely, as this elastic envelope is stretched, manipulative mechanical energy is added to it, and the fascial colloid becomes more 'sol' and less 'gel'. As a result of the added energy, as well as of a directional contribution in applying it, the underlying structures, including muscles which determine the placement of the body parts in space, and also their relations to each other, come a little closer to the normal.

The contractile nature of fascia is a fairly recent observation. For example, Yahia et al (1993) have noted, 'Histologic studies indicate that the posterior layer of the (lumbodorsal) fascia is able to contract as if it were infiltrated with muscular tissue'.

The implications of this feature become clearer when we observe the variety of planes and directions of attachments of the lumbodorsal fascia as evidenced by the dissections of Barker & Briggs (1999). They have shown the lumbodorsal fascia to have a remarkable structural and functional continuity that extends from the pelvis to the cervical area: 'Both superficial and deep laminae of the posterior layer are more extensive superiorly than previously thought'. It is apparent that there is fibrous continuity throughout the lumbar, thoracic and cervical spine that directly connects with the tendons of the splenius muscles superiorly (see Fig 2.10).

Fascial properties

MET methods, which involve passive and active stretching of shortened and often fibrosed structures, have marked effects on fascial changes such as those described by Rolf, which can have universal involvement in total body function, as indicated by osteopathic physician Angus Cathie's list of the properties of fascia (Cathie 1974). Fascia, he tells us:

- Is richly endowed with nerve endings
- Has the ability to contract and relax elastically
- Provides extensive muscular attachments
- Supports and stabilises all structures, so enhancing postural balance
- Is vitally involved in all aspects of movement
- Assists in circulatory economy, especially of venous and lymphatic fluids
- Will demonstrate changes preceding many chronic degenerative diseases
- Will frequently be associated with chronic passive tissue congestion when such changes occur
- Will respond to tissue congestion by formation of fibrous tissue, followed by increased hydrogen ion concentration in articular and periarticular structures

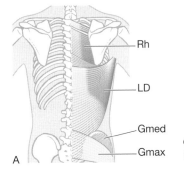

Rh = Rhomboids
LD = Latissimus dorsi
Gmed = Gluteus medius
Gmax = Gluteus maximus

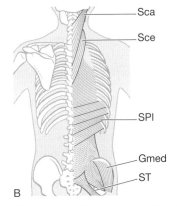

Sca = Splenius capitis
Sce = Splenius cervicis
Gmed = Guteus medius
SPI = Serratus posterior inferior
ST = Sacrotuberous

Figure 2.10 The lumbodorsal fascia has structural and functional continuity that extends from the pelvis to the cervical area. **A** Superficial lamina: Rh = rhomboids, LD = latissimus dorsi, GMed = gluteus medius, GMax = gluteus maximus. **B** Sca = splenius capitis, Sce = splenius cervicis, GMed = gluteus medius, SPI = serratus posterior inferior, ST = sacrotuberous. (Redrawn from Barker & Briggs 1999.)

- Will form specialised 'stress bands' in response to the load demanded of it
- Commonly produces a pain of a burning nature in response to sudden stress-trauma
- Is a major arena of many inflammatory processes
- Is the medium along the fascial planes of which many fluids and infectious processes pass
- Is the tissue which surrounds the CNS.

See also Box 1.5 (previous chapter) in regard to connective tissue and its water content.

Cathie also points out that many 'trigger' points correspond to sites where nerves pierce fascial investments. Stress on the fascia can be seen to

increases in proportion to the velocity of motion applied to them, which makes a gentle touch a fundamental requirement if viscous drag and resistance are to be avoided, when attempting to produce a release.

When stressful forces (either undesirable or therapeutic) are applied to fascia, there is a first reaction in which a degree of slack is allowed to be taken up, followed by what is colloquially referred to as 'creep' – a variable degree of resistance (depending upon the state of the tissues). 'Creep' is an honest term which accurately describes the slow, delayed yet persistent change that occurs in response to a continuously applied load, as long as this is gentle enough to not provoke the resistance of colloidal 'drag'. This highlights the absolute need in applying MET for stretching purposes (as will be described in later chapters) to be slow and gentle, involving 'taking out of slack', followed by unforced stretching, at the pace the tissues allow, if a defensive response is to be avoided.

Since fascia comprises a single body-wide structure, the implications for body-wide repercussions of distortions in that structure are clear. An example of one possible negative influence of this sort can be noted in the fascial divisions within the cranium, the tentorium cerebelli and falx cerebri, which are commonly warped during birthing difficulties (too long or too short a time in the birth canal, forceps delivery, etc.) as noted in craniosacral therapy to affect total body mechanics via the influence on fascia (and therefore the musculature) throughout the body (Brookes 1984).

In line with the work of Brookes, Biedermann (1992, 2001) has described what are termed 'KISS' children (an acronym for **k**inematic **i**mbalances due to **s**uboccipital **s**train), in whom the main clinical feature is torticollis, often combined with an asymmetrical cranium, general postural asymmetry and a range of dysfunctional symptoms. Biedermann notes: '[KISS imbalances] can be regarded as one of the main reasons for asymmetry in posture and consequently asymmetry of the osseous structures of the cranium and the spine'.

Among the many symptoms reported by Biedermann in such children are: torticollis, reduced range of motion of the head/neck, cervical hypersensitivity, opisthotonos, restless-ness, inability to control head movement, and one upper limb under-used (based on statistical records of 263 babies treated in one calendar year up to June 1995).

Biedermann reports that the most effective treatment for such infants is removal of sub-occipital strain by manual treatment, and not by direct treatment of cranial asymmetry as this is considered to be a symptom of the underlying problem (most commonly suboccipital strain). Following appropriate treatment to re-establish full range of upper cervical motion, functional improvement is reported to be common within 2–3 weeks, although normalisation of cranial asymmetry takes many months.

Postural (fascial) patterns

Zink & Lawson (1979) have described what they term 'common compensatory patterns' (CCP) of postural adaptation, determined by fascial compensation and decompensation.

- Fascial *compensation* is seen to commonly involve useful, beneficial and above all, functional adaptations (i.e. no obvious symptoms emerge) on the part of the musculoskeletal system, for example in response to anomalies such as a short leg, or to overuse.

- *Decompensation* describes the same phenomenon, but only in relation to a situation in which adaptive changes are seen to be dysfunctional, to produce symptoms, evidencing a failure of homeostatic adaptation.

By testing the tissue 'preferences' in different areas, and evaluating obvious distortion patterns, it is often possible to classify common compensatory patterns in clinically useful ways:

- *Ideal* (minimal adaptive load transferred to other regions) – more or less equal degrees of normal range rotation are observed.

- *Compensated* patterns which alternate in direction, from area to area (e.g. atlanto-occipital– cervicothoracic–thoracolumbar–lumbosacral), and which represent positive adaptive modifications. The most commonly observed pattern, according to Zink & Lawson, is left–right–left–right – commencing with the atlanto-occipital joint.

- *Uncompensated* patterns that do not alternate are commonly the result of trauma, and represent negative adaptive modifications. The consequences of an uncompensated CCP are that adaptation potential is minimal or absent, and unpredictable responses may be observed when specific changes are introduced via treatment or arise from, for instance, leg length modification (e.g. heel lift) or alterations in occlusion.

Functional evaluation of common compensatory (fascial) patterns

Zink & Lawson (1979) have described methods for testing tissue preference. There are four crossover sites where fascial tensions/restrictions can easily be noted: occipitoatlantal (OA), cervicothoracic (CT), thoracolumbar (TL), lumbosacral (LS). These sites are tested for their rotation (and/or side-bending) preferences.

Zink & Lawson's research showed that most people display alternating patterns of rotatory preference, with about 80% of people showing a CCP of left–right–left–right, 'reading' from the occiptotatlantal region downwards. Zink & Lawson observed that the 20% of people whose compensatory pattern did not alternate commonly had poor health histories.

Treatment of either CCP or uncompensated fascial patterns has the objective of trying as far as is possible to create a symmetrical degree of rotatory motion at the key crossover sites. The treatment methods used to achieve this range from direct muscle energy approaches to indirect positional release techniques. Restoration of an alternating compensatory pattern can be seen as evidence of successful therapeutic intervention.

Observed CCP signs

Defeo & Hicks (1993) have described the observed signs of CCP as follows:

In the common compensatory pattern (CCP), an examiner will note the following observations in the supine patient. The left leg will appear longer than the right. The left iliac crest will appear higher or more cephalad than the right. The pelvis will roll passively easier to the right than to the left because the lumbar spine is sidebent left and rotated right. The sternum is displaced to the left as it courses inferiorly. The left infraclavicular parasternal area is more prominent anteriorly because the thoracic inlet is sidebent right and rotated right. The upper neck rotates easier to the left. The right arm appears longer than the left, when fully extended.

Assessment of tissue preference

NOTE: If a differential assessment as to the location of major areas of dysfunction is being attempted, the procedures outlined below should be performed in both supine and standing. Differential assessment is explained below.

Occipitoatlantal (OA) area

(a) The patient is supine. The practitioner sits at the patient's head, slightly to one side, and faces the corner of the table. One hand (caudal hand) cradles the occiput with opposed index finger and thumb palpating the atlas. The other hand is placed on the patient's forehead. The hand palpating the occiptoatlantal joint evaluates the tissue preference (which way does it move most easily without force?) as the area is slowly rotated left and then right.

Or, seated or standing at the head of the table, both hands are used to take the neck into maximal unstressed flexion (to lock segments below C2) and the rotational preference is assessed.

(b) When the patient is standing, the head neck is placed in full flexion and rotation left and right, of the head on the neck, are evaluated for the preferred direction (range) of movement.

Cervicothoracic (CT) area

(a) The patient is supine and the practitioner places his hands so that they lie, palms upward, beneath the scapulae. The practitioner's forearms and elbows should be in touch with the table surface. Leverage can be introduced by one arm at a time as the practitioner's weight is introduced towards the floor through one elbow and then the other, easing the patient's scapulae anteriorly. This allows a safe and relatively stress-free assessment to be made of the freedom with which one side and then the other moves, producing a rotation at the cervicothoracic junction. Rotational preference can easily be ascertained.

(b) The patient is seated or standing in a relaxed posture with the practitioner behind, with hands placed to cover the medial aspects of the upper trapezius so that his fingers rest over the clavicles and thumbs rest on the transverse processes of the T1/T2 area. The hands assess the area being palpated for its 'tightness/looseness' preferences as a slight degree of rotation left and then right is introduced at the level of the cervicothoracic junction. If there was a preference for the OA area to rotate left, then there should ideally be a preference for right rotation at the CT junction.

Thoracolumbar (TL) area

(a) The patient is supine or prone. The practitioner stands at waist level facing cephalad and places his hands over the lower thoracic structures, fingers along lower rib shafts laterally. Treating the structure being palpated as a cylinder, the hands test the preference for the lower thorax to rotate around its central axis, one way and then the other. The preferred TL rotation direction should be compared with those of OA and CT test results. Alternation in these should be observed if a healthy adaptive process is occurring.

(b) With the patient standing, the practitioner stands behind and with hands over the lower thoracic structures, fingers along lower rib shafts laterally, tests the preference for the lower thorax to rotate around its central axis, one way and then the other.

Lumbosacral (LS) area

(a) The patient is supine. The practitioner stands below waist level facing cephalad and places his hands on the anterior pelvic structures, using the contact as a 'steering wheel' to evaluate tissue preference as the pelvis is rotated around its central axis, seeking information as to its 'tightness/

looseness' preferences. Alternation with previously assessed preferences should be observed if a healthy adaptive process is occurring.

(b) The patient is standing and the practitioner, standing behind, places his hands on the pelvic crest, and rotates the pelvis around its central axis, to identify its rotational preference.

NOTE: By holding tissues in their 'tight' or bind directions, and introducing an isometric contraction, changes may be encouraged.

Questions the practitioner should ask himself following the assessment exercise

1. Was there an 'alternating' pattern to the tissue preferences, and was this the same when supine and when standing?

2. Or was there a tendency for the tissue preference to be in the same direction in all, or most of, the four areas assessed?

3. If the latter was the case, was this in an individual whose health is more compromised than average (in line with Zink & Lawson's observations)?

4. What therapeutic methods would produce a more balanced degree of tissue preference?

Differential assessment, based on findings of supine and standing Zink tests (Liem 2004)

- If the rotational preferences alternate when supine, and display a greater tendency to not alternate (i.e. they rotate in the same directions) when standing, a dysfunctional adaptation pattern that is 'ascending' is most likely, i.e. the major dysfunctions lie in the lower body, pelvis or lower extremities.

- If the rotational pattern remains the same when supine and standing this suggests that the adaptation pattern is primarily 'descending', i.e. the major dysfunctional patterns lie in the upper body, cranium or jaw.

Example of sport-induced compensation (see also Ch. 11)

Kuchera and associates (Kuchera et al 1990) have shown that in healthy collegiate volunteers a significant correlation exists between a history of trauma and the type of athletic activity pursued, most notably in the golf team who displayed a rotation to the right around the right oblique sacral axis.

The volunteers were subjected to a variety of assessments, including palpatory structural analysis, anthropomorphic measurements and radiographic series, as well as photographic centre of gravity analyses. Well-compensated patterns of fascia were noted in those who had a low incidence of back pain but, conversely, a higher incidence of non-compensated patterning related to back pain within the previous year. Subjects reporting a significant history of psoas muscle problems were found to have a high incidence of non-compensated fascial patterning.

'Looseness and tightness' as part of the biomechanical model

Robert Ward (1997) discusses the 'loose–tight' model as a concept that helps the practitioner to appreciate three-dimensionality, as the body, or part of it, is palpated/assessed. This assessment may involve large or small areas in which interactive asymmetry produces areas or structures which are 'tight and loose' relative to each other. Ward illustrates this with the following examples:

- A sacroiliac/hip that is tight on one side and loose on the other
- A tight SCM alongside loose scalenes on the same side
- One shoulder region tight and the other loose.

The terms 'ease' and 'bind' are also used to describe these loose–tight phenomena. Assessment of the 'tethering' of tissues, and of the subtle qualities of 'end-feel' in soft tissues and joints, are prerequisites for appropriate treatment being applied, whether this is of a direct or indirect nature, or whether it is active or passive.

Indeed, the awareness of these features (end-feel, tight–loose, ease–bind) may be the determining factor as to which therapeutic approaches are introduced, and in what sequence. These barriers (tight and loose) can also be seen to refer to the obstacles that are identified in preparation for direct methods such as MET (where the barrier of

restriction is engaged and movement is towards bind, tightness) and indirect methods, such as strain/counterstrain (where movement is towards ease, looseness) (Jones 1982).

Is 'tight' always undesirable?

Clinically, it is always worth considering whether restriction barriers ought to be released, in case they are offering some protective benefit. As an example, van Wingerden (1997) reports that both intrinsic and extrinsic support for the sacroiliac joint derive in part from hamstring (biceps femoris) status. Intrinsically, the influence is via the close anatomical and physiological relationship between biceps femoris and the sacrotuberous ligament (they frequently attach via a strong tendinous link). He states that: 'Force from the biceps femoris muscle can lead to increased tension of the sacrotuberous ligament in various ways. Since increased tension of the sacrotuberous ligament diminishes the range of sacroiliac joint motion, the biceps femoris can play a role in stabilization of the SIJ [sacroiliac joint]' (Vleeming et al 1989).

Van Wingerden also notes that in low-back patients forward flexion is often painful, as the load on the spine increases. This happens whether flexion occurs in the spine or via the hip joints (tilting of the pelvis). If the hamstrings are tight and short they effectively prevent pelvic tilting. 'In this respect, an increase in hamstring tension might well be part of a defensive arthrokinematic reflex mechanism of the body to diminish spinal load.'

If such a state of affairs is longstanding, the hamstrings (biceps femoris) will shorten (see discussion of the effects of stress on postural muscles in this and later chapters), possibly influencing sacroiliac and lumbar spine dysfunction. The decision to treat tight ('tethered') hamstring should therefore take account of why it is tight, and consider that in some circumstances it is offering beneficial support to the SIJ, or that it is reducing low-back stress.

Lewit and 'tight–loose' thinking

Lewit (1996) notes that pain is often located on the 'loose' side when there is an imbalance in which a joint or muscle (group) on one side of the body differs from the other. 'A "tight and loose complex," i.e. one side is restricted and the other side is hypotonic, is frequently noted. Shifting [Lewit is referring to stretching of fascial structures] is examined and treated in a craniocaudal or caudo-cranial direction on the back, but it should be assessed and treated in a circular manner around the axis of the neck and the extremities.'

Pain and the tight–loose concept

Pain is more commonly associated with tight and bound/tethered structures, which may be due to local overuse/misuse/abuse factors, to scar tissue, to reflexively induced influences, or to centrally mediated neural control. When a tight tissue is then asked to either fully contract, or fully lengthen, pain is often experienced.

Paradoxically, as pointed out by Lewit above, pain is also often noted in the loose rather than in the tight areas of the body, which may involve hypermobility and ligamentous laxity at the loose joint or site. These (lax, loose) areas are vulnerable to injury and prone to recurrent dysfunctional episodes (low back, SI joint, TMJ, etc.) (Muller et al 2003).

Myofascial trigger points may develop in either tight or loose structures, but usually appear more frequently and are more stressed in those which are tethered, restricted, tight (Travell & Simons 1992). Myofascial trigger points will continue to evolve if the aetiological factors which created and/or sustained them are not corrected and, unless the trigger points are deactivated, they will help to sustain the dysfunctional postural patterns which subsequently emerge.

Three-dimensional patterns

Areas of dysfunction will usually involve vertical, horizontal and 'encircling' (also described as cross-over, spiral or 'wrap-around') patterns of involvement. Ward (1997) offers a 'typical' wrap-around pattern associated with a tight left low-back area (which ends up involving the entire trunk and cervical area), as tight areas evolve to compensate for loose, inhibited, areas (or vice versa):

- Tightness in the posterior left hip, SI joint, lumbar erector spinae and lower rib cage

- Looseness on the right low back
- Tightness in the lateral and anterior rib cage on the right
- Tight left thoracic inlet, posteriorly
- Tight left craniocervical attachments (involving jaw mechanics).

The evolution of musculoskeletal dysfunction (Lewit 1974, Janda 1985, Guyton 1987)

The normal response of muscle to any form of stress is to increase in tone (Barlow 1959, Selye 1976). Some of the stress factors which negatively influence musculoskeletal soft tissue structure or function, producing irritation, increased muscle tension and pain, are listed in Box 2.3 (see also Fig. 2.11).

A chain reaction will evolve as any one, or combination of, the stress factors listed in Box 2.3, or additional stress factors, cumulatively demand increased muscular tone in those structures obliged to compensate for, or adapt to them, resulting in the following events:

Box 2.3   Stress factors leading to musculoskeletal dysfunction (see Fig. 2.11)

- Acquired postural imbalances (Rolf 1977)
- 'Pattern of use' stress (occupational, recreational, etc.)
- Inborn imbalance (short leg, short upper extremity, small hemipelvis, fascial distortion via birth injury, etc.)
- The effects of hyper- or hypomobile joints, including arthritic changes
- Repetitive strain from hobby, recreation, sport, etc. (overuse)
- Emotional stress factors (Barlow 1959)
- Breathing pattern disorders/upper chest breathing patterns
- Trauma (abuse), inflammation and subsequent fibrosis
- Disuse, immobilisation
- Reflexogenic influences (viscerosomatic, myofascial and other reflex inputs) (Beal 1983)
- Climatic stress such as chilling
- Nutritional imbalances (vitamin C deficiency reduces collagen efficiency for example) (Pauling 1976)
- Infection

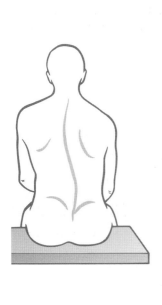 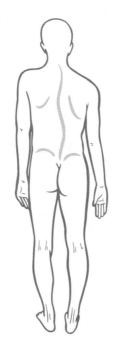 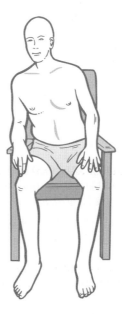

Figure 2.11 Examples of common congenital structural imbalances which result in sustained functional/postural stress – small hemipelvis, short leg and short upper extremity.

- The muscles antagonistic to the hypertonic muscles become weaker (inhibited) – as may the hypertonic muscles themselves.

- The stressed muscles develop areas of relative hypoxia and ultimately ischaemia while, simultaneously, there will be a reduction in the efficiency with which metabolic wastes are removed.

- The combined effect of toxic build-up (largely the by-products of the tissues themselves) (Cyriax 1962) and oxygen deprivation leads to irritation, sensitivity and pain, which feeds back into the loop, so creating more hypertonicity and pain. This feedback loop becomes self-perpetuating.

- Oedema may also be a part of the response of the soft tissues to stress.

- If inflammation is part of the process, fibrotic changes in connective tissue may follow.

- Neural structures in the area may become facilitated, and therefore hyper-reactive to stimuli, further adding to the imbalance and dysfunction of the region (see discussion, later in this chapter, of myofascial trigger points and other areas of facilitation).

- Initially, the soft tissues involved will show a reflex resistance to stretch and after some weeks (some say less, see Van Buskirk's view earlier in this chapter, p 36) a degree of fibrous infiltration may appear as the tissues under greatest stress mechanically, and via oxygen lack, adapt to the situation.

- The tendons and insertions of the hypertonic muscles will also become stressed, and pain and localised changes will begin to manifest in these regions. Tendon pain and periosteal discomfort are noted (Lewit & Simons 1984).

- If any of the hypertonic structures cross joints, and many do, these become crowded and some degree of imbalance will manifest as abnormal movement patterns evolve (with antagonistic and synergistically related muscles being excessively hypertonic and/or hypotonic, for example), leading ultimately to joint dysfunction.

- Localised reflexively active structures (trigger points) will emerge in the highly stressed, most ischaemic, tissues, and these will themselves become responsible for the development of pain and additional dysfunction at distant target sites, typically inhibiting antagonist muscles (Travell & Simons 1983, 1992, Lewit & Simons 1984).

- Because of excessive hypertonic activity there will be energy wastage and a tendency to fatigue – both locally and generally (Gutstein 1955).

- Functional imbalances will occur, for example involving respiration, when chain reactions of hypertonicity and weakness impact on this vital function (Lewit 1980, Garland 1994).

- Overbreathing commonly leads to an increased anxiety level that results in even more rapid breathing (Zvolensky & Eifert 2001).

- Breathing pattern disorders (the extreme form of which is hyperventilation) automatically speed up levels of anxiety and apprehension, which may be sufficient to alter motor control and to markedly influence balance control (Aust & Fischer 1997).

- Affected muscles tend to become involved in 'chain reactions' of dysfunction. A process develops in which some muscles will be used inappropriately as they learn to compensate for other structures which are weak or restricted, leading to adaptive movements, and loss of the ability to act synergistically as in normal situations (see notes on crossed syndromes later in this chapter, and also Liebenson's comments in Ch. 8) (Janda 1985).

- Over time, the central nervous system learns to accept altered patterns of use as being normal, adding further to the complication of recovery since rehabilitation will now demand a relearning process as well as the more obvious structural (shortness) and functional (inhibition/weakness) corrections (Knott & Voss 1968).

Examples

Postural strain and repetitive activites lead almost inevitably to problems such as carpal tunnel syndrome (CTS), thoracic outlet syndrome (TOS) and other chronic pain patterns (Middaugh et al 1994). Some examples include:

- Peper et al (1994) showed that computer users and typists unconsciously tense upper trapezius, scalene and forearm muscles whenever they use a keyboard. They also display a tendency towards increased respiration rates and thoracic breathing, so overusing accessory breathing muscles such as scalenes and upper trapezius.

- Skubick et al (1993) demonstrated that carpal tunnel syndrome (CTS) is commonly linked to excessive activity in the sternocleidomastoid muscles, together with the cervical paraspinal muscles. They also noted that many patients with CTS also demonstrated increased activity in the forearm flexor–extensor muscles of the painful arm.

Fitness, weakness, strength and hypermobility influences

While much of the emphasis in the rationale of use of MET relates to hypertonic structures, it would be folly to neglect to mention the converse – hypotonia. Kraus (1970) and Nixon & Andrews (1996) have presented evidence of the negative influence of relative lack of fitness (deconditioning) on the evolution of low-back pain.

Whether through acquired lack of fitness, reflex inhibition, or more seriously, inborn hypermobility, the fact is that lack of tone contributes enormously to musculoskeletal problems, imbalances and changes in functional sequence patterns, and generally causes a good deal of compensating overuse by synergistic or related muscles (Janda 1960, Fahrni 1966).

Janda (1986a) describes weakness in muscles which relate to altered movement patterns, resulting from 'changed motor regulation and motor performance'. Structural and functional factors can be involved in a variety of complex ways: 'A motor defect [weakness] of a neurological origin can almost always be considered as a result of the combination of a direct structural (morphological) lesion of some motor neurons and of inhibition effects. Both causes may occur even in the same neuron'.

Deterioration of muscle function can be demonstrated by three syndromes, according to Janda:

- Hypotonia, which can be determined by inspection and palpation

- Decrease in strength, which can be determined by testing (although, according to Janda, evaluation of strength is 'difficult and inaccurate as it is often impossible to differentiate the function of individual muscles').

- Changed sequence of activation in principal movement patterns, which can be more easily observed and evaluated if they are well understood (see also Ch. 5).

Ligaments and muscles which are hypermobile do not adequately protect joints and therefore fail to prevent excessive ranges of motion from being explored. Without this stability, overuse and injury stresses evolve and muscular overuse is inevitable, and indeed, hypermobility has been shown to be a major risk factor in the evolution of low-back pain (Muller et al 2003).

Janda (1986a) observes that in his experience, 'In races in which hypermobility is common there is a prevalence of muscular and tendon pain, whereas typical back pain or sciatica are rare'.

Significant ethnic differences in the presence of hypermobility have been noted. Al-Rawi et al (1985), supported by subsequent research by Hudson et al (1995), showed that prevalence rates of hypermobility vary markedly depending upon the population being examined, and range between 5% in Caucasian adults to rates as high as 38% in younger Middle Eastern women.

Interestingly, breathing pattern disorders have been found to be much more common in hypermobile individuals – often associated with chronic pain syndromes such as fibromyalgia (Bulbena et al 1993, Martin-Santos et al 1998).

Logically, the excessive work rate of muscles which are adopting the role of 'pseudoligaments' leads to tendon stress and muscle dysfunction, increasing tone in the antagonists of whatever is already weakened and complicating an already complex set of imbalances, including altered patterns of movement (Beighton et al 1983, Janda 1984).

Characteristics of altered movement patterns

Among the key alterations which are demonstrable in patterns of altered muscle movement are:

- The start of a muscle's activation is delayed, resulting in an alteration in the order in which a sequence of muscles is activated.

- Non-inhibited synergists or stabilisers often activate earlier in the sequence than the inhibited, weak muscle.

- There is an overall decrease in activity in the affected muscle, which in extreme cases can result in EMG readings showing it to be almost completely silent. This can lead to a misinterpretation that muscle strength is totally lacking when in fact, after proper facilitation, it may be capable of being activated towards more normal function. (Janda calls these changes 'pseudoparesis'.)

- An anomalous response is possible from such muscles since, unlike the usually beneficial activation of motor units seen in isometric training, such work against resistance can actually decrease even further the activity of pseudoparetic muscles (similar to the effect seen in muscles which are antagonists of the muscles in spasm in poliomyelitis).

- Some muscles are more likely to be affected by hypotonia, loss of strength and the effects of altered movement patterns. Janda points to tibialis anticus, peronei, vasti, long thigh adductors, the glutei, the abdominal muscles, the lower stabilisers of the scapulae, the deep neck flexors.

Among the causes of such changes in mainly phasic muscles are the effects of reciprocal inhibition by tight muscles, and in such cases, Janda comments, 'Stretching and achievement of normal length of the tight muscles disinhibits the pseudoparetic muscles and improves their activity'.

The phenomenon of increased tone is the other side of the picture.

What does increased bind/tone actually represent? (Box 2.4)

Janda (1989) notes that the word 'spasm' is commonly used without attention to various functional causes of hypertonicity and he has divided this phenomenon into five variants:

1. Hypertonicity of limbic system origin, which may be accompanied by evidence of stress, and be associated with, for example, tension-type headaches.

2. Hypertonicity of a segmental origin, involving interneuron influence. The muscle is likely to be spontaneously painful, and will probably be painful to stretch and will certainly have weak (inhibited) antagonists.

3. Hypertonicity due to uncoordinated muscle contraction resulting from myofascial trigger point activity. The muscle will be painful spontaneously if triggers are active. There may only be increased tone in part of the muscle, which will be hyperirritable while neighbouring areas of the same muscle may be inhibited.

4. Hypertonicity resulting from direct pain irritation, such as might occur in torticollis. This muscle would be painful at rest, not only when palpated, and would demonstrate electromyographic evidence of increased activity even at rest. This could be described as reflex spasm due to nociceptive influence, as discussed earlier in this chapter.

5. Overuse hypertonicity results in muscles becoming increasingly irritable, with reduced range of motion, tightness and pain only on palpation.

Thus increased tone of functional origin can result from pain sources, from trigger point activity, from higher centres or CNS influences, and from overuse.

Liebenson (1990a) suggests that each type of hypertonicity requires different therapeutic approaches, ranging from adjustment (joint manipulation), through use of soft tissue and rehabilitation and facilitation approaches. The many different MET variations offer the opportunity to influence all stages of dysfunction, as listed above – the acute, the chronic and everything in between – as will become clear in our evaluation of the methods.

Clearly we all adapt and (de)compensate at our own rates, depending upon multiple variables ranging from our inherited tendencies, genetic make-up and nutritional status, to the degree, variety and intensity of the stressors confronting us, past and present.

Adding to the complexity of these responses is another variable: the fact that there are predictable and palpable differences in the responses of the soft tissues to stress – some muscles becoming progressively weak, while others become progressively hypertonic (Janda 1978) or actually lengthen (Norris 1999).

Different stress response of muscles

There are different ways of describing how muscles respond to the stressful demands of overuse, misuse, abuse and disuse. A number of models have emerged in which respected clinicians and researchers take quite different standpoints in the way they interpret the functional characteristics of muscles.

There are descriptions of the muscles of the body relating to whether they are 'postural or phasic', 'mobiliser or stabiliser', 'superficial or deep', 'polyarticular or monoarticular', and whether, as a result of their nature, they respond to 'stress' by shortening, weakening, lengthening, altering their firing patterns, atrophying or hypertrophying, or indeed whether some muscles are capable of a combination of such responses.

It seems that, in order to make sense of these complexities, it is necessary to characterise and categorise the constituent features of complicated organisations such as the musculoskeletal system. The problem is that there is no consensus as to how to perform the act of categorisation.

One popular model is that first promulgated by Janda (1978) and Lewit (1974) that describes 'postural' and 'phasic' muscles and their behaviour. This was the model used in the first edition of this text, and is described below as a part of an attempt to present readers with information in order that they should be able to investigate this confusion over semantics for themselves.

Postural and phasic muscles

The research and writings of prominent workers in physical medicine, such as Lewit (1974), Korr

Box 2.4 Muscle spasm, tension, atrophy (Walsh 1992, Liebenson 1996)

- Muscles are often said to be short, tight, tense, or in spasm; however, these terms are used very loosely.
- Muscles experience either neuromuscular, viscoelastic, or connective tissue alterations or combinations of these.
- A tight muscle could have either increased neuromuscular tension or connective tissue modification (e.g. fibrosis).

Spasm (tension with EMG elevation)
- Muscle spasm is a neuromuscular phenomenon relating either to an upper motor neuron disease or an acute reaction to pain or tissue injury.
- Electromyographic (EMG) activity is increased in these cases.
- Examples include spinal cord injury, reflex spasm (such as in a case of appendicitis) or acute lumbar antalgia with loss of flexion relaxation response (Triano & Schultz 1987).
- Long-lasting noxious (pain) stimulation has been shown to activate the flexion withdrawal reflex (Dahl et al 1992).
- Using electromyographic evidence, Simons has shown that myofascial trigger points can 'cause reflex spasm and reflex inhibition in other muscles, and can cause motor incoordination in the muscle with the trigger point' (Simons 1994).

Contracture (tension of muscles without EMG elevation)
- Increased muscle tension can occur without a consistently elevated EMG (as, for example, in trigger points in which muscle fibres fail to relax properly).
- Muscle fibres housing trigger points have been shown to have different levels of EMG activity within the same functional muscle unit.
- Hyperexcitability, as shown by EMG readings, has been demonstrated in the nidus of the trigger point, which is situated in a taut band (which shows no increased EMG activity) and has a characteristic pattern of

reproducible referred pain (Hubbard & Berkoff 1993). When pressure is applied to an active trigger point, EMG activity is found to increase in the muscles to which sensations are being referred ('target area') (Simons 1994).

Increased stretch sensitivity
- Increased sensitivity to stretch can lead to increased muscle tension.
- This can occur under conditions of local ischaemia, which have also been demonstrated in the nidus of trigger points, as part of the 'energy crisis' which, it is hypothesised (see Ch. 6), produces them (Mense 1993, Simons 1994).
- Liebenson (1996) confirms that 'local ischemia is a key factor involved in increased muscle tone. Under conditions of ischemia groups III and IV muscle afferents become more sensitive to stretch'.
- These same afferents also become sensitised in response to a build-up of metabolites when sustained mild contractions occur, such as happens in prolonged, slumped sitting (Johansson 1991).
- Mense (1993) suggests that a range of dysfunctional events emerge from the production of local ischaemia which can occur as a result of venous congestion, local contracture and tonic activation of muscles by descending motor pathways.
- Sensitisation (which is in all but name the same phenomenon as facilitation, discussed more fully in Ch. 6) involves a change in the stimulus–response profile of neurons, leading to a decreased threshold as well as increased spontaneous activity of types III and IV primary afferents.
- Schiable & Grubb (1993) have implicated reflex discharges from (dysfunctional) joints in the production of such neuromuscular tension.
- According to Janda (1991), neuromuscular tension can also be increased by central influences due to limbic dysfunction.

(1980), Janda (1978), Basmajian (1978), Liebenson (1996) and others, suggest that muscles which have predominantly stabilising functions will shorten when stressed, while others which have more active 'moving', or phasic functions, will not shorten but will become weak (inhibited).

The muscles which shorten are said to be those which have a primarily postural rather than phasic

(active, moving) role and it is possible to learn to conduct, in a relatively short space of time, an assessment sequence in which the majority of these can be identified as being either relatively short or fairly 'normal' (Chaitow 1991a).

Janda (1978) informs us that postural muscles have a tendency to shorten, not only under pathological conditions but also often under normal circumstances. He has noted, using electromyographic instrumentation, that 85% of the walking cycle is spent on one leg or the other, and that this is the most common postural position for man. Those muscles which enable this position to be satisfactorily adopted (one-legged standing) are genetically older; they have different physiological, and probably biochemical, qualities compared with phasic muscles which normally weaken and exhibit signs of inhibition in response to stress or pathology.

Later in this chapter other models in which muscles are grouped or characterised differently will be examined. Before that, orthopaedic surgeon Gordon Waddell's (1998) opinion is worth recording:

Different muscles contain varying proportions of slow and fast muscle fibres. Slow fibres maintain posture; they activate more easily, are capable of more sustained contraction, and tend to become shortened and tight. Fast or phasic fibres give dynamic, voluntary movement; they fatigue more rapidly and tend to weakness. Postural and phasic muscles are often antagonistic ... . Hypertrophy and atrophy occur at the same time in antagonistic muscles, which may lead to changes in resting length, with contracture of the postural muscles and stretching of the phasic muscles.

Box 2.5 Postural muscles that shorten under stress

Gastrocnemius, soleus, medial hamstrings, short adductors of the thigh, hamstrings, psoas, piriformis, tensor fascia lata, quadratus lumborum, erector spinae muscles, latissimus dorsi, upper trapezius, sternomastoid, levator scapulae, pectoralis major and the flexors of the arms

Postural muscles

Those postural muscles which have been noted as responding to stress by shortening are listed in Box 2.5. The scalenes are a borderline set of muscles – they start life as phasic muscles but can become, through overuse/abuse (asthma for example), more postural in their function (Fig. 2.12 A and B).

Can postural muscles and phasic muscles change from one form into the other?

While Lewit and Janda (Lewit 1999) have suggested that postural muscles under stress will shorten, and phasic muscles similarly stressed will weaken, it is now becoming clear that the function of a muscle can modify its structure. This helps to explain some mysteries – for example why the scalenes are sometimes short, and sometimes weak, and sometimes both, and yet are classified generally as phasic muscles, and sometimes as 'equivocal' (maybe postural and maybe phasic).

Lin et al (1994), writing in *The Lancet*, examined motor muscle physiology in growing children, reviewing current understanding of the postural/phasic muscle interaction. Muscles, Lin observed, are considered to be developmentally static, which is surprising considering in vitro information relating to the development and adaptability of muscles derived from mammals. For example, Buller (1960) showed that a committed muscle fibre type could be transformed from slow twitch to fast twitch, and vice versa, in cross-innervation experiments, confirming that impulse traffic down the nerve conditions the fibre type.

The implication of this research is that if a group of muscles such as the scalenes are dedicated to movement (which they should be) and not to stabilisation (which they may have to be if 'postural' stresses are imposed), they can become postural in type, and so will develop a tendency to shorten if stressed. This is precisely what seems to happen in people with chronic upper-chest breathing patterns or asthma.

Characteristics of postural and phasic muscles

The characteristics which identify a muscle as belonging to one or other of these two groups, in this particular model, are given in Table 2.1.

Embedded in the descriptions of these muscle groupings in some of the writing about them is the assumption that postural muscles have a predominance of type I fibres, and phasic muscles type II. All muscles comprise both red (type I) and white (type II), slow and fast, fibres which produce both postural and phasic functions; however, the

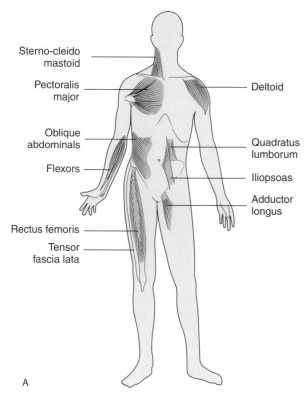

Figure 2.12A The major postural muscles of the anterior aspect of the body.

Labels (anterior):
Sterno-cleido mastoid, Pectoralis major, Oblique abdominals, Flexors, Rectus femoris, Tensor fascia lata, Deltoid, Quadratus lumborum, Iliopsoas, Adductor longus

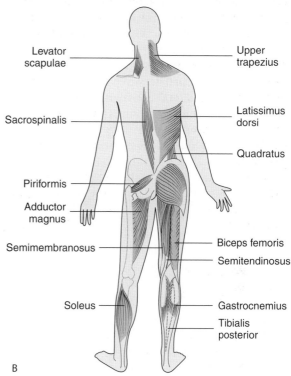

Figure 2.12B The major postural muscles of the posterior aspect of the body.

Labels (posterior):
Levator scapulae, Sacrospinalis, Piriformis, Adductor magnus, Semimembranosus, Soleus, Upper trapezius, Latissimus dorsi, Quadratus, Biceps femoris, Semitendinosus, Gastrocnemius, Tibialis posterior

classification of a muscle into either a 'postural' or 'phasic' group is made on the basis of their *predominant* activity, their major functional tendency.

Norris (personal communication, 1999) states:

Gastrocnemius is a mobiliser or 'task muscle' [see discussion of stabiliser/mobiliser categorisations later in this chapter], and has a predominance of type II fibres in most people. However, training may affect the appearance of muscle as a type I or type II. For example hard fast calf training will selectively recruit the type II fibres and cause them to hypertrophy. The muscle now acts as if it had more type II fibres (because they are bigger and more 'practised' at recruitment). Although the actual fibre number is unchanged it appears functionally to the clinician (not using EMG) that it has. The change can therefore be one of hypokinetics or hyperkinetics.

Put more simply, function modifies structure, and this may be the result of use patterns, as in the gastrocnemius example, or of positional (postural) adaptation, as in the effect on suboccipital musculature resulting from chronic 'chin-poke' posture, related to sterrnocleidomastoid shortness.

Rehabilitation implications

Janda suggests that before any attempt is made to strengthen weak muscles, any hypertonicity in

Table 2.1 Postural/phasic muscle characteristics

	Postural muscles	Phasic muscles
Type	Slow twitch – red	Fast twitch – white
Respiration	Anaerobic	Aerobic
Function	Static/supportive	Phasic/active
Dysfunction	Shorten	Weaken
Treatment	Stretch/relax	Facilitate/strengthen

their antagonists should be addressed by appropriate treatment which relaxes (and if appropriate lengthens) them – for example, by stretching using MET. Relaxation of hypertonic muscles leads to an automatic restoration of tone to their antagonists, once inhibitory hypertonic effects have been removed. Should a hypertonic muscle also be weak, it commonly regains strength following stretch/relaxation (Janda 1978).

Commenting on this phenomenon, chiropractic rehabilitation expert Craig Liebenson (1990b) states:

> *Once joint movement is free, hypertonic muscles relaxed, and connective tissue lengthened, a muscle-strengthening and movement coordination program can begin. It is important not to commence strengthening too soon because tight, overactive muscles reflexively inhibit their antagonists, thereby altering basic movement patterns. It is inappropriate to initiate muscle strengthening programs while movement performance is disturbed, since the patient will achieve strength gains by use of 'trick' movements.*

Liebenson discusses these and other treatment and rehabilitation topics more fully in Ch. 8.

Skiers' muscles as an example

Just how common such imbalances are was illustrated by Schmid (1984), who studied the main postural and phasic muscles in eight members of the male Olympic ski teams from Switzerland and Liechtenstein. He found that among this group of apparently superbly fit individuals, fully six of the eight members had demonstrably short right iliopsoas muscles, five also had left iliopsoas shortness, and the majority also displayed weakness of the rectus abdominis muscles (see Ch. 11 for more on muscle changes in athletes).

A number of other muscle imbalances were noted, and the conclusion was that athletic fitness offers no more protection from muscular dysfunction than does a sedentary lifestyle (possibly quite the contrary!).

Liebenson (1990b) has discussed the work of Sommer (1985), who found that competitive basketball and volleyball players frequently produce patellar tendinitis and other forms of knee dys-

function, due to the particular stresses they endure because of muscular imbalances. Their ability to jump is often seriously impaired by virtue of shortened psoas and quadriceps muscles with associated weakness of gluteus maximus. This imbalance leads to decreased hip extension and hyperextension of the knee joint. Once muscular balance is restored, a more controlled jump is possible, as is a reduction in reported fatigue. The element of fatigue should not be forgotten in this equation, since hypertonic muscles are working excessively both to perform their functions and often to compensate for weakness in associated muscles.

Evjenth & Hamberg (1984) succinctly summarise:

> 'Every patient with symptoms involving the locomotor system, particularly symptoms of pain and/or constrained movement, should be examined to assess joint and muscle function. If examination shows joint play to be normal, but reveals shortened muscles or muscle spasm, then treatment by stretching [and by implication MET] is indicated.'

Stabilisers and mobilisers (Box 2.6)

British physiotherapist researcher Chris Norris (2000b) comments on the postural/phasic model:

> *The terms postural and phasic, used by Jull and Janda (1987), can be misleading. In their categorisation, the hamstring muscles are placed in the postural grouping while the gluteals are placed in the phasic grouping. The reaction described for these muscles is that the postural group (represented by the hamstrings in this case) tend to tighten, are biarticular, have a lower irritability threshold, and a tendency to develop trigger points. This type of action would suggest a phasic (as opposed to tonic) response, and is typical of a muscle used to develop power and speed in sport for example, a task carried out by the hamstrings. The so called 'phasic group' is said to lengthen, weaken, and be uniarticular, a description perhaps better suited to the characteristics of a muscle used for postural holding. The description of the muscle responses described by Jull and Janda (1987) is accurate, but the terms postural and phasic do not seem to adequately describe the groupings.*

The issue of 'naming' what is observed, in terms of muscle behaviour, seems to be a key feature of the debate. Norris (2000b) suggests that mobiliser muscles are more or less the same, in most of their characteristics, as Janda's postural muscles. Similarly, stabilisers are equated with phasic muscles. Apart from the apparent semantic contradiction (i.e. it is hard to liken a 'stabiliser' to 'phasic' activity), this suggests that the intrinsic model is accurate, whatever the names ascribed to the muscle categories. Some muscles do tend to shorten, and some do tend to weaken (and in some cases lengthen), whatever names we give them.

The language discrepancy between the mobiliser/stabiliser and the postural/phasic designations of muscles does not, however, exhaust the complications facing practitioners trying to make sense of modern research. They also have to contend with words and terms such as deep/superficial, global/local, monoarticular/polyarticular.

Global and local muscles

Bergmark (1989) and Richardson et al (1999) have categorised muscles in yet another way. They describe some muscles as *local* ('central') and others as being *global* ('guy rope'). Global muscles are likened to the ropes supporting a ship's mast. In this model central muscles are seen as lying deep, or as possessing deep components which attach to the spine. Global muscles are seen as having the capacity to control the spine's resistance to bending, as well as being able to influence spinal alignment, balancing and accommodating to the forces imposed on the spine:

- *Global muscles*: anterior portion of the internal obliques, external obliques, rectus abdominis, the lateral fibres of the quadratus lumborum and the more lateral portions of the erector spinae (Bogduk & Twomey 1991).

- *Local muscles*: multifidi, intertrasversarii, interspinales, transversus abdominis, the posterior portion of the internal oblique, the medial fibres of quadratus lumborum and the more central portion of the erector spinae.

Richardson et al (1999) describe (discussing low-back pain) the essentially practical nature of their

---

Box 2.6 Mobiliser and stabiliser characteristics (Richardson et al 1992, 1999)

Mobiliser features	Stabiliser features
Fusiform	Aponeurotic
Fast twitch	Slow twitch
Produce angular rotation	Maintain joint balance
Relatively small proprioceptive role	Major proprioceptive role
Produce torque and power activities	Antigravity endurance tasks
Phasic activity	Tonic activity
Concentric muscle functions	Eccentric and isometric functions
Fatigue easily	Resistant to fatigue
Often superficial	Often more deeply placed
Activated at 30–40% MVC (maximum voluntary contraction)	Activated above 40% MVC
Tighten and shorten	Selectively weaken and lengthen

Examples of these muscle designations

Mobilisers (which selectively shorten and tighten):

- Rectus abdominis

- Lateral fibres external oblique
- Erector spinae
- Gastrocnemius/soleus
- Iliocostalis
- Hamstrings
- Upper trapezius
- Adductors of the thigh
- Levator scapulae
- Iliopsoas
- Suboccipitals
- Rectus femoris
- Pectoralis major and minor

Stabilisers (which selectively weaken and lengthen):

- Gluteus medius and maximus
- Vastus medius oblique

- Transversus abdominis
- Internal obliques
- Multifidus
- Serratus anterior
- Deep neck flexors
- Lower trapezius
- Quadratus lumborum (see notes on this controversial muscle in this chapter and in Box 4.8)

---

focus on the 'local' and 'global' characterisation model:

Basically, there are two broad approaches for improving the spinal protection role of the muscles which can be gleaned from anatomical and

biomechanical studies on lumbopelvic stabilization. The first utilizes the principle of minimizing
forces applied to the lumbar spine during functional activities. The second is to ensure that the
deep local muscle system is operating to stabilize
the individual spinal segments.

This model is therefore essentially pragmatic:
'Lighten the stress load and improve stabilising
function' would summarise its objectives, and few
clinicians would argue with these.

Identification of those muscles under-performing
in their stabilisation roles (usually deep rather
than superficial), followed by re-education of the
appropriate use of these, plays a major part in the
protocols which emerge from this approach. Little
attention is described as being paid to overactive
antagonists that might be inhibiting underactive
deep muscles. However, as well as a brief
encouragement to deal with ergonomic factors,
these authors do state that:

Global [i.e. superficial] muscle function can cause
potentially harmful effects if there is overactivity
in certain muscles of this system. Methods of
treatment aimed at decreasing any unnecessary
activity in these muscles will assist in minimizing harmful forces. Logically this could only
be safely pursued if the protective function of the
deep-local muscles was being reestablished at the
same time.

Clinical question   Should short, tight structures,
whatever name they are given, be treated first, or
should the weakened structures (whatever they
are named), receive primary attention, or should a
synchronised approach that deals with both sides
of the equation be adopted?

Readers will make their own choices and it is
probable that any of these choices would have
positive outcomes in particular circumstances;
however, the primary author suggests (based on
clinical experience rather than objective evidence)
that as a general rule, shortened, hypertonic structures should receive primary attention.

Dual role of certain muscles

In the mobiliser/stabiliser model some muscles
seem to act as both. Norris (2000b) states:

The quadratus lumborum has been shown to be
significant as a stabiliser in lumbar spine
movements (McGill et al 1996) while tightening
has also been described (Janda 1983). It seems
likely that the muscle may act functionally
[differently] in its medial and lateral portions,
with the medial portion being more active as a
stabiliser of the lumbar spine and the lateral more
active as a mobiliser. Such sub-division is seen
in a number of other muscles, for example the
gluteus medius where the posterior fibres are
more posturally involved (Jull 1994); the internal
oblique where the posterior fibres attaching to the
lateral raphe are considered stabilisers (Bergmark
1989); the external oblique where the lateral fibres
work during flexion in parallel with the rectus
abdominis (Kendall et al 1993).

Does this debate influence MET?

Of particular interest in application of MET, as
described in this text, is the observation (see
Box 2.6), that postural/mobiliser muscles activate
with contractions below 30% of maximum voluntary contraction (MVC). Hoffer & Andreasson
(1981) demonstrated that efforts below 25% MVC
provide maximal joint stiffness. More importantly,
McArdle et al (1991) have shown that a prolonged
tonic holding contraction and a low MVC (under
30–40% MVC) selectively recruits tonic (postural)
fibres, the very structures that will have shortened
and which are (probably) in need of lengthening.
This vital information will be noted again in the
technique segments of the book. The debate as to
the degree of the ideal degree of force needed in
isometric contractions is taken further in Ch. 5.

Easing the confusion

This text remains faithful to the model described
by Janda and others in describing muscles as being
either *postural* or *phasic*. This does not mean rejec-
tion of alternative concepts (such as stabiliser/
mobiliser, global/local, etc.) as described by Norris,
Richardson and others. It is simply that, although
renaming something may serve a purpose in
research terms, it does not seem to offer any
particular advantage clinically in relation to the
identification of shortness or weakness, or of the
appropriate application of MET to such structures.

Chiropractic rehabilitation expert Craig Liebenson (personal communication, 1999) suggests a way in which the clinician can avoid the possibility of confusion. Simply define particular muscles as 'having a tendency to shortening or weakening'. Whether they are classified as postural or phasic, or as mobilisers or stabilisers, then becomes irrelevant to what needs doing.

Norris (2000b) supports the possibility of confusion arising out of attempts at muscle categorisation:

Any relatively simplistic categorisation of muscle is fraught with problems. The danger with muscle imbalance categorisation is that practitioners will expect set changes to occur and fail to adequately assess a patient. When this occurs, important deviations from the 'imbalance norm' can be missed and treatment outcomes will be impaired. Although muscle imbalance categorisation can usefully assist the astute practitioner, they are not cast in stone. Assessment will still be required but can be refined to reveal the subtleties of muscle reaction to altered use and pathology.

He points out that if the practitioner can identify that a muscle is weak (i.e. has poor inner range holding), rehabilitation methods are needed to remedy this. Further, if a muscle is inappropriately tight or short, safe methods (such as MET) exist to release and/or lengthen it. And of course once muscle balance has been restored, habitual posture and use patterns need to be addressed.

Box 2.7 offers summaries of some of the patterns which can be associated with imbalances between stabilisers and mobilisers, and possible observational evidence which can be confirmed by tests (Norris 1995a–e, 1998; see also Chs 5 and 8 for functional assessments, and Boxes 2.8 and 2.9 and Fig. 2.13A–C in this chapter).

Where do joints fit into the picture?

Janda has an answer to this emotive question when he says that it is not known whether dysfunction of muscles causes joint dysfunction or vice versa (Janda 1988). He points out, however, that since clinical evidence abounds that joint mobilisation (thrust or gentle mobilisation) influences the muscles that are in anatomic or functional relationships with the joint, it may well be that normalisation of the excessive tone of the muscles is what is providing the benefit, and that, by implication, normalisation of the muscle tone by other means (such as MET) would provide an equally useful basis for a beneficial outcome and joint normalisation. Since reduction in muscle spasm/contraction commonly results in a reduction in joint pain, the answer to many such problems would seem to lie in appropriate soft tissue attention.

Liebenson (1990b) takes a view with a chiropractic bias: 'The chief abnormalities of [musculoskeletal] function include muscular hypertonicity and joint blockage. Since these abnormalities are functional rather than structural they are reversible in nature ... once a particular joint has

---

Box 2.7 Patterns of imbalance

Patterns of imbalance as some muscles weaken and lengthen, and synergists become overworked, while antagonists shorten (see this chapter for cross syndromes, and Ch. 5 for Janda's functional tests for muscle imbalance):

Lengthened or underactive stabiliser	Overactive synergist	Shortened antagonist
1. Gluteus medius	TFL, quadratus lumborum, piriformis	Thigh adductors
2. Gluteus maximus	Iliocostalis lumborum and hamstrings	Iliopsoas, rectus femoris
3. Transverse abdominis	Rectus abdominis	Iliocostalis lumborum
4. Lower trapezius	Levator scapulae/upper trapezius	Pectoralis major
5. Deep neck flexors	SCM	Suboccipitals
6. Serratus anterior	Pectoralis major/minor	Rhomboids
7. Diaphragm		Scalenes, pectoralis major

Box 2.8 Observation

Observation can often provide evidence of an imbalance involving cross-patterns of weakness/lengthening and shortness (see this chapter for cross syndromes, and Ch. 5 for Janda's functional tests for muscle imbalance). For example:

Muscle inhibition/weakness/ lengthening	Observable sign
Transverse abdominis	Protruding umbilicus
Serratus anterior	Winged scapula
Lower trapezius	Elevated shoulder girdle ('Gothic' shoulders)
Deep neck flexors	Chin 'poking'
Gluteus medius	Unlevel pelvis on one-legged standing
Gluteus maximus	Sagging buttock(s)

Tests can be used to assess muscle imbalance.

Postural inspection provides a quick screen, muscle length tests, movement patterns, and inner holding endurance times (see Box 2.9).

Box 2.9 Inner range holding (endurance) tests (see Fig. 2.13)

'Inner holding isometric endurance' tests can be performed for muscles which have a tendency to lengthen, in order to assess their ability to maintain joint alignment in a neutral zone. Usually a lengthened muscle will demonstrate a loss of endurance when tested in a shortened position. This can be tested by the practitioner passively pre-positioning the muscle in a shortened position and assessing the duration of time that the patient can hold the muscle in the shortened position. There are various methods used, including:
- Ten repetitions of the holding position for 10 seconds at a time.
- Alternatively, a single 30-second hold can be requested.
- If the patient cannot hold the position actively from the moment of passive pre-positioning, this is a sign of inappropriate antagonist muscle shortening.
- Norris (1999) states that: 'Optimal endurance is indicated when the full inner range position can be held for 10 to 20 seconds. Muscle lengthening is present if the limb falls away from the inner range position immediately.'

Norris (1999) describes examples of inner range holding tests for:

Iliopsoas (see Ch. 4, Fig. 4.7)
- Patient is seated.
- Practitioner lifts one leg into greater hip flexion so that foot is well clear of floor.
- Patient is asked to hold this position.

Gluteus maximus
- Patient is prone.
- Practitioner lifts one leg into extension at the hip (knee flexed to 90°).
- Patient is asked to hold the leg in this position.

Posterior fibres of gluteus medius
- Patient is side-lying with uppermost leg flexed at hip and knee so that both the knee and foot are resting on the floor/surface.
- Practitioner places the flexed leg into a position of maximal unforced external rotation at the hip, foot still resting on the floor.
- Patient is asked to maintain this position.

---

lost its normal range of motion, the muscles around that joint will attempt to minimise stress at the involved segment.'

After describing the processes of progressive compensation, as some muscles become hypertonic while inhibiting their antagonists, he continues, 'What may begin as a simple restriction of movement in a joint can lead to the development of muscular imbalances and postural change. This chain of events is an example of what we try to prevent through adjustments of subluxations.'

We are left then with one view which has it that muscle release will frequently normalise joint restrictions, as well as a view which holds the opposite – that joint normalisation sorts out soft tissue problems, leaving direct work on muscles for rehabilitation settings, and for attention if joint mobilisation fails to deal with long-term changes (fibrosis, etc.).

Clinical question   If a joint is restricted or painful should manipulation be the first therapeutic choice, or should soft tissue approaches be used initially, and manipulation only employed if soft tissue treatment fails to normalise the condition?

Training and licensing issues enter into the choices made, as manipulation is only an option if the practitioner is both skilled and licensed to perform it. If that obstacle is removed it seems

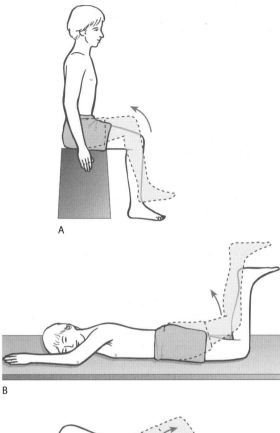

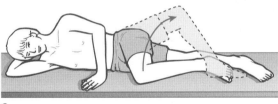

Figure 2.13 **A** Iliopsoas holding test. **B** Gluteus maximus holding test. **C** Posterior fibres gluteus medius holding test.

to be a matter of choice. Scott-Dawkins (1997) reported on a study in which 30 patients with chronic cervical pain were randomised to receive either HVLT or MET manipulation. Each group was treated twice weekly for 3 weeks: 'Patients treated with HVLT experienced a greater immediate relief of pain but at the end of the treatment period there was no difference in pain levels, with pain decreasing in both groups to the same extent.'

This sort of evidence suggests that both views are to some extent correct. However, what emphasis therapists/practitioners give to their prime focus – be it joints or be it soft tissues – the certainty is

that what is required is anything but a purely local view, as Janda helps us to understand.

Patterns of dysfunction

When a chain reaction evolves in which some muscles shorten and others weaken, predictable patterns involving imbalances develop, and Janda has described the so-called upper and lower 'crossed' syndromes (see below and Tables 2.2 and 2.3).

Upper crossed syndrome (Fig. 2.14)

This involves the basic imbalance shown in Table 2.2. As the changes listed in Table 2.2 take place, they alter the relative positions of the head, neck and shoulders as follows:

1. The occiput and C1/2 will hyperextend, with the head being pushed forward.

2. The lower cervical to 4th thoracic vertebrae will be posturally stressed as a result.

3. Rotation and abduction of the scapulae occurs.

4. An altered direction of the axis of the glenoid fossa will develop, resulting in the humerus

Table 2.2 Upper crossed syndrome

Pectoralis major and minor	All tighten and shorten
Upper trapezius	
Levator scapulae	
Sternomastoid	
while	
Lower and middle trapezius	All weaken
Serratus anterior and rhomboids	

Table 2.3 Lower crossed syndrome

Hip flexors	All tighten and shorten
Illiopsoas, rectus femoris	
TFL, short adductors	
Erector spinae group of the trunk	
while	
Abdominal and gluteal muscles	All weaken

needing to be stabilised by additional levator scapula and upper trapezius activity, with additional activity from supraspinatus as well.

The result of these changes is greater cervical segment strain plus referred pain to the chest, shoulders and arms. Pain mimicking angina may be noted plus a decline in respiratory efficiency.

The solution, according to Janda, is to be able to identify the shortened structures and to release (stretch and relax) them, followed by re-education towards more appropriate function.

Lower crossed syndrome (Fig. 2.15)

This involves the basic imbalance shown in Table 2.3. The result of the chain reaction in Table 2.3 is that the pelvis tips forward on the frontal plane, flexing the hip joints and producing lumbar lordosis and stress at L5–S1 with pain and irritation. A further stress commonly appears in the sagittal plane in which quadratus lumborum tightens and gluteus maximus and medius weaken.

When this 'lateral corset' becomes unstable, the pelvis is held in increased elevation, accentuated when walking, resulting in L5–S1 stress in the sagittal plane. One result is low-back pain. The combined stresses described produce instability at the lumbodorsal junction, an unstable transition point at best.

Also commonly involved are the piriformis muscles which in 20% of individuals are penetrated by the sciatic nerve so that piriformis syndrome can produce direct sciatic pressure and pain. Arterial involvement of piriformis shortness produces ischaemia of the lower extremity, and through a relative fixation of the sacrum, sacroiliac dysfunction and pain in the hip.

Part of the solution for an all too common pattern such as this is to identify the shortened structures and to release them, ideally using variations on the theme of MET, followed by re-education of posture and use.

Chain reaction leads to facial and jaw pain

In case it is thought that such imbalances are of merely academic interest, a practical example of the negative effects of the chain reactions described above is given by Janda (1986b) in an article entitled 'Some aspects of extracranial causes of facial pain'. Janda's premise is that temporo-

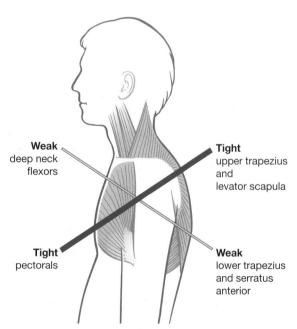

Figure 2.14 The upper crossed syndrome, as described by Janda.

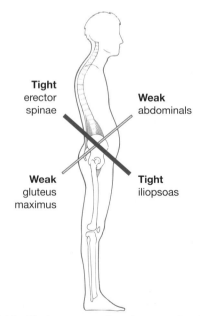

Figure 2.15 The lower crossed syndrome, as described by Janda.

mandibular joint (TMJ) problems and facial pain can be analysed in relation to the patient's whole posture. He has hypothesised that the muscular pattern associated with TMJ problems may be considered as locally involving hyperactivity and tension in the temporal and masseter muscles while, because of this hypertonicity, reciprocal inhibition occurs in the suprahyoid, digastric and mylohyoid muscles. The external pterygoid in particular often develops spasm. This imbalance between jaw adductors and jaw openers alters the ideal position of the condyle and leads to a consequent redistribution of stress on the joint, leading to degenerative changes.

Janda describes the typical pattern of muscular dysfunction of an individual with TMJ problems as involving upper trapezius, levator scapula, scaleni, sternomastoid, suprahyoid, lateral and medial pterygoid, masseter and temporal muscles, all of which show a tendency to tighten and to develop spasm.

He notes that while the scalenes are unpredictable, and while commonly, under overload conditions, they become atrophied and weak, they may also develop spasm, tenderness and trigger points.

The postural pattern in a TMJ patient might involve (see Fig. 2.16, also Fig. 2.15):

1. Hyperextension of knee joints
2. Increased anterior tilt of pelvis
3. Pronounced flexion of hip joints
4. Hyperlordosis of lumbar spine
5. Rounded shoulders and winged (rotated and abducted) scapulae
6. Cervical hyperlordosis
7. Forward thrust of head
8. Compensatory overactivity of upper trapezius and levator scapulae
9. Forward thrust of head resulting in opening of mouth and retraction of mandible.

This series of changes provokes increased activity of the jaw adductor and protractor muscles, creating a vicious cycle of dysfunctional activity. Intervertebral joint stress in the cervical spine follows.

Clinical question What skills are required to ensure that the sort of chain of dysfunction described by Janda can be recognised?

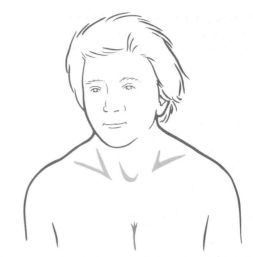

Figure 2.16 A typical pattern of upper thoracic and cervical stress as described by Janda would involve a degree of TMJ stress. Note the 'Gothic shoulders' which result from upper trapezius hypertonicity and shortening.

Training in observation, palpation and assessment skills is clearly an essential foundation, since the sort of evidence Janda offers makes it clear that such patterns first need to be identified before they can be assessed for the role they might be playing in the patient's pain and restriction conditions, and certainly before these can be successfully and appropriately treated. (Liebenson discusses a number of Janda's observation assessment methods in Ch. 8.)

Patterns of change with inappropriate breathing (Fig. 2.17A and B)

Garland (1994) describes the somatic changes which follow from a pattern of hyperventilation, upper chest breathing. When faced with persistent upper chest breathing patterns we should be able to identify reduced diaphragmatic efficiency and commensurate restriction of the lower rib cage as these evolve into a series of changes with accessory breathing muscles being inappropriately and excessively used:

- A degree of visceral stasis and pelvic floor weakness will develop, as will an imbalance between increasingly weak abdominal muscles and increasingly tight erector spinae muscles.

- Fascial restriction from the central tendon via the pericardial fascia, all the way up to the basiocciput, will be noted.

- The upper ribs will be elevated and there will be sensitive costal cartilage tension.

- The thoracic spine will be disturbed by virtue of the lack of normal motion of the articulation with the ribs, and sympathetic outflow from this area may be affected.

- Accessory muscle hypertonia, notably affecting the scalenes, upper trapezius and levator scapulae, will be palpable and observable.

- Fibrosis will develop in these muscles, as will myofascial trigger points.

- The cervical spine will become progressively rigid with a fixed lordosis being a common feature in the lower cervical spine.

- A reduction in the mobility of the 2nd cervical segment and disturbance of vagal outflow from this region is likely.

- Breathing pattern disorders cause loss of functional tone of the diaphragm and core stabilising muscles, such as transversus abdominus (McGill et al 1995, Hodges et al 2001).

More hyperventilation effects

Although not noted in Garland's list of dysfunctions (in which he states 'psychology overwhelms physiology'), we should bear in mind that the other changes which Janda has listed in his upper crossed syndrome (see above) are also likely consequences, including the potentially devastating effects on shoulder function of the altered position of the scapulae and glenoid fossae, as this pattern evolves.

Hyperventilation results in respiratory alkalosis, leading to reduced oxygenation of tissues (including the brain), smooth muscle constriction, heightened pain perception, speeding up of spinal reflexes, increased excitability of the corticospinal system, hyperirritability of motor and sensory axons, changes in serum calcium and magnesium levels, and encouragement of the development of myofascial trigger points – all or any of which, in one way or another, are capable of modifying normal motor control of skeletal musculature (Nixon & Andrews 1996, Mogyoros et al 1997, Seyal et al 1998, Chaitow 2004).

Nixon & Andrews (1996) note the possible effects of hyperventilation on a deconditioned individual: 'Muscular aching at low levels of effort; restlessness and heightened sympathetic activity; increased neuronal sensitivity; and, constriction of smooth-muscle tubes (e.g. vascular, respiratory and gastric-intestinal), can accompany the basic

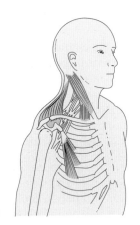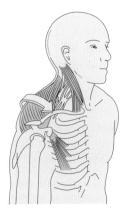

A

Figure 2.17A A progressive pattern of postural and biomechanical dysfunction develops, resulting in, and aggravated by, inappropriate breathing function.

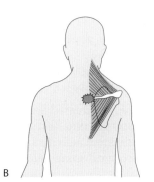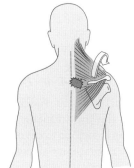

B

Figure 2.17B The local changes in the muscles of an area being stressed in this way will include the evolution of fibrotic changes and myofascial trigger points.

symptom of inability to make and sustain normal levels of effort'.

Also worth noting in relation to breathing function and dysfunction are two important muscles not included in Garland's list: quadratus lumborum and iliopsoas, both of which merge fibres with the diaphragm. Since these are both postural muscles, with a propensity to shortening when stressed, the impact of such shortening, either uni- or bilaterally, can be seen to have major implications for respiratory function, whether the primary feature of such a dysfunction lies in diaphragmatic or in muscular distress.

Garland concludes his listing of somatic changes associated with hyperventilation by saying: 'Physically and physiologically [all of] this runs against a biologically sustainable pattern, and in a vicious cycle, abnormal function (use) alters normal structure, which disallows return to normal function.'

He also points to the likelihood of counselling (for associated anxiety or depression, perhaps) and breathing retraining being far more likely to be successfully initiated if the structural component(s) – as listed – are dealt with in such a way as to minimise the effects of the somatic changes described.

The words of the pioneer osteopathic physician Carl McConnell (1902) remind us of wider implications:

Remember that the functional status of the diaphragm is probably the most powerful mechanism of the whole body. It not only mechanically engages the tissues of the pharynx to the perineum, several times per minute, but is physiologically indispensable to the activity of every cell in the body. A working knowledge of the crura, tendon, and the extensive ramification of the diaphragmatic tissues, graphically depicts the significance of structural continuity and functional unity. The wealth of soft tissue work centering in the powerful mechanism is beyond compute, and clinically it is very practical.

Clinical question   Is it possible to incorporate breathing pattern assessment into a normal musculoskeletal screening protocol?

Observation of the patient's breathing pattern can easily be made a part of a regular manual therapy intake, with basic palpation and assessment methods adding no more than a few minutes to the proceedings (Chaitow et al 2002, Chaitow 2003).

Fascia and the thorax

In both Garland's and McConnell's discussion of respiratory function mention has been made of fascia, the importance of which was indicated earlier in this chapter. An additional early reference to the ubiquitous nature and vital importance of this structure comes from Leon Page (1952), who discusses the involvement of fascia in the thoracic region:

The cervical fascia extends from the base of the skull to the mediastinum and forms compartments enclosing oesophagus, trachea, carotid vessels and provides support for the pharynx, larynx and thyroid gland. There is direct continuity of fascia from the apex of the diaphragm to the base of the skull, extending through the fibrous pericardium upward through the deep cervical fascia and the continuity extends not only to the outer surface of the sphenoid, occipital and temporal bones but proceeds further through the foramina in the base of the skull around the vessels and nerves to join the dura.

Goldthwaite's postural overview

Goldthwaite (1945), in his classic discussion of posture, links a wide array of problems to the absence of balanced posture. Clearly some of what he hypothesises remains conjecture, but we can see just how much impact postural stress can have on associated tissues, starting with diaphragmatic weakness:

The main factors which determine the maintenance of the abdominal viscera in position are the diaphragm and the abdominal muscles, both of which are relaxed and cease to support in faulty posture. The disturbances of circulation resulting from a low diaphragm and ptosis may give rise to chronic passive congestion in one or all of the organs of the abdomen and pelvis, since the local as well as general venous drainage may be impeded by the failure of the diaphragmatic pump to do its full work in the drooped body.

Furthermore, the drag of these congested organs on their nerve supply, as well as the pressure on the sympathetic ganglia and plexuses, probably causes many irregularities in their function, varying from partial paralysis to over-stimulation. All these organs receive fibres from both the vagus and sympathetic systems, either one of which may be disturbed. It is probable that one or all of these factors are active at various times in both the stocky and the slender anatomic types, and are responsible for many functional digestive disturbances. These disturbances, if continued long enough, may lead to diseases later in life. Faulty body mechanics in early life, then, becomes a vital factor in the production of the vicious cycle of chronic diseases and presents a chief point of attack in its prevention ... In this upright position, as one becomes older, the tendency is for the abdomen to relax and sag more and more, allowing a ptosic condition of the abdominal and pelvic organs unless the supporting lower abdominal muscles are taught to contract properly. As the abdomen relaxes, there is a great tendency towards a drooped chest, with narrow rib angle, forward shoulders, prominent shoulder blades, a forward position of the head, and probably pronated feet. When the human machine is out of balance, physiological function cannot be perfect; muscles and ligaments are in an abnormal state of tension and strain. A well-poised body means a machine working perfectly, with the least amount of muscular effort, and therefore better health and strength for daily life.

Note how closely Goldthwaite mirrors the picture Janda paints in his upper and lower crossed syndromes, and 'posture and facial pain' description (described earlier in this chapter).

Clinical question Should observation of patterns such as those described by Goldthwaite be a normal feature of assessment?

Observation is commonly neglected as being too subjective. However, observation offers an early clinical impression of patterns of function, and dysfunction, which can then be subjected to more clinically verifiable assessment methods. Observation of the patient in static and active (gait, etc.) situations can also offer points of

reference, so that when repeated subsequent to, or during, a course of treatment, functional changes can be noted (Greenman 1996).

Korr's trophic influence research

Irwin Korr has spent half a century investigating the scientific background to osteopathic methodology and theory, and among his most important research was that which demonstrated the role of neural structures in delivery of trophic substances (Korr et al 1967, Korr 1986). The various patterns of stress covered in this chapter are capable of drastically affecting this. He states:

Also involved in somatic dysfunction are neural influences that are based on the transfer of specific proteins synthesised by the neuron to the innervated tissue. This delivery is accomplished by axonal transport and junctional traversal. These 'trophic' proteins are thought to exert long-term influences on the developmental, morphologic, metabolic and functional qualities of the tissues – even on their viability. Biomechanical abnormalities in the musculoskeletal system can cause trophic disturbances in at least two ways (1) by mechanical deformation (compression, stretching, angulation, torsion) of the nerves, which impedes axonal transport; and (2) by sustained hyperactivity of neurons in facilitated segments of the spinal cord (see below) which slows axonal transport and which because of metabolic changes, may affect protein synthesis by the neurons. It appears that manipulative treatment would alleviate such impairments of neurotrophic function.

Identification and normalisation of patterns of dysfunction

Observation, palpation, specific assessment and other tests – these are the ways in which such patterns may be identified so that treatment can take account of more than the local dysfunction, and can place the patient's symptoms within the context of whole-body dysfunctional patterns which represent the sum of their present adaptation and compensation efforts.

Patterns of imbalance can be observed in predictable areas, relating to specific forms of dysfunction (headache, thoracic inlet, low back, etc.) and the reader is directed to Liebenson's analysis of this approach to assessment in Ch. 8.

If an imbalance pattern is recognisable, and, within that, emphasis is given to what is restricted or hypertonic and what (within both hypertonic and hypotonic muscles) is reflexively active, as in the case of myofascial trigger points, a therapeutic starting point is possible which leads physiologically towards the normalisation and resolution – if only partially – of the somatic dysfunction patterns currently on display.

When whatever is excessively tense and tight is released and stretched, antagonists should regain tone, and a degree of balance be restored. As local myofascial trigger areas are resolved, so should reflexively initiated pain and sympathetic overactivity be minimised. The stress burden should be lightened, energy be saved, function improved, joint stress reduced and exacerbation of patterns of dysfunction modified.

This is not the end of the story, however, since re-education as to more appropriate use is clearly the ideal long-term objective, if the causes of dysfunction related to misuse, abuse or overuse of the musculoskeletal system are to be addressed. It is suggested that such re-education – whether postural or functional (as in breathing retraining), or sensory-motor rehabilitation where faulty motor patterns are well established – should be more successfully achieved if chronic mechanical restrictions have been minimised.

Liebenson (1990b) comments:

'In rehabilitation it is important to identify and correct overactive or shortened musculature prior to attempting a muscle strengthening regimen ... . The effectiveness of any rehabilitation program is enhanced if hypertonic muscles are relaxed, and if necessary stretched, prior to initiating a strengthening program'

(see Ch. 8 for an introduction to Liebenson's rehabilitation methods).

There are certainly other ways of normalising hypertonicity than use of MET, even if only temporarily, such as use of inhibitory ischaemic compression (Chaitow 1991b), positional release methods (Jones 1982) or joint manipulation (Lewit 1999). Indeed, many experts in manual medicine hold that manipulation of associated joints will automatically and spontaneously resolve soft tissue hypertonicity (Mennell 1952, Janda 1978); however, neither manipulation of joints, nor use of methods which do not in some way stretch the tissues will reduce and encourage towards normal those tissues that have shortened structurally, whereas MET will do so if used appropriately (see Chs 4–7).

The major researchers into myofascial trigger points, Travell & Simons, influenced by the work of Karel Lewit, also suggest that use of MET is an ideal means of normalising these centres of neurological mayhem (Travell & Simons 1992).

Trigger points

It is necessary to include a brief overview of myofascial trigger points in any consideration of patterns of dysfunction.

The reflex patterns – and facilitation

In the body, when an area is stressed repetitively and chronically, the local nerve structures in that area tend to become sensitised, overexcitable, more easily activated, hyperirritable – a process known in osteopathic medicine as facilitation. There are two forms of facilitation, and if we are to make sense of muscle dysfunction, we should understand these.

Segmental facilitation (Korr 1976, Patterson 1976)

Organ dysfunction will result in facilitation of the paraspinal structures at the level of the nerve supply to that organ. If, for example, there is any form of cardiac disease, there will be a 'feedback' of impulses along these same nerves towards the spine, and the paramuscles, at that upper thoracic level, will become hypertonic. If the cardiac problem continues, the area will become facilitated, with the nerves of the area, including those passing to the heart, becoming hyperirritable (Fig. 2.18).

Electromyographic readings of the paraspinal muscles at the upper thoracic level would show this region to be very active compared with segments above and below it, and the muscles alongside the spine at that level would be hypertonic and probably painful to pressure.

Once facilitated, any additional factor, of any sort, whether emotional, physical, chemical, climatic or mechanical, which imposed stress on the person as a whole – not just this particular part of their body – would cause a marked increase in neural activity in the facilitated area and not in the rest of the spinal structures.

Korr has described such an area as a 'neurological lens' – it concentrates the neural activity to the facilitated area, so creating more activity and also a local increase in muscle tone at that level of the spine. Similar segmental (spinal) facilitation occurs in response to any organ problem, usually affecting only the part of the spine from which the nerves to that organ emerge. Other causes of segmental (spinal) facilitation can include biomechanical stress imposed on a part of the spine through injury, overactivity, repetitive stress, poor posture or structural imbalance (short leg for example).

Korr (1978) tells us that when subjects who have had facilitated segments identified 'were exposed to physical, environmental and psychological stimuli

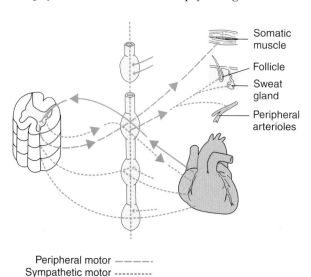

Peripheral motor ‑ ‑ ‑ ‑ ‑
Sympathetic motor ⋯⋯⋯⋯⋯
Visceral afferent ————

Figure 2.18 Schematic representation of the neurological influences involved in the process of facilitation resulting from visceral dysfunction (cardiac disease in this example). Hyperirritable neural feedback to the CNS will result, which influences muscle, skin (both palpable) and venous structures in associated areas, as well as the neural supply to the organ itself.

similar to those encountered in daily life, the sympathetic responses in those segments was exaggerated and prolonged. The disturbed segments behaved as though they were continually in or bordering on a state of "physiologic alarm".'

In assessing and treating somatic dysfunction, the phenomenon of segmental facilitation needs to be borne in mind, since the causes and treatment of these frequently lie outside the scope of practice of manual practitioners and therapists. In many instances, however, appropriate manipulative treatment, including use of MET, can help to 'destress' facilitated areas.

How to recognise a facilitated area

A number of observable and palpable signs indicate an area of segmental (spinal) facilitation. Beal (1983) tells us that such an area will usually involve two or more segments (unless traumatically induced, in which case only single segments may be involved). The paraspinal tissues will palpate as rigid or 'board-like' (Fig. 2.19). With the patient supine and the palpating hands under the patient's paraspinal area to be tested (standing at the head of the table, for example, and reaching under the shoulders for the upper thoracic area), any ceilingward 'springing' attempt on these tissues will result in a distinct lack of elasticity, unlike more normal tissues above or below the facilitated area (Beal 1983).

Korr (1948), Gunn & Milbrandt (1978), Grieve (1986) and Lewit (1999) have all helped to define the palpable and visual signs that accompany facilitated dysfunction (local or segmental):

- A gooseflesh appearance is observable in facilitated areas when the skin is exposed to cool air – the result of a facilitated pilomotor response.

- A palpable sense of 'drag' is noticeable as a light touch contact is made across such areas, due to increased hydrosis (sweat production) resulting from facilitation of the sudomotor reflexes.

- There is likely to be cutaneous hyperaesthesia in the related dermatome, as the sensitivity is increased – for example, to a pin prick – due to facilitation.

Labels for Figure 2.18:
Somatic muscle
Follicle
Sweat gland
Peripheral arterioles

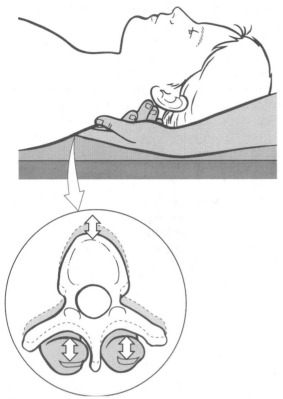

Figure 2.19 Beal's springing assessment for paraspinal rigidity associated with segmental facilitation.

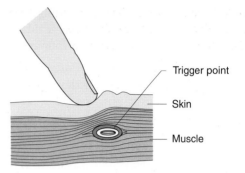

Figure 2.20 Trigger points are areas of local facilitation which can be housed in any soft tissue structure, most usually muscle and/or fascia. Palpation from the skin or at depth may be required to localise these.

- Lewit (1999) has termed these areas *hyperalgesic skin zones*.

- An 'orange peel' appearance is noticeable in the subcutaneous tissues when the skin is rolled over the affected segment, due to subcutaneous trophoedema.

- There is commonly localised spasm of the muscles in a facilitated area, which is palpable segmentally as well as peripherally in the related myotome. This is likely to be accompanied by an enhanced myotatic reflex due to the process of facilitation.

Local (trigger point) facilitation in muscles (Fig. 2.20)

A similar process of facilitation occurs when particularly easily stressed parts of muscle (origins and insertions for example) are overused, abused, misused or disused in any of the many ways discussed earlier in this chapter.

Localised areas of hypertonicity will develop, sometimes accompanied by oedema, sometimes with a stringy feel – but always with a sensitivity to pressure. Many of these localised, palpably painful, tender, sensitive, facilitated points are myofascial trigger points which are not only painful themselves when pressed, but will also when active transmit or activate pain (and other) sensations some distance away from themselves, in 'target' tissues.

In the same manner as the facilitated areas alongside the spine, trigger points are made more active by any stress, of whatever type, impacting on the body as a whole – not just in the area in which they lie. When not actively referring or radiating familiar (recognised as a common symptom by the patient) pain, to a distant area, trigger points are said to be 'latent'. The same signs as described for spinal/segmental facilitation can be observed and palpated in these areas, with 'drag' palpation being among the most rapid means of identifying such local dysfunction.

The leading researchers into pain, Melzack & Wall (1988), have stated that there are few, if any, chronic pain problems which do not have trigger point activity as a major part of the picture, perhaps not always as a prime cause, but almost always as a maintaining feature.

What causes the trigger point to develop?

Janet Travell and David Simons (Travell & Simons 1983, 1992) are the two physicians who, above all others, have helped our understanding of trigger points. Simons has described the evolution of trigger points as follows (Lewit & Simons 1984):

In the core of the trigger lies a muscle spindle which is in trouble for some reason. Visualise a spindle like a strand of yarn in a knitted sweater ... a metabolic crisis takes place which increases the temperature locally in the trigger point, shortens a minute part of the muscle (sarcomere) – like a snag in a sweater, and reduces the supply of oxygen and nutrients into the trigger point. During this disturbed episode an influx of calcium occurs and the muscle spindle does not have enough energy to pump the calcium outside the cell where it belongs. Thus a vicious cycle is maintained and the muscle spindle can't seem to loosen up and the affected muscle can't relax.

Simons has tested his concept and found that, at the core of trigger points, there is an oxygen deficit compared with the muscle tissue which surrounds it. This has been confirmed by studies such as that of Shah et al (2003) who used microdialysis techniques to evaluate histological changes. They noted significant differences in a number of biochemical markers between trigger point sites and normal tissues, as well as the fact that pH was markedly lower in trigger point regions.

Travell has confirmed that the following factors can all help to maintain and enhance trigger point activity: nutritional deficiency (especially vitamin C, B-complex vitamins and iron); hormonal imbalances (low thyroid, menopausal or premenstrual situations for example); infections (bacteria, viruses or yeast); allergies (wheat and dairy in particular); low oxygenation of tissues (aggravated by tension, stress, inactivity, poor respiration) (Simons et al 1999).

Facilitation and the central nervous system

Facilitation, both segmental and local, is a feature of the shortening of muscles, as a whole, or in part. Korr has shown that muscle spindles in areas of dysfunction are hypersensitive to change in muscle length, possibly due to incorrect spinal cord setting of the gamma-neuron control of the intrafusal muscle fibres. If influences from higher centres further exaggerate this high 'gamma-gain', exacerbation of local restriction is likely.

It is only when gamma-gain is restored to normal, possibly via manipulation, that normality is achieved. This scenario may be accompanied by another feature of internal discord in which, because of multiple stresses being imposed on them, musculoskeletal reporting stations (proprioceptors in soft tissues, including skin) are presenting 'garbled' and conflicting information, so making appropriate adaptive responses impossible (Korr 1975).

An example is a situation in which high-gain spindles would be reporting greater than real muscle lengths, and this information was simultaneously being contradicted by reports from joint receptors. The CNS responses to mixed signals would be inappropriate and could lead to increased dysfunction, spasm, etc. This set of events forms the basis of functional and 'strain/counterstrain' methods of soft tissue normalisation (Jones 1981, D'Ambrogio & Roth 1997).

Ultimately nerves subserve the CNS and the brain, and at times this central control mechanism may be responsible for excessive or diminished neural activity. Just as a local muscle area may become hyperirritable if repetitively stressed, forming a trigger point for example, so can the central nervous system, or parts of it, including parts of the brain, become sensitised when bombarded with pain and distress messages, or when biochemically disturbed, allowing it to become more easily irritated, interfering with accurate interpretation of the messages from the body, as well as causing instructions being sent to the body parts to be inappropriate. This 'central sensitisation' process is thought to be a major part of what happens in many chronic pain conditions (Butler 2000).

Fibromyalgia and trigger points

Is the result of widespread trigger point activity, myofascial pain syndrome (MPS) the same as fibromyalgia syndrome (FMS)?

According to a leading researcher into this realm, P. Baldry (1993), the two conditions are similar or identical in that both fibromyalgia and myofascial pain syndrome:

- Are affected by cold weather

- May involve increased sympathetic nerve activity and may involve conditions such as Raynaud's phenomenon

- Have tension headaches and paraesthesia as major associated symptoms

- Are unaffected by anti-inflammatory pain-killing medication whether of the cortisone type or standard formulations.

However, fibromyalgia and myofascial pain syndrome are different in that:

- MPS affects males and females equally, FMS mainly females.

- MPS is usually local to an area such as the neck and shoulders, or low back and legs, although it can affect a number of parts of the body at the same time; FMS is a generalised problem, often involving all four 'corners' of the body at the same time.

- Muscles which contain areas which feel 'like a tight rubber band' are found in around 30% of people with MPS but more than 60% of people with FMS.

- People with FMS have poorer muscle endurance (they get tired faster) than do people with MPS.

- MPS can sometimes be bad enough to cause disturbed sleep; in FMS the sleep disturbance has a more causative role, and is a pronounced feature of the condition.

- MPS produces no morning stiffness whereas FMS does.

- There is not usually fatigue associated with MPS while it is common in FMS.

- MPS can sometimes lead to depression (reactive) and anxiety whereas in a small percentage of FMS cases (some leading researchers believe) these conditions can be the trigger for the start of the condition.

- Conditions such as irritable bowel syndrome, dysmenorrhoea and a feeling of swollen joints are noted in FMS but seldom in MPS.

- Low-dosage tricyclic antidepressant drugs are helpful in dealing with the sleep problems, and many of the symptoms, of FMS, but not of MPS.

- Exercise programmes (cardiovascular fitness) can help some FMS patients, according to experts, but this is not a useful approach in MPS.

The outlook for people with MPS is excellent, since the trigger points usually respond quickly to manipulative (stretching in particular) techniques or acupuncture, whereas the outlook for FMS is less positive, with a lengthy treatment and recovery phase being the norm.

Summary (Rothschild 1991, Block 1993, Goldenberg 1993)

Trigger points are certainly part – in some cases the major part – of the pain suffered by people with muscle pain in general, as well as fibromyalgia, and when they are, MET offers a useful means of treatment, since a trigger point will reactivate if the muscle in which it lies cannot easily reach its normal resting length (see Fig. 2.21).

Summary of trigger point characteristics

- Janet Travell defines trigger points as 'hyper-irritable foci lying within taut bands of muscle which are painful on compression and which refer pain or other symptoms at a distant site'.

- Embryonic trigger points will develop as satellites of existing triggers in the target area, and in time these will produce their own satellites.

- According to Professor Melzack, nearly 80% of trigger points are in exactly the same positions as known acupuncture points, as used in traditional Chinese medicine.

- Painful points which do not refer symptoms to a distant site are simply latent triggers requiring additional stress to create greater facilitation and turn them into active triggers.

- The taut band in which triggers lie will twitch if a finger is run across it, and is tight but not

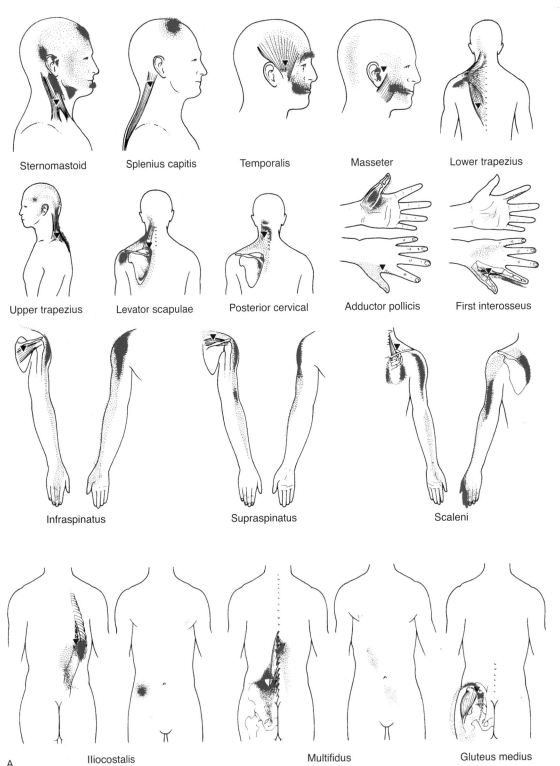

Sternomastoid   Splenius capitis   Temporalis   Masseter   Lower trapezius

Upper trapezius   Levator scapulae   Posterior cervical   Adductor pollicis   First interosseus

Infraspinatus   Supraspinatus   Scaleni

A   Iliocostalis   Multifidus   Gluteus medius

Figure 2.21   A selection of the most commonly found examples of representations of trigger point sites and their reference (or target) areas. Trigger points found in the same sites in different people will usually refer to the same target areas.

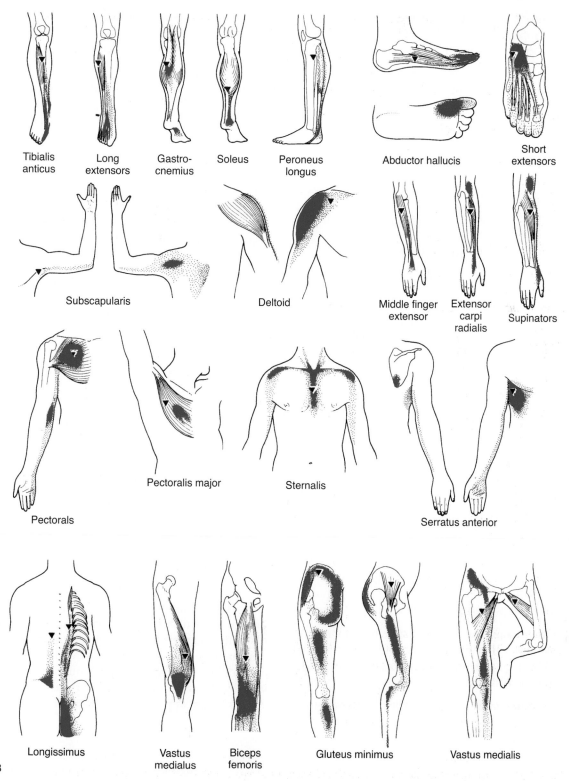

Tibialis anticus

Long extensors

Gastro-cnemius

Soleus

Peroneus longus

Abductor hallucis

Short extensors

Subscapularis

Deltoid

Middle finger extensor

Extensor carpi radialis

Supinators

Pectorals

Pectoralis major

Sternalis

Serratus anterior

Longissimus

Vastus medialus

Biceps femoris

Gluteus minimus

Vastus medialis

B

fibrosed, since it will soften and relax if the appropriate treatment is applied – something fibrotic tissue cannot do.

- Muscles which contain trigger points will often hurt when they are contracted (i.e. when they are working).

- Trigger points are areas of increased energy consumption and lowered oxygen supply due to inadequate local circulation. They will therefore add to the drain on energy and any fatigue being experienced.

- The muscles in which trigger points lie cannot reach their normal resting length (i.e. they are held in a shortened position).

- Until muscles can reach this normal resting length without pain or effort, any treatment of the trigger points will only achieve temporary relief, since they will reactivate when re-stressed sufficiently.

- Stretching of the muscles, using either active or passive methods, is useful in treating both the shortness and the trigger point since this can reduce the contraction (taut band) as well as increasing circulation to the area.

- There are many ways of treating trigger points, including acupuncture, procaine injections, direct manual ischaemic pressure, stretching and ice therapy, some of which (pressure, acupuncture) cause the release of endorphins, which explains one of the ways in which pain is reduced – another involves the substitution of one sensation (pressure, needle) for another in which pain messages are partially or totally blocked from reaching or being registered by the brain.

- Other treatment methods (stretching for example) alter the dynamics of the circulatory imbalance affecting trigger points and appear to deactivate them.

- The target area to which a trigger refers pain will be the same in everyone if the trigger point is in the same position – but this distribution of pain does not relate directly to neural pathways or to acupuncture meridian pathways.

- The way in which a trigger point relays pain to a distant site is thought to involve one of a variety of neurological mechanisms, and probably involves the brain 'mislocating' pain messages which it receives via several different pathways.

- The sites of trigger points lie in parts of muscles (postural or phasic) most prone to mechanical stress, producing circulatory inadequacy and lack of oxygen – among other changes.

- Trigger points become self-perpetuating (a cycle of pain – increased tone – pain) and will never go away unless adequately treated.

Integrated neuromuscular inhibition technique (INIT)

The author (Chaitow 1994) has described an integrated sequence in which, after location of an active (referring symptoms) trigger point, this receives ischaemic compression, followed by positional release (osteopathic functional or strain/counter-strain methods), followed (in the same position of ease) by the imposition by the patient of an isometric contraction which is either stretched subsequently (postfacilitation stretch) or simultaneously (isolytic stretch). This combination of methods effectively deactivates trigger points (see Ch. 7).

Efficient stretching and releasing of whatever soft tissues are short and tight requires an approach which incorporates choices from the variety of different uses of MET as described above. In the following chapters, presentation will be made of sequences of assessment and MET treatment methods for the major postural muscles as identified by the work of Lewit, Janda and others, as well as other applications of variations on the theme of MET.

References

Al-Rawi ZS, Adnan J, Al-Aszawi A et al 1985 Joint mobility among university students in Iraq. British Journal of Rheumatology 24: 326–331

Aust G, Fischer K 1997 Changes in body equilibrium response caused by breathing. A posturographic study with visual feedback. Laryngorhinootologie 76(10): 577–582

Bailey M, Dick L 1992 Nociceptive considerations in treating with counterstrain. Journal of the American Osteopathic Association 92: 334–341

Baldry P E 1993 Acupuncture trigger points and musculoskeletal pain. Churchill Livingstone, London

Barker P, Briggs C 1999 Attachments of the posterior layer of lumbar fascia. Spine 24(17): 1757–1764

Barlow W 1959 Anxiety and muscle tension pain. British Journal of Clinical Practice 13(5): 339–350

Basmajian J 1978 Muscles alive. Williams and Wilkins, Baltimore

Beal M 1983 Palpatory testing of somatic dysfunction in patients with cardiovascular disease. Journal of the American Osteopathic Association 82: 822–831

Beighton P et al 1983 Hypermobility of joints. Springer-Verlag, Berlin

Bennet C 1952 Physics. Barnes and Noble, New York

Bergmark A 1989 Stability of the lumbar spine: a study in mechanical engineering. Acta Orthopaedica Scandinavica 230(suppl): 20–24

Bhatia R 1999 Role of abnormal integrin-cytoskeletal interactions in impaired 1 integrin function in chronic myelogenous leukemia hematopoietic progenitors. Experimental Hematology 27(9): 1384–1396

Biedermann H 1992 Kinematic imbalances due to suboccipital strain. Journal of Manual Medicine 31: 92–95

Biedermann H 2001 Primary and secondary cranial asymmetry in KISS children. In: von Piekartz H, Bryden L (eds) Craniofacial dysfunction and pain. Butterworth-Heinemann, Oxford

Block S 1993 Fibromyalgia and the rheumatisms. Controversies in Clinical Rheumatology 19(1): 61–78

Bogduk N, Twomey L 1991 Clinical anatomy of the lumbar spine, 2nd edn. Churchill Livingstone, Edinburgh

Booth R, Thomason D 1991 Molecular and cellular adaptations of muscle in response to exercise: Perspectives of various models. Physiological Review 71: 541–580

Brookes D 1984 Cranial osteopathy. Thorsons, London

Buchanan C, Marsh R 2002 Effects of exercise on the biomechanical, biochemical and structural properties of tendons. Comparative Biochemistry and Physiology – Part A: Molecular and Integrative Physiology 133(4): 1101–1107

Bulbena A et al 1993 Anxiety disorders in the joint hyper-mobility syndrome. Psychiatry Research 46: 59–68

Buller A 1960 Interactions between motor neurons and muscles. Journal of Physiology (London) 150: 417–439

Butler D 2000 The sensitive nervous system. Noigroup Publications, Adelaide

Cantu R, Grodin A 1992 Myofascial manipulation. Aspen Publications, Maryland

Cathie A 1974 Selected writings. Academy of Applied Osteopathy Yearbook 1974, pp 15–126

Chaitow L 1991a Palpatory literacy. Thorsons/Harper Collins, London

Chaitow L 1991b Soft tissue manipulation. Healing Arts Press, Rochester

Chaitow L 1994 INIT in treatment of pain and trigger points – an introduction. British Journal of Osteopathy 13: 17–21

Chaitow L 2003 Palpation skills and assessment, 2nd edn. Churchill Livingstone, Edinburgh

Chaitow L 2004 Breathing pattern disorders, motor control, and low back pain. Journal of Osteopathic Medicine 7(1): 34–41

Chaitow L, Bradley D, Gilbert C 2002 Multidisciplinary approaches to breathing pattern disorders. Churchill Livingstone, Edinburgh

Chen C, Ingber D 1999 Tensegrity and mechanoregulation: from skeleton to cytoskeleton. Osteoarthritis and Cartilage 7: 81–94

Chicural M, Chen C, Ingber D 1998 Cellular control lies in the balance of forces. Current Opinions in Cellular Biology 10(2): 232–239

Cisler T 1994 Whiplash as a total body injury. Journal of the American Osteopathic Association 94(2): 145–148

Cyriax J 1962 Textbook of orthopaedic medicine. Cassell, London

Dahl J B, Erichsen C J, Fuglsang-Frederiksen A, Kehlet H 1992 Pain sensation and nociceptive reflex excitability in surgical patients and human volunteers. British Journal of Anaesthesia 69: 117–121

D'Ambrogio K, Roth G 1997 Positional release therapy. Mosby, St Louis, Missouri

Defeo G, Hicks L 1993 A description of the common compensatory pattern in relationship to the osteopathic postural examination. Dynamic Chiropractic 11(24)

Deyo R, Weinstein J 2001 Low back pain. New England Journal of Medicine 344(5): 363–369

DiGiovanna E 1991 An osteopathic approach to diagnosis and treatment. Lippincott, Philadelphia

Evjenth O, Hamberg J 1984 Muscle stretching in manual therapy. Alfta Rehab, Sweden

Fahrni H 1966 Backache relieved. Thomas, Springfield

Garland W 1994 Presentation to Respiratory Function Congress, Paris, 1994

Goldenberg D 1993 Fibromyalgia, chronic fatigue syndrome and myofascial pain syndrome. Current Opinions in Rheumatology 5: 199–208

Goldthwaite J 1945 Essentials of body mechanics. Lippincott, Philadelphia

Greenman P 1989 Principles of manual medicine. Williams and Wilkins, Baltimore

Greenman P 1996 Principles of manual medicine, 2nd edn. Williams and Wilkins, Baltimore

Grieve G 1986 Modern manual therapy. Churchill Livingstone, London

Gunn C, Milbrandt W 1978 Early and subtle signs in low back sprain. Spine 3: 267–281

Gutstein R 1955 A review of myodysneuria (fibrositis). American Practitioner and Digest of Treatments 6(4): 570–577

Guyton A 1987 Basic neuroscience, anatomy and physiology. W B Saunders, Philadelphia

Hodges P, Heinjnen I, Gandevia S 2001 Postural activity of the diaphragm is reduced in humans when respiratory demand increases. Journal of Physiology 537(3): 999–1008

Hoffer J, Andreasson C 1981 Inefficient muscular stabilisation of the lumbar spine associated with low back pain. Spine 21: 2640–2650

Hubbard D R, Berkoff G M 1993 Myofascial trigger points show spontaneous needle EMG activity. Spine 18: 1803–1807

Hudson N et al 1995 Diagnostic associations with hypermobility in new rheumatology referrals. British Journal of Rheumatology 34: 1157–1161

Isaacson J 1980 Living anatomy – an anatomic basis for osteopathic theory. Journal of the American Osteopathic Association 79(12): 752–759

Janda V 1960 Postural and phasic muscles in the pathogenesis of low back pain. In: Proceedings XI Congress Rehabilitation International, Dublin

Janda V 1978 Muscles – central nervous motor regulation and back problems. In: Korr I (ed) Neurobiological mechanisms in manipulative therapy. Plenum Press, New York

Janda V 1983 Muscle function testing. Butterworths, London

Janda V 1984 Low back pain – trends, controversies. Presentation, Turku, Finland, 3–4 September 1984

Janda V 1985 Pain in the locomotor system. In: Glasgow E (ed) Aspects of manipulative therapy. Churchill Livingstone, London

Janda V 1986a Muscle weakness and inhibition in back pain syndromes. In: Grieve G (ed) Modern manual therapy of the vertebral column. Churchill Livingstone, Edinburgh

Janda V 1986b Some aspects of extracranial causes of facial pain. Journal of Prosthetic Dentistry 56(4): 484–487

Janda V 1988 In: Grant R (ed) Physical therapy of the cervical and thoracic spine. Churchill Livingstone, New York

Janda V 1989 Differential diagnosis of muscle tone in respect of inhibitory techniques. Presentation, Physical Medicine Research Foundation, 21 September 1989

Janda V 1991 Muscle spasm – a proposed procedure for differential diagnosis. Manual Medicine 1001: 6136–6139

Johansson H 1991 Pathophysiological mechanisms involved in genesis and spread of muscular tension. A hypothesis. Medical Hypotheses 35: 196

Jones L 1964 Spontaneous release by positioning. The DO 4: 109–116

Jones L 1981 Strain and counterstrain. American Academy of Osteopathy, Newark

Jones L 1982 Strain and counterstrain. Academy of Applied Osteopathy, Boulder

Jull G 1994 Active stabilisation of the trunk. Course notes, Edinburgh

Jull G, Janda V 1987 Muscles and motor control in low back pain: assessment and management. In: Twomey L (ed) Physical therapy of the low back. Churchill Livingstone, New York

Kaltenborn F 1985 Mobilization of the extremity joints. Olaf Norlis Bokhandel, Oslo

Kendall F P, McCreary E K, Provance P G 1993 Muscles: testing and function, 4th edn. Williams and Wilkins, Baltimore

Knott M, Voss D 1968 Proprioceptive neuromuscular facilitation. Hoeber, New York

Komendatov G 1945 Proprioceptivnije reflexi glaza i golovy u krolikov. Fiziologiceskij Zurnal 31: 62

Komura T, Prokopow P, Nagano A 2004 Evaluation of the influence of muscle deactivation on other muscles and joints during gait motion. Journal of Biomechanics 37(4): 425–436

Korr I 1947 The neural basis of the osteopathic lesion. Journal of the American Osteopathic Association 48: 191–198

Korr I 1948 The emerging concept of the osteopathic lesion. Journal of the American Osteopathic Association 48: 127–138

Korr I 1975 Proprioceptors and somatic dysfunction. Journal of the American Osteopathic Association 74: 638–650

Korr I 1976 Spinal cord as organiser of the disease process. Academy of Applied Osteopathy Yearbook 1976, Newark, Ohio

Korr I 1978 Sustained sympatheticotonia as a factor in disease. In: Korr I (ed) The neurobiological mechanisms in manipulative therapy. Plenum Press, New York

Korr I 1980 Neurobiological mechanisms in manipulation. Plenum Press, New York

Korr I 1986 Somatic dysfunction, osteopathic manipulative treatment, and the nervous system. Journal of the American Osteopathic Association 86(2): 109–114

Korr I, Wilkinson P, Chornock F 1967 Axonal delivery of neuroplasmic components to muscle cells. Science 155: 342–354

Kraus H 1970 Clinical treatment of back and neck pain. McGraw Hill, New York

Kuchera M et al 1990 Athletic functional demand and posture. Journal of the American Osteopathic Association 90(9): 843–844

Latey P 1996 Feelings, muscles and movement. Journal of Bodywork and Movement Therapies 1(1): 44–52

Lewit K 1974 Functional pathology of the motor system. In: Proceedings of the Fourth Congress of the International Federation of Manual Medicine, Prague

Lewit K 1980 Relation of faulty respiration to posture with clinical implications. Journal of the American Osteopathic Association 79(8): 525–529

Lewit K 1996 Role of manipulation in spinal rehabilitation. In: Liebenson C (ed) Rehabilitation of the spine. Williams and Wilkins, Baltimore

Lewit K 1999 Manipulation in rehabilitation of the motor system. Butterworths, London

Lewit K, Simons D 1984 Myofascial pain – relief by post-isometric relaxation. Archives of Physical Medicine and Rehabilitation 65: 462–466

Liebenson C 1990a Muscular relaxation techniques. Journal of Manipulative and Physiological Therapeutics 12(6): 446–454

Liebenson C 1990b Active muscular relaxation techniques (part 2). Journal of Manipulative and Physiological Therapeutics 13(1): 2–6

Liebenson C 1996 Rehabilitation of the spine. Williams and Wilkins, Baltimore

Lieber R 1992 Skeletal muscle structure and function. Williams and Wilkins, Baltimore, pp 95–100

Liem T 2004 Cranial osteopathy principles and practice. Churchill Livingstone/Elsevier, Edinburgh, pp 340–342

Lin J P et al 1994 Physiological maturation of muscles in childhood. Lancet (June): 1386–1389

McArdle W, Katch F, Katch V 1991 Exercise physiology, energy, nutrition and human performance, 3rd edn. Lea Febiger, Philadelphia

McConnell C 1902 Yearbook of the Osteopathic Institute of Applied Technique 1902, pp 75–78

McGill S, Sharratt M, Seguin J 1995 Loads on spinal tissues during simultaneous lifting and ventilatory challenge. Ergonomics 38(9): 1772–1792

McGill S M, Juker, D, Kropf P 1996 Quantitative intramuscular myoelectric activity of quadratus lumborum during a wide variety of tasks. Clinical Biomechanics 11: 170–172

Martin-Santos R et al 1998 Association between joint hypermobility syndrome and panic disorders. American Journal of Psychiatry 155: 1578–1583

Mathews P 1981 Muscle spindles. In: Brooks V (ed) Handbook of physiology. American Physiological Society, Bethseda

Melzack R, Wall P 1988 The challenge of pain. Penguin, New York

Mennell J 1952 The science and art of manipulation. Churchill Livingstone, London

Mense S 1993 Nociception from skeletal muscle in relation to clinical muscle pain. Pain 54: 241–290

Middaugh S et al 1994 Muscle overuse and posture as factors in the development and maintenance of chronic musculoskeletal pain. In: Grzesiak R, Ciccone D (eds) Psychological vulnerability to chronic pain. Springer, New York, pp 55–89

Mogyoros I, Kiernan K, Burke D et al 1997 Excitability changes in human sensory and motor axons during hyperventilation and ischaemia. Brain 120(2): 317–325

Muller K et al 2003 Hypermobility and chronic back pain. Manuelle Medizin 41: 105–109

Myers T 1997 The anatomy trains. Journal of Bodywork and Movement Therapies 1(2): 91–191

Myers T 1998 A structural approach. Journal of Bodywork and Movement Therapies 2(1): 14–20

Myers T 2001 Anatomy trains: myofascial meridians for manual and movement therapists. Churchill Livingstone, Edinburgh

Neuberger A et al 1953 Metabolism of collagen. Biochemistry Journal 53: 47–52

Nixon P, Andrews J 1996 A study of anaerobic threshold in chronic fatigue syndrome (CFS). Biological Psychology 43(3): 264

Nordhoff L 2000 Cervical trauma following motor vehicle collisions. In: Murphy D (ed) Conservative management of cervical spine syndromes. McGraw Hill, New York

Norris C M 1995a Spinal stabilisation. 1. Active lumbar stabilisation – concepts. Physiotherapy 81(2): 61–64

Norris C M 1995b Spinal stabilisation. 2. Limiting factors to end-range motion in the lumbar spine. Physiotherapy 81(2): 64–72

Norris C M 1995c Spinal stabilisation. 3. Stabilisation mechanisms of the lumbar spine. Physiotherapy 81(2): 72–79

Norris C M 1995d Spinal stabilisation. 4. Muscle imbalance and the low back. Physiotherapy 81(3): 127–138

Norris C M 1995e Spinal stabilisation. 5. An exercise program to enhance lumbar stabilisation. Physiotherapy 81(3): 138–146

Norris C M 1998 Sports injuries, diagnosis and management, 2nd edn. Butterworths, London

Norris C M 1999 Functional load abdominal training. Journal of Bodywork and Movement Therapies 3(3): 150–158

Norris C 2000a Back stability. Human Kinetics, Champaign, Illinois

Norris C 2000b The muscle designation debate. Journal of Bodywork and Movement Therapies 4(4): 225–241

Page L 1952 Academy of Applied Osteopathy Yearbook

Patterson M 1976 Model mechanism for spinal segmental facilitation. Academy of Applied Osteopathy Yearbook 1976, Newark, Ohio

Pauling L 1976 The common cold and 'flu. Freeman, London

Peper E et al 1994 Prevent computer user injury with biofeedback: Assessment and training protocol. In: Electromyography applications in physical therapy, Volume 9: Repetitive strain injury. Thought Technology Ltd, West Chazy, NY

Prior T 1999 Biomechanical foot function: a podiatric perspective (part 2). Journal of Bodywork and Movement Therapies 3(3): 169–184

Richardson C, Jull G, Toppenburg R, Comerford C 1992 Techniques for active lumbar stabilisation for spinal protection. Australian Journal of Physiotherapy 38(2): 106–112

Richardson C, Jull G, Hodges P, Hides J 1999 Therapeutic exercise for spinal segmental stabilisation in low back pain. Churchill Livingstone, Edinburgh

Rolf I 1962 Structural dynamics. British Academy of Osteopathy Yearbook 1962, Maidstone

Rolf I 1977 Rolfing – the integration of human structures. Harper and Row, New York

Rothschild B 1991 Fibromyalgia – an explanation. Comprehensive Therapy 17(6): 9–14

Ruwhof C et al 2000 Mechanical stress-induced cardiac hypertrophy: mechanisms and signal transduction pathways. Cardiovascular Research 47(1): 23–37

Sandman K 1984 Psychophysiological factors in myofascial pain. Journal of Manipulative and Physiological Therapeutics 7(4): 237–242

Scariati P 1991 Myofascial release concepts. In: DiGiovanna E (ed) An osteopathic approach to diagnosis and treatment. Lippincott, London

Schamberger W 2002 The malalignment syndrome. Churchill Livingstone, Edinburgh, p 410

Schiable H G, Grubb B D 1993 Afferent and spinal mechanisms of joint pain. Pain 155: 5–54

Schmid H 1984 Muscular imbalances in skiers. Manual Medicine (2): 23–26

Scott-Dawkins C 1997 Comparative effectiveness of adjustments versus mobilizations in chronic mechanical neck pain. In: Proceedings of the Scientific Symposium. World Chiropractic Congress, Tokyo, June 1997

Selye H 1976 The stress of life. McGraw-Hill, New York

Seyal M, Mull B, Gage B 1998 Increased excitability of the human corticospinal system with hyperventilation. Electroencephalography and Clinical Neurophysiology/Electromyography and Motor Control 109(3): 263–267

Shah J et al 2003 A novel microanalytical technique for assaying soft tissue demonstrates significant quantitative biochemical differences in 3 clinically distinct groups: normal, latent, and active. Archives of Physical Medicine and Research 84(9): Abstract 17

Simons D 1994 Ch 28. In: Vecchiet L, Albe-Fessard D, Lindblom U, Giamberardino M (eds) New trends in referred pain and hyperalgesia, pain research and clinical management, vol 7. Elsevier Science Publishers, Amsterdam

Skubick D, Clasby R, Donaldson S et al 1993 Carpal tunnel syndrome as an expression of muscular dysfunction in the neck. Journal of Occupational Rehabilitation 3: 31–44

Sommer H 1985 Patellar chodropathy and apicitis – muscle imbalances of the lower extremity. Butterworths, London

Stedman 1998 Stedman's electronic medical dictionary. Version 4. Williams and Wilkins, Baltimore

Swartz M A, Tschumperlin D J, Kamm R D, Drazen J M 2001 Mechanical stress is communicated between different cell types to elicit matrix remodeling. Proceedings National Academy of Sciences USA 98: 6180–6185

Travell J, Simons D 1983 Myofascial pain and dysfunction – the trigger point manual, vol 1. Williams and Wilkins, Baltimore

Travell J, Simons D 1992 The trigger point manual, vol 2. Williams and Wilkins, Baltimore

Triano J, Schultz A B 1987 Correlation of objective measure of trunk motion and muscle function with low-back disability ratings. Spine 12: 561

Van Buskirk R 1990 Nociceptive reflexes and the somatic dysfunction. Journal of the American Osteopathic Association 90(9): 792–809

van Wingerden J-P 1997 The role of the hamstrings in pelvic and spinal function. In: Vleeming A, Mooney V, Dorman T, Snijders C, Stoekart R (eds) Movement, stability and low back pain. Churchill Livingstone, New York

Vleeming A, Mooney A, Dorman T, Snijders C, Stoekart R 1989 Load application to the sacrotuberous ligament: influences on sacroiliac joint mechanics. Clinical Biomechanics 4: 204–209

Waddell G 1998 The back pain revolution. Churchill Livingstone, Edinburgh

Waersted M, Eken T, Westgaard R 1993 Psychogenic motor unit activity – a possible muscle injury mechanism studied in a healthy subject. Journal of Musculoskeletal Pain 1(3/4): 185–190

Walsh E G 1992 Muscles, masses and motion: the physiology of normality, hypotonicity, spasticity, and rigidity. MacKeith Press, Blackwell Scientific Publications, Oxford

Walther D 1988 Applied kinesiology. SDC Systems, Pueblo

Ward R 1997 Foundations of osteopathic medicine. Williams and Wilkins, Baltimore

Wohl G, Boyd S, Judex S et al 2000 Functional adaptation of bone to exercise and injury. Journal of Science Medicine in Sport 3: 313–324

World Health Organization 1981 Third report on rehabilitation. WHO, Geneva

Yahia L, Pigeon P et al 1993 Viscoelastic properties of the human lumbodorsal fascia. Journal of Biomedical Engineering 15: 425–429

Zink G, Lawson W 1979 Osteopathic structural examination and functional interpretation of the soma. Osteopathic Annals 7(12): 433–440

Zvolensky M, Eifert G 2001 A review of psychological factors/processes affecting anxious responding during voluntary hyperventilation and inhalations of carbon dioxide-enriched air. Clinical Psychology Review 21(3): 375–400

How to use MET

3

CHAPTER CONTENTS

Palpation skills 78

Ease and bind 78

Goodridge's ease–bind palpation exercise, part 1 79

Goodridge's ease–bind palpation exercise, part 2 80

Basic exercise in MET using postisometric relaxation
(PIR) in acute context 82

Basic exercise in MET using postisometric relaxation
(PIR) followed by stretch, in a chronic context 82

Reciprocal inhibition 83

Basic exercise in MET using reciprocal inhibition
in acute and chronic contexts 83

**MET – some common errors and
contraindications 84**

Patient errors during MET 84

Practitioner errors in application of MET 84

Contraindications and side-effects of MET 84

Breathing and MET 86

Degree of effort with isometric contraction 86

MET variations 87

Strength testing – Mitchell's view 87

Janda's view 87

Ruddy's methods – 'pulsed MET' 89

Isotonic concentric strengthening MET methods 90

Isotonic eccentric alternatives 90

Strengthening a joint complex with isokinetic MET 91

Reduction of fibrotic changes with isolytic
(isotonic eccentric) MET 92

Summary of choices for MET in treating
muscle problems 92

Joints and MET 93

Self-treatment 94

When should MET be applied to a muscle? 95

Evaluation 95

**Muscle energy technique – summary
of variations 96**

1. Isometric contraction – using reciprocal inhibition
(in acute setting, without stretching) 96

2. Isometric contraction – using postisometric
relaxation (in an acute setting, without stretching) 96

3. Isometric contraction – using postisometric
relaxation (in a chronic setting, with stretching,
also known as postfacilitation stretching) 97

4. Isometric contraction – using reciprocal inhibition
(chronic setting, with stretching) 97

5. Isotonic concentric contraction
(for toning or rehabilitation) 100

6. Isotonic eccentric contraction
(isolytic, for reduction of fibrotic change,
to introduce controlled microtrauma) 102

7. Isotonic eccentric contraction (slowly performed)
for strengthening weak postural muscles and
preparing their antagonists for stretching 104

8. Isokinetic (combined isotonic and isometric
contractions) 106

Muscle maps 107

References 107

Chapter 1 described a number of variations on the theme of MET (and stretching) as described by clinicians such as Karel Lewit, Vladimir Janda, Philip Greenman, Craig Liebenson, Aaron Mattes, Edward Stiles, Robert McAtee and others.

In this chapter, suggestions are given as to how to begin to learn the application of MET methods, both for muscles and for joints (specific muscle by muscle and particular joint descriptions of MET treatment can be found in later chapters). Additionally there will be examples of the use of pulsed MET (repetitive mini-contractions based on the work of T. J. Ruddy, 1962) in facilitating proprioceptive re-education of weak and shortened structures.

Chapter 5 will describe a suggested sequence for the evaluation/assessment of the major postural (or *mobiliser*) muscles of the body – for relative shortness – along with details of suggested MET approaches for normalising, stretching and relaxing those muscles, much of the material based on the work of experts such as those mentioned above.

But can the words and suggestions of authorities and 'experts' be sufficient grounds for using therapeutic methods in particular ways, without supportive primary research evidence?

In recent times, authority-based descriptions have become less trusted, as the demand for evidence-based medicine and therapy advances. To meet this requirement, Ch. 4 describes the increasingly broad body of evidence there is for the variations in MET methodology, advocated in this text. However, the fact remains that at this time there exist areas of MET methodology that are only lightly supported by research validation.

The reader therefore needs to decide whether to wait for future evidence as to just why and how MET produces its apparent benefits most effectively, or whether, based on clinical and anecdotal reporting, together with the body of evidence that already exists, to trust the quoted authorities. Whichever option is chosen, a primary requirement for the practitioner is the identification, by means of assessment, of a need for the use of MET, or an alternative means of releasing, relaxing and/or stretching, shortened or restricted tissues. Is there an identifiable restriction that requires such treatment?

This brings us to the need for sound palpation skills.[1]

Palpation skills

Ease and bind

The concept and reality of tissues providing the palpating hands or fingers with a sense of states of relative tension, or 'bind', as opposed to states of relaxation or 'ease', is one which the beginner needs to grasp, and that the advanced practitioner probably takes for granted. There can never be enough focus on these two characteristics, which allow the tissues to speak as to their current degree of comfort or distress. In the previous chapter the 'loose–tight' concept was discussed. Ward (1997) states that 'Tightness suggests tethering, while looseness suggests joint and/or soft tissue laxity, with or without neural inhibition'.

Osteopathic pioneer H. V. Hoover (1969) described ease as a state of equilibrium, or 'neutral', which the practitioner senses by having at least one completely passive 'listening' contact (either the whole hand or a single of several fingers or thumb) in touch with the tissues being assessed. Bind is, of course, the opposite of ease, and can most easily be noted by lightly palpating the tissues surrounding, or associated with, a joint, as this is taken towards the end of its range of movement – its resistance barrier (Box 3.1).

Greenman (1996) states:

> *The examiner must be able to identify and characterize normal and abnormal ranges of movement, as well as normal and abnormal barriers to movement, in order to make an accurate assessment of tissue status. Most joints allow motion in multiple planes, but for descriptive purposes barriers to movement are described within one plane of motion, for a*

---

[1] In this text the practitioner is presented as being male (because the lead author is), whereas the patient/client is described variously as male or female. It is hoped that this gender bias regarding the practitioner does not offend the reader, since no offence is intended.

Box 3.1 Barriers

When measuring the range of motion of a joint, the structures surrounding the joint itself – joint capsules, ligaments and physical structures of the articulation – provide resistance to the overall range of motion of the joint. In addition to this, the skin and subcutaneous connective tissue also play a part in restriction of a joint's motion (Shellock & Prentice 1985, Gajdosik 1991). Johns and Wright (1962) have shown that the passive torque that is required to move a joint is contributed by the joint capsule (47%), tendon (10%), muscle (41%), and skin (2%).

A variety of different terms can be used to describe what is perceived when a restriction barrier is reached or engaged. These terms frequently relate to the type of tissue providing the restriction, and to the nature of the restriction. For example:

- Normal end of range for soft tissues is felt as a progressive build-up of tension, leading to a gradually reached barrier, as all slack is removed.
- If a fluid restriction (oedema, congestion, swelling) causes reduction in the range of motion, the end-feel will be 'boggy', yielding yet spongy.
- If muscle physiology has changed (hypertonicity, spasm, contracture), the end-feel will be a tight, tugging sensation.
- If fibrotic tissue is responsible for a reduction in range, end-feel will be rapid and harsh but with a slight elasticity remaining.
- In hypermobile individuals, or structures, the end-feel will be loose and the range greater than normal.
- If bony tissue is responsible for a reduction in range (arthritis for example), end-feel will be sudden and hard without any elasticity remaining.
- Pain may also produce a restriction in range, and the end-feel resulting from sudden pain will be rapid and widespread, as surrounding tissues protect against further movement.

The barrier used in MET treatment is a 'first sign of resistance' barrier, in which the very first indication of the onset of 'bind' is noted.

This is the place at which further movement would produce stretching of *some* fibres of the muscle(s) involved.

This is where MET isometric contractions, whether these involve the agonists or antagonists, commence in acute (and joint) problems, and short of which contractions should commence in chronic problems.

single joint. The total range of motion from one extreme to the other is limited by the anatomical integrity of the joint and its supporting ligaments, muscles and fascia, and somewhere within the total range of movement is found a neutral point of balance.

This is the point of 'maximum ease' which the exercise described below attempts to identify.

In order to 'read' hypertonicity (bind), and the opposite, a relaxed (ease) state, palpation skills need to be refined. As a first step, Goodridge (1981) suggested the following test, which examines medial hamstring and short adductor status. This exercise offers the opportunity for becoming comfortable with the reality of ease and bind in a practical manner.[2]

Test for palpation of ease and bind during assessment of adductors of the thigh (Fig. 3.1A and B; see also Fig. 1.3)

Goodridge (1981) described a basic method for beginning to become familiar with MET. Before starting this exercise, ensure that the patient/model lies supine, so that the non-tested leg is abducted slightly, heel over the end of the table. The leg to be tested should be close to the edge of the table. Ensure that the tested leg is in the anatomically correct position, knee in full extension and with no external rotation of the leg, which would negate the test.

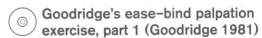 **Goodridge's ease–bind palpation exercise, part 1 (Goodridge 1981)**

1. The practitioner slowly eases the straight leg into abduction. 'After grasping the supine patient's foot and ankle, in order to abduct the lower limb, the practitioner closes his eyes

---

[2] This test and its interpretation, and suggested treatment, using MET (should shortness be noted), will be fully explained in Ch. 5, but in this setting it is being used as an exercise for the purposes of the practitioner becoming familiar with the sense of 'ease and bind', and not for actually testing the muscles involved for dysfunction.

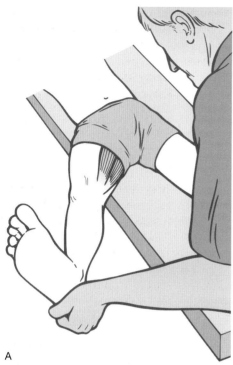

A

Figure 3.1A Assessment of 'bind'/restriction barrier with the first sign of resistance in the adductors (medial hamstrings) of the right leg. In this example, the practitioner's perception of the transition point, where easy movement alters to demand some degree of effort, is regarded as the barrier.

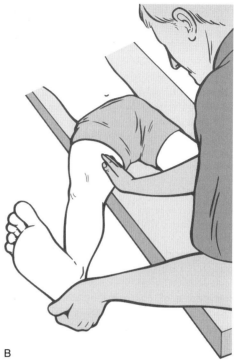

B

Figure 3.1B Assessment of 'bind'/restriction barrier with the first sign of resistance in the adductors (medial hamstrings) of the right leg. In this example, the barrier is identified when the palpating hand notes a sense of bind in tissues which were relaxed (at ease) up to that point.

during the abduction, and feels, in his own body, from his hand through his forearm, into his upper arm, the beginning of a sense of resistance.'

2. 'He stops when he feels it, opens his eyes, and notes how many degrees in an arc the patient's limb has traveled.'

What Goodridge (1981) is trying to establish is that the practitioner senses the *very beginning, the first sign,* of the end of the range of free movement, where easy, 'free-floating' motion ceases, and effort on the part of the practitioner moving the part, begins. This barrier is not a pathological one, but represents the first sign of resistance, the place at which tissues require some degree of passive effort

to move them. This is also the place at which the first signs of bind should be palpated (see part 2 of this exercise).

It is suggested that the process described by Goodridge be attempted several (indeed many) times, so that the practitioner gets a sense of where resistance begins.

The exercise is then performed again as described below.

Goodridge's ease–bind palpation exercise, part 2

The patient lies close to the edge of the table on the side of the leg being tested. The practitioner stands between the patient's partially abducted leg and the table, facing the head of the table, so that all control of the tested leg is achieved by using the lateral (non-table-side) hand, which holds and supports the leg at the ankle. The other (table-side) hand rests passively on the inner thigh, palpating the muscles which are being tested (adductors and medial hamstrings).

This palpating hand (often described as the 'listening' hand in osteopathy) must be in touch with the skin, moulded to the contours of the tissues being assessed, but should exert no pressure, and should be completely relaxed.

As in part 1 of this exercise, abduction of the tested leg is introduced by the non-table-side hand/arm, until the first sign of resistance is noted by the hand which is providing the motive force (i.e. the one holding the leg). As this point of resistance is approached, a tightening of the tissues ('a sense of bind') in the mid-inner thigh should be noted under the palpating hand.

If this sensation is not clear, then the leg should be taken back towards the table, and slowly abducted again, but this time it should be taken past the point where easy movement is lost, and effort begins, and towards its end of range. Here 'bind' will certainly be sensed.

As the leg is taken back towards the midline once more, a softening, a relaxation, an 'ease', will be noted in these same tissues.

The same sequence should then be performed with the other leg, so that the practitioner becomes increasingly familiar with the sense of these two extremes (ease and bind).

It is important to try to note the very moment at which the transition from ease to bind (and bind to ease) occurs, whether movement is into abduction or back towards the table.

Normal excursion of the straight leg into abduction is around 45°, and by testing both legs, as described, it is possible to evaluate whether the inner thigh muscles are tight and short on both sides, or whether one is and the other is not. Even if both are tight and short, one may be more restricted than the other. This is the one to treat first using MET.

NOTE: When learning to assess the first sign of resistance barrier, by applying parts 1 and 2 of this

exercise, the contralateral ASIS should be observed, to see whether or not the resistance barrier has been passed. The pelvis (ASIS) will be seen to move in response to any movement that introduces a degree of stretch into the tissues being evaluated as the assessment is being performed, i.e. once the barrier has been passed, preceded by a feeling of 'effort' in part 1, and of 'bind' in part 2.

MET exercise

It is suggested that before using MET clinically you should perform palpation exercises relating to ease and bind (as described above) on many other muscles, as they are being both actively and passively moved, until skill in reading this change in tone has been acquired. In the example described above, once you feel that the beginnings of bind in the adductors can be ascertained by palpation, and having decided which leg to treat, you can attempt simple use of MET.

The point at which the very first sign of bind was noted (or where the hand carrying the leg felt the first sign that effort was required during abduction) is the resistance barrier (see also Box 3.1, above). In subsequent chapters this barrier will be referred to many times. It is the place where an MET isometric contraction is commenced, in some applications of the methods (notably PIR – see below). It is also the place which is mentally/ visually marked if the practitioner wishes to start a contraction from an easier mid-range position, but which is necessary to note as the place at which resistance *was* a feature, before the isometric contraction.

Identification and appropriate use of the first sign of the barrier of resistance (i.e. where bind is first noted) is a fundamental part of the successful use of MET, along with other key features which include the degree of effort to be used by the patient, how long this should be maintained, and whether subsequently (after the contraction) the tissues should be taken to a new barrier, or through the old one, to introduce passive stretching, and most importantly how long stretches should be held for maximum benefit.

The following exercises in MET variations include the key features emphasised by some of the leading clinicians who have contributed to MET modern methodology.

Chapter 4 offers a background to current research evidence that validates some of these variables.

Basic exercise in MET using postisometric relaxation (PIR) in acute context

- The patient's limb is positioned at the point at which resistance was first perceived during abduction.

- The patient/model is asked to use no more than 20% of available strength to attempt to take the leg gently back towards the table (i.e. to adduct the leg) against firm, unyielding resistance offered by the practitioner.

- In this example the patient is trying to take the limb away from the barrier, while the practitioner holds the limb firmly at (towards) the barrier (as explained previously, this would be described as a practitioner-direct method).

- The patient/model will be contracting the agonists, the muscles which require release (and which, once released, should allow greater and less restricted abduction).

- As the patient/model induces and holds the contraction she may be asked to hold an inhaled breath.

- The isometric contraction should be introduced slowly, and resisted without any jerking, wobbling or bouncing.

- Maintaining the resistance to the contraction should produce no strain in the practitioner.

- The contraction should be held for between 7 and 10 seconds. In the 'neurological' model that attempts to explain the MET mechanism (see Ch. 4) this is the length of time it is thought necessary for the 'load' on the Golgi tendon organs to neurologically influence the intrafusal fibres of the muscle spindles, inhibiting muscle tone and providing the opportunity for the muscle to be taken to a new resting length/resistance barrier without effort, or to stretch it through the barrier of resistance, if this is appropriate (see below) (Scariati 1991).

- An instruction is given to the patient, 'Release your effort, slowly and completely', while the practitioner maintains the limb at the same resistance barrier.

- The patient/model is asked to breathe in and out, and to completely relax, and as she exhales, the limb is gently guided to the new resistance barrier, where bind is once more sensed (the range should almost always be able to be increased by a significant degree).

- After use of the isometric contraction (which induces postisometric relaxation (PIR) in the previously contracted tissues) there exists a latency period of some 10 to 20 seconds during which the muscle can be taken to its new resting length, or stretched more easily than would have been the case before the contraction (Guissard et al 1988, Moore & Kukulka 1991) suggest that this latency period is no more than 10 seconds.

The exercise can be repeated, precisely as described above, to see whether even more release is possible, working from the new resistance barrier to whatever new range is gained following each successive contraction. This approach represents an example of Lewit's PIR method, as described in Ch. 1 (Lewit 1999), and is ideal for releasing tone and relaxing spasm, particularly in acute conditions.

Basic exercise in MET using postisometric relaxation (PIR) followed by stretch, in a chronic context

Where fibrosis is a feature, or when treating chronic conditions, a more vigorous approach can be used in order to actually stretch the muscle(s), rather than simply taking them to a new barrier. This would be closer to Janda's (1993) approach ('postfacilitation stretch' as described in Ch. 1), which calls for the commencing of the contraction from a more relaxed, mid-range position, rather than at the actual barrier.

- Janda suggested stretching the tissues *immediately* following cessation of the contraction, and holding the stretch for at least 10 seconds, before allowing a rest period of up to half a minute. As explained in Ch. 4 a more lengthy holding period for the stretch is probably more appropriate (see below).

- Janda also suggested the procedure be repeated if necessary.

Modification of Janda's approach

- The recommendation for use of MET for chronic fibrotic tissues, based on the lead author's experience, is that following a contraction of between 7 to 10 seconds, commencing from a mid-range position rather than at a barrier, using more than 20% but not more than 35% of the patient's available strength (Janda asks for full strength), a short (2–3 seconds) rest period is allowed for complete postisometric relaxation (PIR), before stretch is introduced, which takes the tissues to a point *just beyond* the previous barrier of resistance.

- It is useful to have the patient gently assist in taking the (now) relaxed area towards and through the barrier. Patient participation in movement towards stretch activates the antagonists, and therefore reduces the danger of a stretch reflex (Mattes 1990).

- The stretch is held for 30 seconds.

- The procedure of contraction, relaxation, followed by patient assisted stretch is repeated (ideally with a rest period between contractions) until no more gain in length of restricted tissues is being achieved (usually after 2 or 3 repetitions).

The differences between Janda's and Lewit's use of PIR

- Lewit starts at, and Janda short of, the restriction barrier.

- Janda utilises a longer and stronger contraction.

- Janda suggests taking the tissues beyond, rather than just to, the new barrier of resistance (with or without patient assistance).

Janda's approach is undoubtedly successful but carries with it a possibility of very mildly traumatising the tissues (albeit that this is an approach only recommended for chronic and not acute situations). The stronger contraction which he suggests, and the rapid introduction of stretching following the contraction, are the areas which it is suggested should be modified (as described above) with little loss of successful outcome, and with a greater degree of comfort.

Reciprocal inhibition

An alternative physiological mechanism, reciprocal inhibition (RI), is thought by some to produce a very similar latency ('refractory') period to that produced by PIR (Kuchera & Kuchera 1992).

RI is advocated for acute problems, especially where the muscle(s) requiring release are traumatised or painful, and which cannot easily or safely be called on to produce sustained contractions such as those described in the notes on PIR above.

To use RI, the tissues requiring treatment should be placed just short of their resistance barrier (as identified by palpation) (Liebenson 1989). This requirement relates to two factors:

1. The greater ease of initiating a contraction from a mid-range position as opposed to the relative difficulty of doing so when at an end of range.

2. Reduced risk of inducing cramp from a mid-range position, particularly in lower extremity structures such as the hamstrings, and especially if longer or stronger contractions than the norm (±20% strength, 7–10 seconds) are being used.

Basic exercise in MET using reciprocal inhibition in acute and chronic contexts

The example involves abduction of the limb (i.e. shortened adductors), as outlined above:

- The first sense of restriction/bind is evaluated as the limb is abducted, at which point the limb is returned a fraction towards a mid-range position (by a few degrees only).

- From this position the patient/model is asked to attempt to *abduct* the leg themselves, using no more than 20% of strength, taking it towards the restriction barrier, while the practitioner resists this effort (as discussed earlier, this would be described as a patient-direct method).

- Following the end of the contraction, the patient/model is asked to 'release and relax', followed by inhalation and exhalation and further relaxation, at which time the limb is guided by the practitioner *to* (in acute problem) or *through* (in chronic problem) the new barrier *with* (if chronic) or *without* (if acute) the patient's/model's assistance.

MET – some common errors and contraindications

Greenman (1989) summarises several of the important component elements of MET as follows. There is a patient-active muscle contraction:

1. From a controlled position
2. In a specific direction
3. Met by practitioner applied distinct counterforce
4. Involving a controlled intensity of contraction.

The common errors which he notes include those listed below.

Patient errors during MET

(Commonly based on inadequate instruction from the practitioner!)

1. Contraction is too strong (remedy: give specific guidelines, e.g. 'use only 20% of strength', or whatever is more appropriate).

2. Contraction is in the wrong direction (remedy: give simple but accurate instructions).

3. Contraction is not sustained for long enough (remedy: instruct the patient/model to hold the contraction until told to ease off, and give an idea ahead of time as to how long this will be).

4. The individual does not relax completely after the contraction (remedy: have them release and relax and then inhale and exhale once or twice, with the suggestion 'now relax completely').

To this list the author would add:

5. Starting and/or finishing the contraction too hastily. There should be a slow build-up of force and a slow letting go; this is easily achieved if a rehearsal is carried out first to educate the patient into the methodology.

Practitioner errors in application of MET

These include:

1. Inaccurate control of position of joint or muscle in relation to the resistance barrier (remedy: have a clear image of what is required and apply it).

2. Inadequate counterforce to the contraction (remedy: meet and match the force in an *isometric* contraction; allow movement in an *isotonic* concentric contraction; and overcome the contraction in an *isolytic* manoeuvre or slow eccentric isotonic contraction – see Chs 1 and 5).

3. Counterforce is applied in an inappropriate direction (remedy: ensure precise direction needed for best results).

4. Moving to a new position too hastily after the contraction (there is usually at least 10 seconds of refractory muscle tone release during which time a new position can easily be adopted – haste is unnecessary and may be counterproductive) (Moore & Kukulka 1991).

5. Inadequate patient instruction is given (remedy: get the instructions right so that the patient can cooperate). Whenever force is applied by the patient in a particular direction,

and when it is time to release that effort, the instruction must be to do so gradually. Any rapid effort may be self-defeating.

6. The coinciding of the forces at the outset (patient and practitioner), as well as at release is important. The practitioner must be careful to use enough, but not too much, effort, and to ease off at the same time as the patient.

7. The practitioner fails to maintain the stretch position for a period of time that allows soft tissues to begin to lengthen (ideally 30 seconds, but certainly not just a few seconds).

Contraindications and side-effects of MET

If pathology is suspected, no MET should be used until an accurate diagnosis has been established. Pathology (osteoporosis, arthritis, etc.) does not rule out the use of MET, but its presence needs to be established so that dosage of application can be modified accordingly (amount of effort used, number of repetitions, stretching introduced or not, etc.).

As to side-effects, Greenman (1989) explains:

All muscle contractions influence surrounding fascia, connective tissue ground substance and interstitial fluids, and alter muscle physiology by reflex mechanisms. Fascial length and tone is altered by muscle contraction. Alteration in fascia influences not only its biomechanical function, but also its biochemical and immunological functions. The patient's muscle effort requires energy and the metabolic process of muscle contraction results in carbon dioxide, lactic acid and other metabolic waste products that must be transported and metabolised. It is for this reason that the patient will frequently experience some increase in muscle soreness within the first 12 to 36 hours following MET treatment. Muscle energy procedures provide safety for the patient since the activating force is intrinsic and the dosage can be easily controlled by the patient, but it must be remembered that this comes at a price. It is easy for the inexperienced practitioner to overdo these procedures and in essence to overdose the patient.

DiGiovanna (1991) states that side-effects are minimal with MET:

MET is quite safe. Occasionally some muscle stiffness and soreness after treatment. If the area being treated is not localised well or if too much contractive force is used pain may be increased. Sometimes the patient is in too much pain to contract a muscle or may be unable to cooperate with instructions or positioning. In such instances MET may be difficult to apply.

Side-effects will be limited if MET is used in ways that:

- Stay within the very simple guideline which states categorically *cause no pain when using MET.*

- Stick to light (20% of strength) contractions.

- Do not stretch over-enthusiastically, but only take muscles a short way past the restriction barrier when stretching.

- Have the patient assist in this stretch.

No side-effects are likely, apart from the soreness mentioned above, and this is a normal feature of most manual methods of treatment.

While the lead author advocates that the above recommendations be kept as a guideline for all therapists and practitioners exploring the MET approach, not all texts advocate a completely painless use of stretching and the contrary view needs to be recorded.

Sucher (1990), for example, suggests that discomfort is inevitable with stretching techniques, especially when self-applied at home: 'There should be some discomfort, often somewhat intense locally ... however, symptoms should subside within seconds or minutes following the stretch.'

Kottke (1982) says, 'Stretching should be past the point of pain, but there should be no residual pain when stretching is discontinued.'

Clearly what is noted as pain for one individual will be described as discomfort by another, making this a subjective exercise. Hopefully, sufficient emphasis has been given to the need to keep stretching associated with MET light, just past the restriction barrier, and any discomfort tolerable to the patient.

Breathing and MET

Many of the guidelines for application of isometric contraction call for patient participation over and above their 'muscle energy' activity, most notably involving respiratory synkinesis, the holding of a breath during the contraction/effort and the release of the breath as the new position or stretch is passively or actively adopted (Lewit et al 1998, Lewit 1999). Is there any valid evidence to support this apparently clinically useful element of MET methodology?

There is certainly 'common practice' evidence, for example in weight training, where the held breath is a feature of the harnessing and focusing of effort, and in yoga practice, where the released breath is the time for adoption of new positions. Fascinating as such anecdotal material might be, it is necessary to explore the literature for evidence which carries more weight, and fortunately this is available in abundance.

Cummings & Howell (1990) have looked at the influence of respiration on myofascial tension and have clearly demonstrated that there is a mechanical effect of respiration on resting myofascial tissue (using the elbow flexors as the tissue being evaluated). They also quote the work of Kisselkova & Georgiev (1976), who reported that resting EMG activity of the biceps brachii, quadriceps femoris and gastrocnemius muscles 'cycled with respiration following bicycle ergonometer exercise, thus demonstrating that non-respiratory muscles receive input from the respiratory centres'. The conclusion was that 'these studies document both a mechanically and a neurologically mediated influence on the tension produced by myofascial tissues, which gives objective verification of the clinically observed influence of respiration on the musculoskeletal system, and validation of its potential role in manipulative therapy'.

So there is an influence, but what variables does it display? Lewit helps to create subdivisions in the simplistic picture of 'inhalation enhances effort' and 'exhalation enhances movement', and a detailed reading of his book *Manipulative Therapy in Rehabilitation of the Motor System* (Lewit 1999)

is highly recommended for those who wish to understand the complexities of the mechanisms involved. Among the simpler connections which Lewit (1999) discusses, and for which evidence is provided, are the following:

- The abdominal muscles are assisted in their action during exhalation, especially against resistance.
- Movement into flexion of the lumbar and cervical spine is assisted by exhalation.
- Movement into extension (i.e. straightening up from forward bending; bending backwards) of the lumbar and cervical spine is assisted by inhalation.
- Movement into extension of the thoracic spine is assisted by exhalation (try it and see how much more easily the thoracic spine extends as you exhale than when you inhale).
- Thoracic flexion is enhanced by inhalation.
- Rotation of the trunk in the seated position is enhanced by inhalation and inhibited by exhalation.
- Neck traction (stretching) is easier during exhalation, but lumbar traction (stretching) is eased by inhalation and retarded by exhalation.

Many individuals find controlled breathing and holding of the breath distressing, in which case these aspects of MET should be avoided altogether.

The lead author suggests that breathing assistance to isometric contractions should only be employed if it proves helpful to the patient, and in specific situations. For example, in the case of the scalene muscles, a held inhalation automatically produces an isometric contraction. Therefore in treating these muscles with MET a held breath would seem to be potentially useful.

Degree of effort with isometric contraction

Most MET contractions should be light and only rarely, when large muscle groups are involved, might it be necessary for there to be contractions involving up to 50% of a patient's strength. Among the reasons for suggesting lighter contractions are the practical ones of a lessened degree of difficulty for the practitioner in controlling the forces involved, as well as greater comfort and reduced likelihood of pain being produced when contractions are not strong.

It has also been suggested that recruitment of phasic muscle fibres occurs when an effort in excess of 30–35% of strength is used (Liebenson 1996). If this is a valid position, and since in most instances it is the postural fibres which will have shortened and require stretching, little advantage would be seem to be offered by inducing PIR, reduced tone, in phasic fibres. There would therefore seem to be greater advantage in using mild contractions, rather than increasing the force of a contraction.

In Ch. 1 it was noted that Goodridge & Kuchera (1997) were of the opinion that 'Localization of force is more important than intensity', and this opinion is supported by the lead author. For more on this topic see also Ch. 4, where there is discussion of the work of Schmitt et al (1999) who in contradiction to this viewpoint suggest that progressively *increasing* degrees of isometric effort offers optimal results.

MET variations

Strength testing – Mitchell's view

Before applying MET to an apparently short muscle, Mitchell et al suggest (1979) that it, and its pair, should be assessed for relative strength. If the muscle that requires lengthening tests as weaker than its pair, they call for the reasons for this relative weakness to be evaluated and treated. For example an overactive antagonist, or a myofascial trigger point, might be producing inhibition (Lucas et al 2004), and either of these factors should be dealt with so that the muscle due to receive MET attention is strengthened before being stretched.

Mitchell et al (1979) suggest that MET is best applied to a short, strong muscle. Goodridge (1981) concurs with this view, and states that:

When a left-right asymmetry in range of motion exists, in the extremities that asymmetry may be due to either a hypertonic or hypotonic condition. Differentiation is made by testing for strength, comparing left and right muscle groups. If findings suggest weakness is the cause of asymmetry in range of motion, the appropriate muscle group is treated to bring it to equal strength with its opposite number, before range of motion is retested to determine whether shortness in a muscle group may also contribute to the restriction.

One common reason for a muscle testing as 'weak' (compared with norms, or with its pair) involves increased tone in its antagonist, which would automatically inhibit the weaker muscle. One approach to restoring relative balance might therefore involve the antagonists to any muscle which tests as weak receiving attention first – possibly using MET – to reduce excessive tone and/or to initiate stretching. Following MET treatment of those muscles found to be short and/or hypertonic, subsequent assessment may show that previously weak or hypotonic antagonists have strengthened but still require toning. This can be achieved using isotonic contractions, or Ruddy's methods (see below), or some other form of rehabilitation.

Reference to strength testing will be made periodically in descriptions of MET application to particular muscles in Ch. 5, whenever this factor seems important clinically.

Janda's view

Janda (1993) provides evidence of the relative lack of accuracy involved in strength testing, preferring instead functional assessment, including tests for relative shortness in particular muscles, considered in the context of overall musculoskeletal function, as a means of deciding what needs attention. This seems to be close to the 'loose–tight' concept discussed in Ch. 2 (Ward 1997). Janda effectively dismisses the idea of using strength tests to any degree in evaluating functional imbalances (Kraus 1970, Janda 1993), when he states:

Individual muscle strength testing is unsuitable because it is insufficiently sensitive and does not take into account evaluation of coordinated activity between different muscle groups. In addition, in patients with musculoskeletal syndromes, weakness in individual muscles may be indistinct, thus rendering classical muscle testing systems unsatisfactory. This is probably one of the reasons why conflicting results have been reported in studies of patients with back pain.

Janda is also clear in his opinion that weak, shortened muscles will regain tone if stretched appropriately.

Mitchell and Janda and 'the weakness factor'

Mitchell et al's (1979) recommendation regarding strength testing prior to use of MET complicates the approach advocated by the author, which is to use indications of overactivity or stress, or, even more importantly, signs of mal-coordination and imbalance, as clues to a postural (mobiliser) muscle being short. 'Functional' tests, such as those devised by Janda, and described by Liebenson in Ch. 8, or objective evidence of dysfunction (using one of the many such tests for shortness described in Ch. 5) can be used to provide such evidence.

Put simply:

- If a postural (mobiliser, see Ch. 2) muscle is overused, misused, abused or disused, it will modify by shortening. Evidence of overactivity, inappropriate firing sequences and/or excessive tone, all suggest that such a muscle is dysfunctional and probably short (Janda 1990, Tunnell 1997, Hammer 1999).

- If such a distressed muscle falls within one of the groups described in Ch. 2 as postural or mobiliser, then it may be considered to have shortened.

- The degree of such shortening may then be assessed using palpation and basic tests, as described in Ch. 5.

Additional evidence of a need to use MET-induced stretching can be derived from palpatory or assessment evidence of the presence of fibrosis and/or myofascial trigger point activity, or of inappropriate electromyographic (EMG) activity (should such technology be available).

Ideally therefore, some observable and/or palpable evidence of functional imbalance will be available which can guide the therapist/practitioner as to the need for MET, or other interventions, in particular muscles.[3] For example, in testing for overactivity, and by implication shortness, in quadratus lumborum (QL), an attempt may be made to assess the muscle firing sequence involved in raising the leg laterally in a side-lying position. There is a 'correct' and an 'incorrect' (or balanced and unbalanced) sequence according to Jull & Janda (1987). If the latter is noted, stress is proved and, since this is a postural muscle (or at least the lateral aspect of it is, see discussion of QL in Ch. 2), shortness can be assumed and stretching indicated.

Each clinican needs to decide whether or not to introduce Mitchell's (1979) element of strength testing into any assessment protocol involving possible use of therapeutic stretching such as MET. The recommendation by Mitchell and colleagues (1979) that muscle strength be taken into account before MET is used will not be detailed in each paired muscle discussed in the text, and is highlighted here (and in a few specific muscles where these noted authors and clinicians place great emphasis on its importance) in order to remind the reader of the possibility of its incorporation into the methodology of MET use.

The lead author has not found that application of weakness testing (as part of the work-up before deciding on the suitability or otherwise of MET use for particular muscles) significantly improves results. He does, however, recognise that in individual cases it might be a useful approach, but considers that systematic weakness testing may be left until later in a treatment programme, after dealing with muscles which show evidence of shortness.

Strength testing methodology

In order to test a muscle for strength a standard procedure is carried out as follows:

- The area should be relaxed and not influenced by gravity.

---

[3] This topic is discussed further in Ch. 8, which is devoted to Liebenson's views on rehabilitation and which further discusses aspects of Janda's functional tests. Some of Janda's, as well as Lewit's, functional assessments are also included in the specific muscle evaluations given in Ch. 5.

- The area/muscle/joint should be positioned so that whatever movement is to be used can be comfortably performed.

- The patient should be asked to perform a concentric contraction that is evaluated against a scale, as outlined in Box 3.2.

The degree of resistance required to prevent movement is a subjective judgement, unless mechanical resistance and/or electronic measurement is available. For more detailed understanding of muscle strength evaluation, texts such as Janda's *Muscle Function Testing* (Janda 1983) are recommended.

Ruddy's methods – 'pulsed MET'

In the 1940s and 50s, osteopathic physician T. J. Ruddy developed a method which utilised a series of rapid pulsating contractions against resistance, which he termed 'rapid rhythmic resistive duction'. As described in Ch. 1, it was in part this work that Fred Mitchell Snr used as his base for the development of MET, along with PNF methodology. Ruddy's method (Ruddy 1962) called for a series of muscle contractions against resistance, at a rhythm a little faster than the pulse rate. This approach can be applied in all areas where isometric contractions are suitable, and is particularly useful for self-treatment following instruction from a skilled practitioner.

According to Greenman (1996), who studied with him, 'He [Ruddy] used these techniques in the cervical spine and around the orbit in his practice as an [osteopathic] ophthalmologist-otorhinolaryngologist'.

Box 3.2 Scale for evaluation of concentric contractions (Janda 1983)

Grade 0	No contraction/paralysis
Grade 1	No motion noted but contraction felt by palpating hand
Grade 2	Some movement possible on contraction, if gravity influence eliminated ('poor')
Grade 3	Motion possible against gravity's influence ('fair')
Grade 4	Movement possible during contraction against resistance ('good')

For the sake of convenience the lead author has abbreviated the title of Ruddy's work from 'rapid rhythmic resistive duction', to 'pulsed MET'. The simplest use of this approach involves the dysfunctional tissue/joint being held at its resistance barrier, at which time the patient, ideally (or the practitioner if the patient cannot adequately cooperate with the instructions), against the resistance of the practitioner, introduces a series of rapid (2 per second), very small contraction efforts towards the barrier.

The barest initiation of effort is called for with, to use Ruddy's words, 'no wobble and no bounce'. The use of this 'conditioning' approach involves contractions that are 'short, rapid and rhythmic, gradually increasing the amplitude and degree of resistance, thus conditioning the proprioceptive system by rapid movements'.

In describing application of pulsed MET to the neck (in a case of vertigo) Ruddy gave instruction as to the directions in which the series of resisted efforts should be made. These, he said, should include 'movements ... in a line of each major direction, forwards, backwards, right forward and right backwards or along an antero-posterior line in four directions along the multiplication "X" sign, also a half circle, or rotation right and left'.

If reducing joint restriction, or elongation of a soft tissue, is the objective then, following each series of 20 mini-contractions, the slack should be taken out of the tissues, and another series of contractions should be commenced from the new barrier, possibly in a different direction – which can and should be varied according to Ruddy's guidelines, to take account of all the different elements in any restriction. Despite Ruddy's suggestion that the amplitude of the contractions be increased over time, the effort itself must never exceed the barest initiation (and then ceasing) of an isometric contraction.

The benefits are likely, Ruddy suggests, to include improved enhanced oxygenation and improved venous and lymphatic circulation through the area being treated. Furthermore, he believed that the method influences both static and kinetic posture because of the effects on proprioceptive and interoceptive afferent pathways, and that this can assist in maintenance of 'dynamic equilibrium', which involves 'a balance in chemical, physical, thermal, electrical and tissue fluid homeostasis'.

In a setting in which tense, hypertonic, possibly shortened musculature has been treated by stretching, it may prove useful to begin facilitating and strengthening the inhibited, weakened antagonists by means of Ruddy's methods. This is true whether the hypertonic muscles have been treated for reasons of shortness/hypertonicity alone, or because they accommodate active trigger points within their fibres, or because of clear evidence of joint restriction of soft tissue origin.

The introduction of a pulsating muscle energy procedure such as Ruddy's, involving these weak antagonists, therefore offers the opportunity for:

- Proprioceptive re-education
- Strengthening facilitation of weak antagonists
- Further inhibition of tense agonists (possibly in preparation for stretching)
- Enhanced local circulation and drainage
- In Liebenson's words (1996), 'reeducation of movement patterns on a reflex, subcortical basis'.

Ruddy's work was a part of the base on which Mitchell Snr, and others, constructed MET, and his work is worthy of study and application since it offers, at the very least, a useful means of modifying the employment of sustained isometric contraction, and has particular relevance to acute problems and safe self-treatment settings. Examples of Ruddy's method will be described in later chapters.

Isotonic concentric strengthening MET methods

Contractions which occur against resistance that is then overcome, allow toning and strengthen of the muscle(s) involved in the contraction. For example:

- The practitioner positions the limb, or area, so that a muscle group will be at resting length, and thus will develop a strong contraction.
- The practitioner explains the direction of movement required, as well as the intensity

and duration of that effort. The patient strongly contracts the muscle with the objective of moving the muscle through a complete range, rapidly (in about 2 seconds).

- The practitioner offers counterforce that is slightly less than that of the patient's contraction, and maintains this throughout the contraction. This is repeated several times, with a progressive increase in practitioner's counterforce (the patient's effort in the strengthening mode is always close to maximal).
- Where weak muscles are being toned using these isotonic methods, the practitioner allows the concentric contraction of the muscles (i.e. offers only partial resistance to the contractile effort).
- Such exercises should always involve practitioner effort which is less than that applied by the patient. The subsequent isotonic concentric contraction of the weakened muscles should allow approximation of the origins and insertions to be achieved under some degree of control by the practitioner.
- Isotonic efforts are usually suggested as being of short duration, ultimately employing maximal effort on the part of the patient.
- The use of concentric isotonic contractions to tone a muscle or muscle group can be expanded to become an isokinetic, whole joint movement (see below).

Isotonic eccentric alternatives

Norris (1999) suggests that there is evidence that when rapid movement is used in isotonic concentric activities it is largely phasic, type II, fibres that are being recruited. In order to tone postural (type 1) muscles that may have lost their endurance potential, *eccentric isotonic exercises*, *performed slowly*, are more effective. Norris states: 'Low resistance, slow movements should be used ... eccentric actions have been shown to be better suited for reversal of serial sarcomere adaptation.'

Rapidly applied isometric eccentric manoeuvres ('isolytic') are described later in this chapter.

Example of a slow eccentric isotonic stretch (SEIS)

Rationale: In the case of an individual with hamstring hypertonicity accompanied by inhibited quadriceps, a slow eccentric isotonic stretch (SEIS) of the quadriceps would both tone these and reciprocally inhibit the hamstrings, allowing subsequent stretching of the hamstrings to be more easily achieved.

- The patient is supine with hip and knee of the leg to be treated, flexed. (*Note:* it is sometimes easier to perform this manoeuvre with the patient prone.)

- The practitioner extends the flexed knee to its first barrier of resistance, palpating the tissues proximal to the knee crease for first sign of 'bind'.

- The patient is asked to resist, using a little more than half available strength, the attempt the practitioner will make to slowly flex the knee fully.

- An instruction should be given which makes clear the objective, 'I am going to slowly bend your knee, and I want you to partially resist this, but to let it slowly happen'.

After performing the slow isotonic stretch of the quadriceps the hamstring should be retested for length and ease of straight leg raising, and if necessary, the hamstrings should be taken into a stretched position and held for 30 seconds before repeating the procedure.

Strengthening a joint complex with isokinetic MET

A variation on the use of simple isotonic concentric contractions, as described above, is to use isokinetic contraction (also known as progressive resisted exercise). In this method the patient, starting with a weak effort but rapidly progressing to a maximal contraction of the affected muscle(s), introduces a degree of resistance to the *practitioner's* effort to put a joint, or area, through a full range of motion. An alternative or subsequent exercise involves the practitioner partially resisting the patient's active movement of a joint through a rapid series of as full a range of movements as possible.

Mitchell et al (1979) describe an isokinetic exercise as follows: 'The counterforce is increased during the contraction to meet changing contractile force as the muscle shortens and its force increases.' This approach is described as being especially valuable in improving efficient and coordinated use of muscles, and in enhancing the tonus of the resting muscle. 'In dealing with paretic muscles, isotonics (in the form of progressive resistance exercise) and isokinetics, are the quickest and most efficient road to rehabilitation.'

The use of isokinetic contraction is reported to be a most effective method of building strength, and to be superior to high repetition, lower resistance exercises (Blood 1980). It is also felt that a limited range of motion, with good muscle tone, is preferable (to the patient) to normal range with limited power. Thus the strengthening of weak musculature in areas of limited mobility is seen as an important contribution, towards which isokinetic contractions may assist.

Isokinetic contractions not only strengthen (largely phasic, type II) fibres, but have a training effect which enables them to subsequently operate in a more coordinated manner. There is often a very rapid increase in strength. Because of neuromuscular recruitment, there is a progressively stronger muscular effort as this method is repeated. Contractions and accompanying mobilisation of the region should take no more than 4 seconds for each repetition, in order to achieve maximum benefit with as little fatiguing as possible of either the patient or the practitioner. Prolonged contractions should be avoided (DiGiovanna 1991).

The simplest and safest applications of isokinetic methods involve small joints such as those in the extremities, largely because they are more easily controlled by the practitioner's hands. Spinal joints are more difficult to mobilise and to control when muscular resistance is being utilised at close to full strength.

The options for achieving increased tone and strength via these methods therefore involves a choice between a partially resisted isotonic contraction, or the overcoming of such a contraction, at the same time as the full range of movement is being introduced. Both of these options can involve virtually maximum contraction of the muscles by the patient. Home treatment of such conditions is possible via self-treatment, as in other MET methods.[4]

DiGiovanna (1991) suggests that isokinetic exercise increases the work which a muscle can subsequently perform more efficiently and rapidly than either isometric or isotonic exercises.

To summarise:

- To tone weak phasic (stabiliser, see Ch. 2) muscles, perform concentric isotonic exercises using full strength, rapidly (4 seconds maximum).

- To tone weak postural (mobiliser, see Ch. 2) muscles, slowly perform eccentric isotonic (i.e. SEIS above) exercises using increasing degrees of effort.

- In order to tone postural fibres, slow speed, eccentric resistance is most effective (Norris 1999).

Reduction of fibrotic changes with isolytic (isotonic eccentric) MET

As discussed above, when a patient initiates a contraction, and it is overcome by the practitioner, this is termed an 'isotonic *eccentric* contraction' (e.g. when a patient tries to flex the arm and the practitioner overrides this effort and straightens it during the contraction of the flexor muscles). In such a contraction the origins and insertions of the muscles (and therefore the joint angles) are separated, despite the patient's effort to approximate them.

When such a procedure is peformed rapidly this is termed an isolytic contraction, in that it involves the stretching and to an extent the breaking down (sometimes called 'controlled microtrauma') of fibrotic tissue present in the affected muscles.

Microtrauma is inevitable, and this form of 'controlled' injury is seen to be useful especially in relation to altering the interface between elastic and non-elastic tissues – between fibrous and non-fibrous tissues. Mitchell (Mitchell et al 1979) states that: 'Advanced myofascial fibrosis sometimes requires this "drastic" measure, for it is a powerful stretching technique.'

[4] Both isotonic concentric and eccentric contractions take place during the isokinetic movement of a joint.

'Adhesions' of this type are broken down by the application of force by the practitioner which is just a little greater than that of the patient. Such procedures can be uncomfortable, and patients should be advised of this, as well as of the fact that they need only apply sufficient effort to ensure that they remain comfortable. Limited degrees of effort are therefore called for at the outset of isolytic contractions.

However, in order to achieve the greatest degree of stretch (in the condition of myofascial fibrosis for example), it is necessary for the largest number of fibres possible to be involved in the isotonic eccentric contraction. There is an apparent contradiction to usual practice in that, in order to achieve as large an involvement as possible, the degree of contraction should be a maximal one, likely to produce pain which, while undesirable in most manual treatment, may be deemed necessary in a given instance.

Additionally, in many situations the procedure involving a maximal contraction might be impossible to achieve if a large muscle group (e.g. hamstrings) is involved, especially if the patient is strong and the practitioner slight, or at least inadequate to the task of overcoming the force of the contracting muscle(s). In such a situation less than optimal contraction is called for, repeated several times perhaps, but confined to specific muscles where fibrotic change is greatest (e.g. tensor fascia lata), and to patients who are not frail, painsensitive, or in other ways unsuitable for what is a vigorous MET method.

Unlike SEIS, which have the aim of strengthening weak postural (mobiliser) muscles, and which are performed slowly (as discussed earlier in this chapter), isolytic contractions aimed at stretching fibrotic tissues are performed rapidly.

Summary of choices for MET in treating muscle problems

To return to Goodridge's introduction to MET (see earlier in this chapter) – using the adductors as our target tissues we can now see that a number of choices are open to the practitioner once the objective has been established, for example to lengthen shortened adductor muscles.

If the objective is to lengthen shortened adductors, on the right, several methods could be used:

- With the right leg of the supine patient abducted to its first barrier of resistance, the patient could contract the *right abductors*, against equal practitioner counterforce, in order to relax the adductors by reciprocal inhibition. This would be followed by stretching of the adductors.

- Instead of this the patient could contract the *right adductors*, against equal practitioner counterforce, in order to achieve post isometric relaxation. This would be followed by stretching of the adductors.

- In another alternative, if chronic fibrosis is a feature, the patient, with the leg at the abduction barrier, could contract the *right adductors* while the practitioner offered greater counterforce, thus *rapidly* overcoming the isotonic contraction (producing a fast eccentric isotonic, or isolytic, contraction), introducing microtrauma to fibrotic tissues in the adductors. This could be followed by further stretching of the adductors. (*Note:* This isolytic approach is not recommended as a procedure unless the patient is robust and prepared for a degree of microtrauma and soreness for some days following treatment.)

- To use the methodology of SEIS the leg would be taken to its abduction barrier, with the patient instructed to attempt to maintain it in that position as the practitioner slowly returns it to the midline. This would tone the inhibited abductors and inhibit the overtight adductors. This would be followed by stretching of the adductors past their restriction barrier.

- Or the limb could be abducted to the restriction barrier where Ruddy's 'pulsed MET' could be introduced, with the practitioner offering counterforce as the patient 'pulses' towards the barrier 20 times in 10 seconds.

In all of these methods the shortened muscles would have been taken to their appropriate barrier before commencing the contraction – either at the first sign of resistance if PIR and movement to a new barrier was the objective, or in a mid-range (just short of the first sense of 'bind') position if RI or a degree of postfacilitation stretching was considered more appropriate.

For an isolytic stretch, or for the SEIS approach, the contraction commences from the resistance barrier, as do all isokinetic and 'Ruddy' activities.

If the objective were to strengthen weakened adductors, on the right:

- Since these are defined as postural (mobiliser) muscles, the patient could be asked to *slowly* adduct the limb from its barrier, as the operator allowed the patient's effort to overcome resistance, so toning the muscle while it was contracting.

The essence of muscle energy methods then is the harnessing of the patient's own muscle power.

The next prerequisite is the application of counterforce, in an appropriate and predetermined manner. In isometric methods this counterforce must be unyielding. No test of strength must ever be attempted. Thus the patient should never be asked to 'try as hard as he can' to move in this or that direction. It is important before commencing that this instruction, and the rest of the procedure, be carefully explained, so that the patient has a clear idea of his role.

The direction, degree of effort required, and duration, must all be clear, as must any associated instructions regarding respiratory or visual synkinesis (breathing patterns and eye movements) methods, if these are being used (see self-treatment examples of this below).

Joints and MET

MET uses muscles and soft tissues for its effects; nevertheless, the impact of these methods on joints is clearly profound since it is impossible to consider joints independently of the muscles which support and move them. For practical purposes, however, an artificial division is made in the text of this book, and in Ch. 6 there will be specific focus given to topics such as MET in treatment of joint restriction and dysfunction; preparing joints for manipulation with MET; as well as the vexed question of the primacy of muscles or joints in dysfunctional settings.

The opinions of experts such as Hartman, Stiles, Evjenth, Lewit, Janda, Goodridge and Harakal will be outlined in relation to these and other joint-related topics.

A chiropractic view is provided in Ch. 8, which includes rehabilitation implications of, but which also touches on the treatment protocol which chiropractic expert Craig Liebenson suggests in relation to dysfunctional imbalances which involve joint restriction/blockage.

In Chs 9, 10 and 11 a variety of other professional variations are described, including the use of MET in physical therapy, massage therapy and athletic training contexts.

Self-treatment

Lewit (1991) is keen to involve patients in home treatment, using MET. He describes this aspect thus:

Receptive patients are taught how to apply this treatment to themselves, as autotherapy, in a home programme. They passively stretched the tight muscle with their own hand. This hand next provided counter pressure to voluntary contraction of the tight muscle (during inhalation) and then held the muscle from shortening, during the relaxation phase. Finally, it supplied the increment in range of motion (during exhalation) by taking up any slack that had developed.

How often should self-treatment be prescribed?

Gunnari & Evjenth (1983) recommend frequent applications of mild stretching or, if this is not possible, more intense but less frequent self-stretching at home. They state that: 'Therapy is more effective if it is supplemented by more frequent self-stretching. In general, the more frequent the stretching, the more moderate the intensity; less frequent stretching, such as that done every other day, may be of greater intensity.'

Self-treatment methods are not suitable for all regions (or for all patients) but there are a large number of areas which lend themselves to such methods. Use of gravity as a counterpressure source is often possible in self-treatment. For

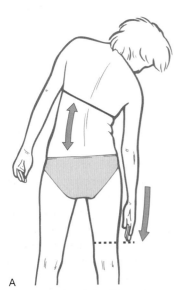

Figure 3.2A MET self-treatment for quadratus lumborum. Patient assesses range of side-bending to the right.

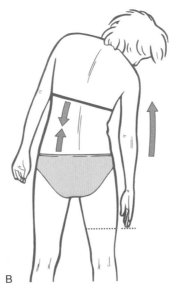

Figure 3.2B Patient contracts quadratus lumborum by straightening slightly, thereby introducing an isometric contraction against gravity.

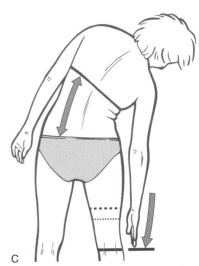

Figure 3.2C After 7–10 seconds, the contraction is released and the patient will be able to side-bend further, stretching quadratus lumborum towards its normal resting length.

example, in order to stretch quadratus lumborum (see Fig. 3.2A–C), the patient stands, legs apart and side-bending, in order to impose a degree of stretch to the shortened muscle. By inhaling and slightly easing the trunk towards an upright position, against the weight of the body, which gravity is pulling towards the floor, and then releasing the breath at the same time as trying to side-bend further towards the floor, a lengthening of quadratus will have been achieved.

Lewit (1999) suggests, in such a procedure, that the movement against gravity be accompanied by movement of the eyes in the direction away from which bending is taking place, while the attempt to bend further – after the contraction – should be enhanced by looking in the direction towards which bending is occurring. Use of eye movements in this way facilitates the effects. Several attempts by the patient to induce greater freedom of movement in any restricted direction by means of such simple measures should achieve good results.

The use of eye movements relates to the increase in tone that occurs in muscles as they prepare for movement when the eyes move in a given direction. Thus, if the eyes look down there will be a general increase in tone (slight, but measurable) in the flexors of the neck and trunk. In order to appreciate the influence of eye movement on muscle tone the reader might experiment by fixing their gaze to the left as an attempt is made to turn the head to the right. This should be followed by gazing right and simultaneously turning the head to the right. The evidence from this simple self-applied example should be convincing enough to create an awareness of what the patients eyes are doing during subsequent stretching procedures!

The principles of MET are now hopefully clearer, and the methods seen to be applicable to a large range of problems.

Rehabilitation, as well as first-aid, and some degree of normalisation of both acute and chronic soft tissue and joint problems are all possible, given correct application. Combined with NMT, this offers the practitioner additional tools for achieving safe and effective therapeutic interventions.

When should MET be applied to a muscle?

When should MET (PIR, RI or postfacilitation stretch) be applied to a muscle to relax and/or stretch it?

1. When it is demonstrably shortened – unless the shortening is attributable to associated joint restriction, in which case this should receive primary attention, possibly also involving MET (see Ch. 5).

2. When it contains areas of shortening, such as are associated with myofascial trigger points or palpable fibrosis. It is important to note that trigger points evolve within stressed (hypertonic) areas of phasic, as well as postural muscles, and that these tissues will require stretching, based on evidence which shows that trigger points reactivate unless shortened fibres in which they are housed are stretched to a normal resting length as part of a therapeutic intervention (Simons et al 1999).

3. When periosteal pain points are palpable, indicating stress at the associated muscle's origin and/or insertion (Lewit 1999).

4. In cases of muscular imbalance, in order to reduce hypertonicity when weakness in a muscle is attributable, in part or totally, to inhibition deriving from a hypertonic antagonist muscle (group).

Evaluation

It is seldom possible to totally isolate one muscle in an assessment, and reasons other than muscle shortness can account for apparent restriction (intrinsic joint dysfunction for example). Other methods of evaluation as to relative muscle shortness are also called for, including direct palpation.

The 'normal' range of movements of particular muscles should be taken as guidelines only, since individual factors will often determine that what is 'normal' for one person is not so for another.

Wherever possible, an understanding is called for of functional patterns which are observable, for example in the case of the upper fixators of the shoulder/accessory breathing muscles. If a pattern of breathing is observed which indicates a predominance of upper chest involvement, as opposed to diaphragmatic, this in itself would indicate that this muscle group was being 'stressed' by overuse. Since stressed postural (mobiliser) muscles will shorten, an automatic assumption of shortness can be made in such a case regarding the scalenes, levator scapulae, etc. (see Ch. 2 for a fuller discussion of Janda's evidence for this and for Garland's description of structural changes relating to this pattern of breathing).

Once again let it be clear that the various tests and assessment methods suggested in Ch. 5, even when utilising evidence of an abnormally short range of motion, are meant as indicators, rather than proof, of shortness. As Gunnari & Evjenth (1983) observe: 'If the preliminary analysis identifies shortened muscles, then a provisional trial treatment is performed. If the provisional treatment reduces pain and improves the affected movement pattern, the preliminary analysis is confirmed, and treatment may proceed.'

Evidence would then be clinical rather than research based. The lead author regrets that in the current climate of 'evidence-based medicine', evidence of benefit and patient satisfaction seems undervalued.

Muscle energy technique – summary of variations

NOTE: See Ch. 4 for discussion of research evidence that supports some of the mechanisms and protocols proposed in these summaries. In many instances these protocols are based purely on clinical experience, with no independent validation available as to the value of particular aspects of the methodology, ranging from positioning, degree of force employed, choice of use of agonist and/or antagonist, number of repetitions, length of stretching period, etc.

1. Isometric contraction – using reciprocal inhibition (in acute setting, without stretching)

Indications

- Relaxing acute muscular spasm or contraction

- Mobilising restricted joints
- Preparing joint for manipulation.

Contraction starting point   For acute muscle, or any joint problem, commence at 'easy' restriction barrier (first sign of resistance towards end of range).

Modus operandi   The patient is attempting to push towards the barrier of restriction against the practitioner/therapist's precisely matched counterforce, therefore antagonist(s) to affected muscle(s) are being employed in an isometric contraction, so obliging shortened muscles to relax via reciprocal inhibition.

Forces   Practitioner/therapist's and patient's forces are matched. Initial effort involves approximately 20% of patient's strength (or less); this can be increased on subsequent contractions if appropriate.

Duration of contraction   Initially 7–10 seconds, increasing in subsequent contractions if greater effect required, and if no pain is induced by the effort.

Action following contraction   The tissues (muscle/joint) are taken to their new restriction barrier without stretch after ensuring complete relaxation. Movement to the new barrier should be performed on an exhalation.

Repetitions   Repeat three times or until no further gain in range of motion is possible.

REMINDER: When using MET in an acute setting no stretching is involved, merely attempts to reduce excessive tone.

2. Isometric contraction – using postisometric relaxation (in an acute setting, without stretching)

Indications

- Relaxing acute muscular spasm or contraction
- Mobilising restricted joints
- Preparing joint for manipulation.

Contraction starting point   At resistance barrier.

Modus operandi   The affected muscles (the agonists) are used in the isometric contraction, therefore the shortened muscles subsequently relax via postisometric relaxation. If there is pain on contraction this method is contraindicated and the previous method (use of antagonist) is employed. The practitioner/therapist is attempting to push towards the barrier of restriction against the patient's precisely matched counter-effort.

Forces   Practitioner/therapist's and patient's forces are matched. The initial effort involves approximately 20% of patient's strength; increasing on subsequent contractions is appropriate. Increase of the duration of the contraction may be more effective than any increase in force.

Duration of contraction   Initially 7–10 seconds, increasing in subsequent contractions if greater effect required.

Action following contraction   The tissues (muscle/joint) are taken to their new restriction barrier without stretch after ensuring patient has completely relaxed. Movement to new barrier should be performed on an exhalation.

Repetitions   Repeat three times or until no further gain in range of motion is possible.

REMINDER: When using MET in an acute setting no stretching is involved, merely attempts to reduce excessive tone.

3. Isometric contraction – using postisometric relaxation (in a chronic setting, with stretching, also known as postfacilitation stretching)

Indications

- Stretching chronic or subacute restricted, fibrotic, contracted soft tissues (fascia, muscle) or tissues housing active myofascial trigger points.

Contraction starting point   Short of the resistance barrier.

Modus operandi   The affected muscles (agonists) are used in the isometric contraction, therefore the shortened muscles subsequently relax via postisometric relaxation, allowing an easier stretch

to be performed (see discussion in Ch. 4). The practitioner/therapist is attempting to push towards the barrier of restriction, against the patient's precisely matched counter-effort.

Forces   The practitioner/therapist's and patient's forces are matched. Initial effort involves approximately 30% of patient's strength; an increase to no more than 40% on subsequent contractions may be appropriate.

Duration of contraction   Initially 7–10 seconds.

CAUTION: Longer, stronger contractions may predispose towards onset of cramping and so should be used with care.

Action following contraction   There should be a rest period of 5 seconds or so, to ensure complete relaxation before commencing the stretch. On an exhalation the area (muscle) is taken to its new restriction barrier, and a small degree beyond, painlessly, and held in this position for at least 30 and up to 60 seconds. The patient should, if possible, participate in assisting in the move to, and through, the barrier, effectively further inhibiting the structure being stretched and retarding the likelihood of a myotatic stretch reflex.

Repetitions   Repeat three times or until no further gain in range of motion is possible, with each isometric contraction commencing from a position just short of the restriction barrier.

4. Isometric contraction – using reciprocal inhibition (chronic setting, with stretching)

Indications

- Stretching chronic or subacute restricted, fibrotic, contracted soft tissues (fascia, muscle) or tissues housing active myofascial trigger points

- This approach is chosen if contracting the agonist is contraindicated because of pain.

Contraction starting point   A little short of the resistance barrier.

Modus operandi   The antagonist(s) to the affected muscles are used in the isometric contraction, therefore the shortened muscles subsequently

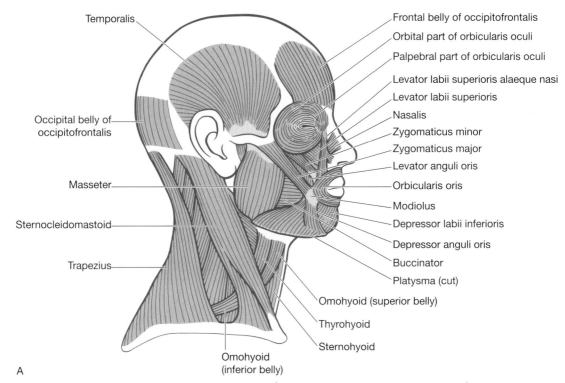

Figure 3.3A The superficial muscles of the head and neck. (Redrawn from *Gray's Anatomy*, 38th edn.)

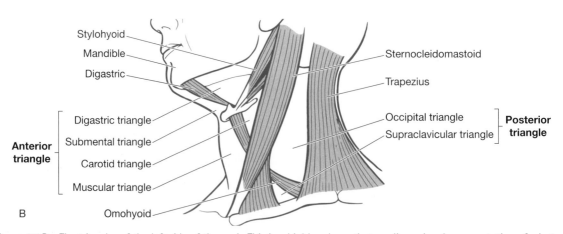

Figure 3.3B The triangles of the left side of the neck. This is a highly schematic two-dimensional representation of what in reality are non-planar trigones distributed over a waisted column. (Redrawn from *Gray's Anatomy*, 38th edn.)

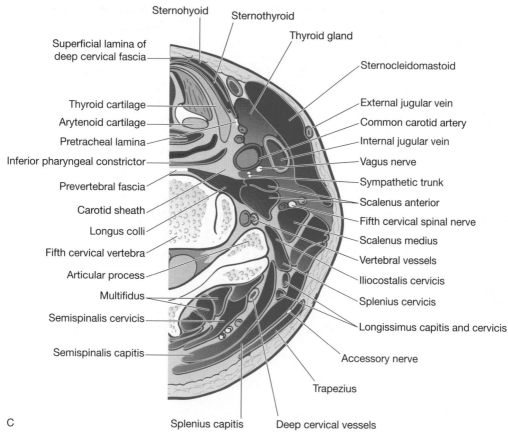

Sternohyoid   Sternothyroid

Thyroid gland

Superficial lamina of
deep cervical fascia

Sternocleidomastoid

Thyroid cartilage
Arytenoid cartilage
Pretracheal lamina
Inferior pharyngeal constrictor
Prevertebral fascia
Carotid sheath
Longus colli
Fifth cervical vertebra
Articular process
Multifidus
Semispinalis cervicis
Semispinalis capitis

External jugular vein
Common carotid artery
Internal jugular vein
Vagus nerve
Sympathetic trunk
Scalenus anterior
Fifth cervical spinal nerve
Scalenus medius
Vertebral vessels
Iliocostalis cervicis
Splenius cervicis
Longissimus capitis and cervicis

Accessory nerve

Trapezius

C   Splenius capitis   Deep cervical vessels

Figure 3.3C Transverse section through the left half of the neck to show the arrangement of the deep cervical fascia. (Redrawn from *Gray's Anatomy*, 38th edn.)

relax via reciprocal inhibition, allowing an easier stretch to be performed. The patient is attempting to push towards the barrier of restriction, against the practitioner/therapist's precisely matched counter-effort.

Forces   The practitioner/therapist's and patient's forces are matched. Initial effort involves approximately 30% of patient's strength: however, an increase on subsequent contractions is appropriate.

CAUTION: Longer, stronger contractions may predispose towards onset of cramping and so should be carefully introduced.

Duration of contraction   Initially 7–10 seconds, increasing to up to 15 seconds in subsequent contractions if greater effect required.

Action following contraction   There should be a rest period of 5 seconds or so, to ensure complete relaxation before commencing the stretch. On an exhalation the area (muscle) is taken to its new restriction barrier, and a small degree beyond, painlessly, and held in this position for at least 30, and up to 60 seconds. The patient should, if possible, participate in assisting in the move to, and through, the barrier, effectively further inhibiting the structure being stretched and retarding the likelihood of a myotatic stretch reflex.

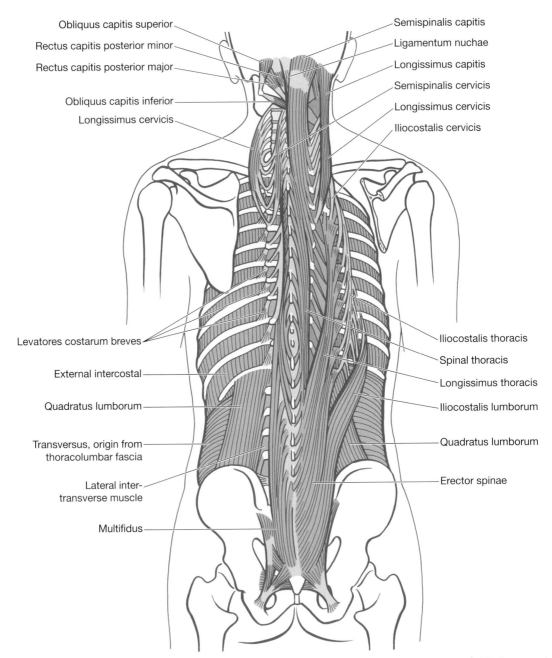

Figure 3.4 The deep muscles of the back. On the left side erector spinae and its upward continuations (with the exception of longissimus cervicis, which has been displaced laterally) and semispinalis capitis have been removed. (Redrawn from *Gray's Anatomy*, 38th edn.)

Repetitions Repeat three times or until no further gain in range of motion is possible, with each isometric contraction commencing from a position short of the barrier.

5. Isotonic concentric contraction (for toning or rehabilitation)

Indications

- Toning weakened musculature.

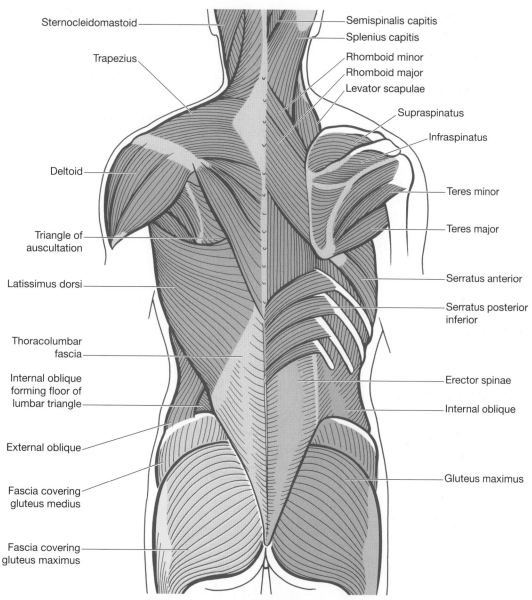

Figure 3.5 Superficial muscles of the back of the neck and trunk. On the left only the skin, superficial and deep fasciae (other than gluteofemoral) have been removed; on the right, sternocleidomastoid, trapezius, latissimus dorsi, deltoid and external oblique have been dissected away. (Redrawn from *Gray's Anatomy*, 38th edn.)

Contraction starting point   In a mid-range easy position.

Modus operandi   The affected muscle is allowed to contract, with some (constant) resistance from the practitioner/therapist.

Forces   The patient's effort overcomes that of the practitioner/therapist since the patient's force is greater than the practitioner/therapist resistance. The patient uses maximal effort available, but force is built slowly, not via sudden effort. The practitioner/therapist maintains a constant degree of resistance.

Duration   3–4 seconds.

Repetitions   Repeat five to seven times, or more if appropriate.

6. Isotonic eccentric contraction (isolytic, for reduction of fibrotic change, to introduce controlled microtrauma)

Indications

- Stretching tight fibrotic musculature.

Contraction starting point   At the restriction barrier.

Modus operandi   The muscle to be stretched is contracted by the patient and is prevented from doing so by the practitioner/therapist, by means of superior practitioner/therapist effort, so that the contraction is rapidly overcome and reversed, introducing stretch into the contracting muscle.

The process should take no more than 4 seconds. Origin and insertion do not approximate. The muscle should be stretched to, or as close as possible to, full physiological resting length.

Forces   The practitioner/therapist's force is greater than that of the patient. Less than maximal patient force should be employed at first. Subsequent contractions build towards this, if discomfort is not excessive.

Duration of contraction   2–4 seconds.

Repetitions   Repeat three to five times if discomfort is not excessive.

CAUTION: Avoid using isolytic contractions on head/neck muscles or at all if patient is frail, very pain-sensitive, or osteoporotic. The patient should anticipate soreness for several days in the affected muscles.

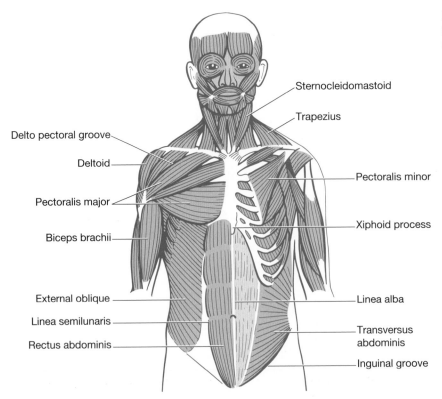

Figure 3.6   Frontal view of the trunk. (Redrawn from *Gray's Anatomy*, 38th edn.)

Sternocleidomastoid

Trapezius

Delto pectoral groove

Deltoid

Pectoralis minor

Pectoralis major

Biceps brachii

Xiphoid process

External oblique

Linea alba

Linea semilunaris

Rectus abdominis

Transversus abdominis

Inguinal groove

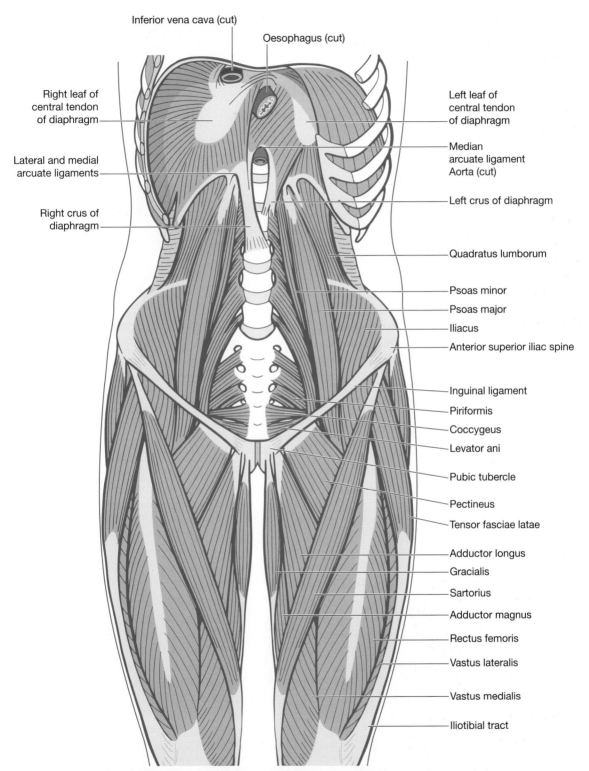

Figure 3.7 View of the abdomen, pelvis and thighs, showing abdominal aspect of the diaphragm, hip flexors and superficial muscles of the thigh. (Redrawn from *Gray's Anatomy*, 38th edn.)

7. Isotonic eccentric contraction (slowly performed) for strengthening weak postural muscles and preparing their antagonists for stretching

Indications

- Strengthening weakened postural muscle
- Preparing tight antagonists to inhibited muscles for stretching.

Contraction starting point　At the restriction barrier.

Modus operandi　The muscle is contracted and is prevented from doing so by the practitioner/therapist, via superior practitioner/therapist effort, so that the contraction is *slowly* overcome and reversed, as the contracting muscle is stretched. The origin and insertion do not approximate but diverge. The muscle should be stretched to its full physiological resting length. This process tones the muscle and inhibits its antagonist(s), and these can subsequently be stretched as in other MET procedures.

Forces　The practitioner/therapist's force is greater than patient's. Less than maximal patient's force should be employed at first. Subsequent contractions build towards this, if discomfort is not excessive.

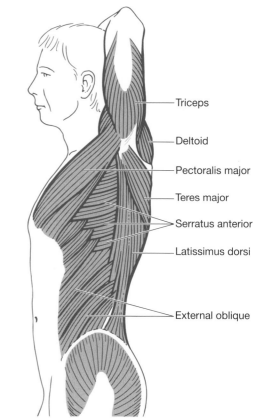

Figure 3.8　Lateral view of the trunk. (Redrawn from *Gray's Anatomy*, 38th edn.)

Triceps
Deltoid
Pectoralis major
Teres major
Serratus anterior
Latissimus dorsi
External oblique

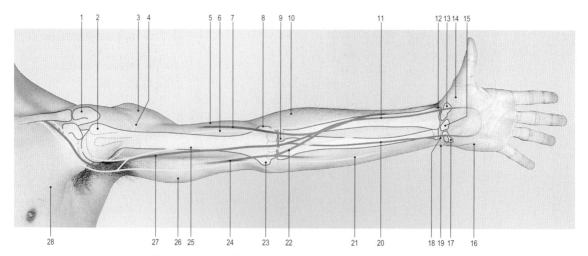

1. Acromion. 2. Greater tubercle (tuberosity). 3. Deltoid. 4. Axillary nerve. 5. Biceps brachii. 6. Radial nerve. 7. Cephalic vein. 8. Lateral epicondyle. 9. Head of radius. 10. Brachioradialis. 11. Radial artery. 12. Styloid process of radius. 13. Scaphoid. 14. Thenar eminence. 15. Lunate. 16. Hypothenar eminence. 17. Triquetrum. 18. Styloid process of ulna. 19. Proximal wrist crease. 20. Ulnar artery. 21. Ulnar nerve. 22. Median cubital vein. 23. Median epicondyle. 24. Basilic vein. 25. Median nerve. 26. Triceps. 27. Brachial artery. 28. Pectoralis major.

Figure 3.9　Anterior view of the arm abducted at the shoulder. (Redrawn from *Gray's Anatomy*, 38th edn.)

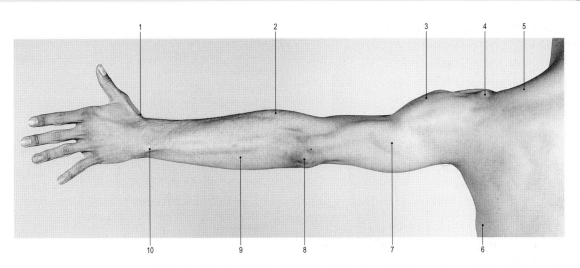

1. Anatomical snuffbox. 2. Brachioradialis. 3. Deltoid. 4. Acromion. 5. Trapezius. 6. Latissimus dorsi. 7. Triceps. 8. Olecranon process. 9. Common extensor muscle group. 10. Extensor carpi ulnaris.

Figure 3.10   Posterior view of the arm abducted at the shoulder. (Redrawn from *Gray's Anatomy*, 38th edn.)

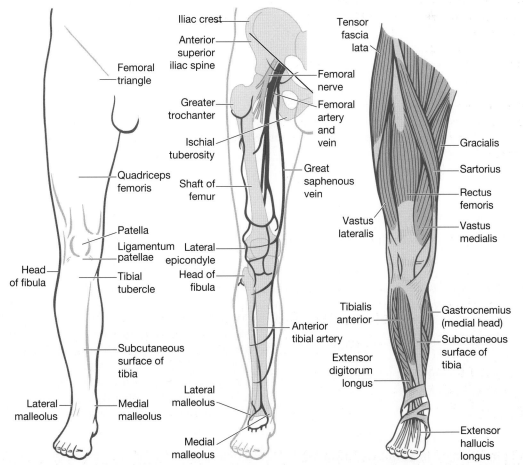

Figure 3.11   Anterior aspect of lower limb to show surface anatomy, bony and soft tissue structures. (Redrawn from *Gray's Anatomy*, 38th edn.)

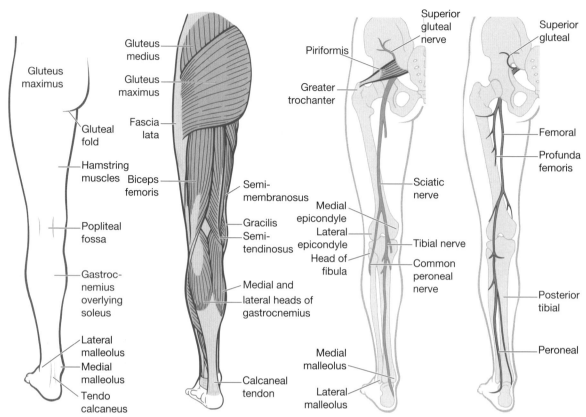

Figure 3.12   Posterior views of the lower limb to show surface anatomy, bony and soft tissue structures and main nerves and arteries. (Redrawn from *Gray's Anatomy*, 38th edn.)

Duration of contraction   5–7 seconds.

Repetitions   Repeat three times if discomfort is not excessive.

🛑 **CAUTION:** Avoid using isotonic eccentric contractions on head/neck muscles involved in rotation, or at all if the patient is frail, very pain-sensitive, or osteoporotic.

8. Isokinetic (combined isotonic and isometric contractions)

Indications

- Toning weakened musculature
- Building strength in all muscles involved in particular joint function

- Training and balancing effect on muscle fibres.

Starting point of contraction   Easy mid-range position.

Modus operandi   The patient resists with moderate and variable effort at first, progressing to maximal effort subsequently, as the practitioner/therapist rapidly puts a joint (ankle or wrist for example) through as full a range of movements as possible. This approach differs from a simple isotonic exercise by virtue of the inclusion of whole ranges of motion, rather than single motions, and because the applied resistance varies, progressively increasing as the procedure progresses.

Forces   The practitioner/therapist's force overcomes the patient's effort to prevent movement.

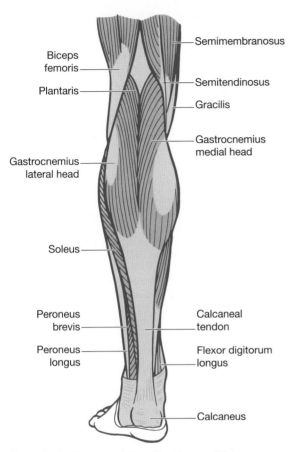

Biceps femoris

Plantaris

Gastrocnemius lateral head

Soleus

Peroneus brevis

Peroneus longus

Semimembranosus

Semitendinosus

Gracilis

Gastrocnemius medial head

Calcaneal tendon

Flexor digitorum longus

Calcaneus

Figure 3.13   Muscles of the left calf: superficial group. (Redrawn from *Gray's Anatomy*, 38th edn.)

First movements (taking an ankle, say, into all its directions of motion) may involve moderate force, progressing to full force subsequently. An alternative is to have the practitioner/therapist (or machine) resist the patient's effort to make all the movements.

Duration of contraction   Up to 4 seconds.

Repetitions   Repeat two to four times.

Muscle maps

Chapter 5 contains descriptions of the MET approaches to individual muscles. It is assumed that before using MET methods a sound grounding will have been achieved in understanding both the anatomy and physiology of the musculoskeletal system.

In almost all instances lengthening, stretching, strategies involves following fibre direction. To assist in application of MET, Figs 3.3–3.13 may enhance awareness of fibre direction.

References

Blood S 1980 Treatment of the sprained ankle. Journal of the American Osteopathic Association 79(11): 689

Cummings J, Howell J 1990 The role of respiration in the tension production of myofascial tissues. Journal of the American Osteopathic Association 90(9): 842

DiGiovanna E 1991 Treatment of the spine. In: DiGiovanna E (ed) An osteopathic approach to diagnosis and treatment. Lippincott, Philadelphia

Gajdosik 1991 Effects of static stretching on short hamstring muscles. Journal of Sports Physical Therapy 14(6): 250–255

Goodridge J 1981 MET – definition, explanation, methods of procedure. Journal of the American Osteopathic Association 81(4): 249

Goodridge J, Kuchera W 1997 Muscle energy treatment techniques. In: Ward R (ed) Foundations of osteopathic medicine. Williams and Wilkins, Baltimore

Greenman P 1989 Principles of manual medicine. Williams and Wilkins, Baltimore

Greenman P 1996 Principles of manual medicine, 2nd edn. Williams and Wilkins, Baltimore

Guissard N et al 1988 Muscle stretching and motorneurone excitability. European Journal of Applied Physiology 58: 47–52

Gunnari H, Evjenth O 1983 Sequence exercise. [Norwegian.] Dreyers Verlag, Oslo

Hammer W 1999 Functional soft tissue examination and treatment by manual methods. Aspen Publications, pp 535–540

Hoover H 1969 A method for teaching functional technique. Yearbook of Academy of Applied Osteopathy 1969, Newark, Ohio

Janda V 1983 Muscle function testing. Butterworths, London

Janda V 1990 Differential diagnosis of muscle tone in respect of inhibitory techniques. In: Paterson J K, Burn L (eds) Back pain, an international review. Kluwer, pp 196–199

Janda V 1993 Assessment and treatment of impaired movement patterns and motor recruitment. Presentation to Physical Medicine Research Foundation, Montreal, 9–11 October, 1993

Johns R J, Wright Y 1962 Relative importance of various tissues in joint stiffness. Journal of Applied Physiology 17: 824–828

Jull G, Janda V 1987 Muscles and motor control in low back pain: assessment and management. In: Twomey L, Grieve G (eds) Physical therapy of the low back. Churchill Livingstone, Edinburgh, pp 253–278

Kisselkova, Georgiev J 1976 Journal of Applied Physiology 46: 1093–1095

Kottke F 1982 Therapeutic exercise to maintain mobility. In: Krusen's handbook of physical medicine and rehabilitation, 3rd edn. W B Saunders, Philadelphia

Kraus H 1970 Clinical treatment of back and neck pain. McGraw Hill, New York

Kuchera W A, Kuchera M L 1992 Osteopathic principles in practice. Kirksville College of Osteopathic Medicine Press, Missouri

Lewit K 1991 Manipulative therapy in rehabilitation of the motor system. Butterworths, London

Lewit K 1999 Manipulative therapy in rehabilitation of the motor system, 3rd edn. Butterworths, London

Lewit K, Janda V, Veverkova M 1998 Respiratory synkinesis – polyelectromyographic investigation. Journal of Orthopaedic Medicine 20: 2–6

Liebenson C 1989 Active muscular relaxation methods. Journal of Manipulative and Physiological Therapeutics 12(6): 446–451

Liebenson C 1996 Rehabilitation of the spine. Williams and Wilkins, Baltimore

Lucas K et al 2004 Latent myofascial trigger points: their effects on muscle activation and movement efficiency.

Journal of Bodywork and Movement Therapies 8(3): 160–166

Mattes A 1990 Active and assisted stretching. Mattes, Sarasota

Mitchell F, Moran P, Pruzzo N 1979 An evaluation and treatment manual of osteopathic muscle energy technique. Valley Park, Missouri

Moore M, Kukulka C 1991 Depression of Hoffman reflexes following voluntary contraction and implications for proprioceptive neuromuscular facilitation therapy. Physical Therapy 71(4): 321–329

Norris C 1999 Functional load abdominal training (part 1). Journal of Bodywork and Movement Therapies 3(3): 150–158

Ruddy T J 1962 Osteopathic rhythmic resistive technic. Academy of Applied Osteopathy Yearbook 1962, pp 23–31

Scariati P 1991 Neurophysiology relevant to osteopathic manipulation. In: DiGiovanna E (ed) An osteopathic approach to diagnosis and treatment. Lippincott, Philadelphia

Shellock F G, Prentice W E 1985 Warming-up and stretching for improved physical perfomance and prevention of sports-related injuries. Sports Medicine 2(4): 267–278

Schmitt G D, Pelham T W, Holt L E 1999 From the field. A comparison of selected protocols during proprioceptive neuromuscular facilitation stretching. Clinical Kinesiology 53(1): 16–21

Simons D, Travell J, Simmons L 1999 Myofascial pain and dysfunction: the trigger point manual, vol 1, 2nd edn. Williams and Wilkins, Baltimore

Sucher B 1990 Thoracic outlet syndrome – a myofascial variant (part 2). Journal of the American Osteopathic Association 90(9): 810–823

Tunnell P 1997 Protocol for visual assessments. Journal of Bodywork and Movement Therapies 1(1): 21–27

Ward R 1997 Foundations of osteopathic medicine. Williams and Wilkins, Baltimore

MET: efficacy and research

4

Gary Fryer

CHAPTER CONTENTS

Efficacy of MET	**110**
Myofascial extensibility	110
MET applied to the spine	118
Research into the mechanisms of therapeutic	
effect	**120**
Myofascial extensibility	120
Spinal dysfunction	126
Directions for research	128
References	**129**

A chapter on research in a manual therapy text? Not so many years ago, this would have been seen as a peculiar inclusion. The accepted practice in the past was that an 'authority' would proclaim that their new technique could do this or that, and the faithful would unquestioningly adopt the techniques and all explanations that accompanied them. In possibly no other disciplines is this practice so apparent as in osteopathy and chiropractic, where quotes of A.T. Still and the Palmers are revered, and diagnostic methods of influential technique developers (such as Fred Mitchell Snr, the developer of muscle energy technique (MET)) continue to be widely used (Peace & Fryer 2004), despite growing evidence of poor reliability and validity (Fryer 2000, Gibbons & Tehan 1998).

Why research? Does scientific evidence complement or contradict 'hands on' manual therapy practice? Can research be useful to the understanding and practice of MET? Does research merely prove those things that are self-evident to practitioners 'at the coal face'? The political, economic, and academic environment in relation to health has changed substantially over the last two decades. First and foremost is the need for research to validate the efficacy of manual treatment: increasingly, we are being asked by governments, health authorities, and insurers to *prove* that what we do works. Secondly, there is an academic quest to understand the nature of dysfunction and *why* (or *if*) manual treatment works. Thirdly, and most importantly to practitioners, research enables us to objectively examine and determine the most effective ways to treat our patients. MET, like most manual therapy approaches, has not yet been examined thoroughly enough to meet these goals, but research in this area is growing.

Much of the research relevant to MET comes from the study of related techniques, such as proprioceptive neuromuscular facilitation (PNF) stretching (see Ch. 8), and most of this research has involved the effect of techniques on hamstring muscle extensibility (stretch). There has been limited investigation of MET on spinal range of motion (ROM), and very little research concerning its effect on clinical outcomes in symptomatic individuals. In part, this may be attributed to the fact that MET is not commonly employed as a stand-alone technique (for instance, in the treatment of low-back pain), but frequently administered in combination with other manual approaches. There is, however, an increasing need to examine the effectiveness of MET using valid clinical outcome measures.

Should evidence change the way we practice? There is a justifiable concern among many practitioners that techniques and approaches found to be useful by generations of osteopaths and practitioners from other manual therapy disciplines might be abandoned due to lack of supporting evidence or on the basis of a few unfavourable studies. *Lack of proof* does not equal *disproof*. 'Evidence-based practice' in the strict sense is not currently possible for manual therapists because so much of what we do has not been examined. Scientific evidence should inform us about our practice, and influence our choices and treatment approaches, but it is not possible to base our practice only on manual techniques supported by high-quality evidence. It is unlikely that we will ever have solid evidence for every manual technique we use, due to the research that would be required and the likelihood that techniques may work best combined with other techniques, rather than in isolation. But it is likely that we will have evidence that informs us of what techniques or approaches are most effective for a particular outcome or complaint, and be able to base our treatment around elements from that approach. It would be foolish to abandon techniques with a long history of anecdotal evidence of efficacy but currently lacking in scientific support, for these techniques may well be effective for many patients and conditions. But when there is growing evidence

of *disproof* – such as evidence of no therapeutic benefit, or the lack of reliability and validity of a diagnostic approach – practitioners have an intellectual and ethical duty to reconsider their practice.

The available evidence (outlined below) clearly points to the effectiveness of MET (and related procedures) for increasing muscle extensibility and spinal ROM, although research relating to the most efficacious type of application, mechanism of action and clinical relevance still requires further investigation.

Efficacy of MET

Myofascial extensibility

Most researchers who have examined the effect of isometric-assisted stretching – MET, proprioceptive neuromuscular facilitation (PNF) stretching, postisometric relaxation – have examined the effect of these techniques on the hamstring muscles. The most common forms of isometric stretching referred to in the literature are contract–relax (CR), where the muscle being stretched is contracted and then relaxed, agonist contract–relax (ACR),[1] where contraction of the agonist (rather than the muscle being stretched) actively moves the joint into increased ROM, and contract–relax agonist contract (CRAC), a combination of these two methods (Table 4.1). These techniques are commonly referred to as PNF stretching, but the similarity to MET procedures for lengthening muscles is obvious.

MET and PNF stretching methods have been clearly shown to bring about greater improvements in joint ROM and muscle extensibility than passive, static stretching, both in the short and

---

[1] The term 'agonist contract–relax' may appear confusing to many because the word 'agonist' apparently refers to the motion produced, not the relationship of the contracting muscle to the one being stretched. Hence, when using this technique to stretch the hamstring muscles (i.e. increase knee extension) the contracting muscle is the quadriceps femoris. The quadriceps is the 'agonist' muscle for knee extension (the movement being increased) – hence the name ACR – but is the 'antagonist' of the muscle being stretched (hamstrings), which is confusing to those who believe this technique primarily has effect by producing hamstring relaxation via reciprocal inhibition.

Table 4.1 MET and PNF isometric contraction-assisted stretching techniques

Manual procedure	Procedure applied to increase hamstring muscle extensibility
Contract–relax (CR)	Hamstring muscles are passively stretched, active isometric contraction of the hamstrings against operator resistance, relaxation followed by additional passive stretching
Agonist contract–relax (ACR)	Hamstring muscles are passively stretched, active contraction of the quadriceps muscles to further increase range of motion and hamstring stretching, relaxation followed by additional passive stretching
Contract–relax agonist contract (CRAC)	Hamstring muscles are passively stretched, active isometric contraction of the hamstrings against operator resistance, relaxation followed by additional passive stretching, active contraction of the quadriceps muscles to further increase range of motion and hamstring stretching, relaxation followed by additional passive stretching

long term (Sady et al 1982, Wallin et al 1985, Magnusson et al 1996c, Osternig et al 1990, Feland et al 2001a, Ferber et al 2002b) (Table 4.2). Researchers have used slightly different MET protocols (varying the force and duration of contraction and stretching, and number of repetitions, use of agonist contraction) and different methods of measuring hamstring length (active knee extension, passive knee extension, measurement of passive torque) to assess the effect of techniques on immediate changes to hamstring length. Researchers have reported immediate hamstring length and ROM increases from 3° (Ballantyne et al 2003) to 33° (Magnusson et al 1996c) following MET or similar methods. Due to differences in measurement methodology, however, it is difficult to determine the most efficacious elements of the various treatment protocols, but it appears that ACR and CRAC methods are more effective for increasing ROM than CR.

Immediate effects of contract–relax techniques

Magnusson et al (1996c) compared the immediate effects of hamstring CR with passive stretching on 10 recreational athletes using passive knee extension (PKE) in the seated position as the measure of ROM. In what the authors called the variable angle protocol, the hamstrings of the subjects were stretched to 10° before the point of onset of posterior thigh pain; the subjects were then asked to perform a forceful isometric contraction for 6 seconds. Following the isometric contraction, the hamstring muscle was stretched to the onset of posterior thigh pain, where the joint angle was measured. The procedure was the same for the passive stretching, except the participant rested during the contraction phase. The CR technique produced significantly greater maximum joint angle (33°) than the passive stretch (28°). It is worth noting that only a single contraction was used in the CR technique for this study. Ballantyne et al (2003) also examined the immediate effect of an MET CR technique (5-second moderate force contraction, 3-second stretch and relaxation; performed four times) on hamstring flexibility, and found a significant, but small (3°), increase in supine PKE when stretched to hamstring discomfort.

Spernoga et al (2001) measured the duration of increased hamstring extensibility following a single application of CR. The researchers examined the hamstrings of the right leg of 30 subjects with visible evidence of tightness (limitation of 20° of full extension) using active knee extension (AKE). The hamstrings were passively stretched until a mild stretching sensation was reported by the subject and then held for 7 seconds. The subject then contracted the hamstring muscle maximally for 7 seconds, relaxed for 5 seconds, and then was passively stretched for a further 7 seconds. This procedure was repeated five times. The researchers found that hamstring extensibility remained significantly increased for only 6 minutes. Interestingly, they found that the non-treated leg displayed decreased extensibility after 2 minutes of inactivity, and attributed this to thixotropy (the property of a tissue to become more liquid after motion and return to a stiffer, gel-like state at rest).

The superiority of CR over passive stretching has been demonstrated in volunteers of a more senior age, but not in those older than 65 years.

Table 4.2 Overview of studies that have investigated isometric stretching techniques for increasing hamstring muscle extensibility

Study	Treatment period	Techniques	Measurement	Reported findings
Sady et al (1982)	6 weeks	SS, ballistic S, CR	Passive SLR	CR < SS = ballistic = control
Wallin et al (1985)	60 days	Ballistic S, CR	PKE	CR < BS < baseline
Etnyre & Abraham (1986a)	Single application	SS, CR, CRAC	Passive SLR	CRAC < CR < SS
Osternig et al (1990)	Single application	SS, CR, ACR	PKE	ACR < CR = SS
Cornelius et al (1992)	Single application	SS, CR, ACR, CRAC, ± ice	PKE	CR = ACR = CRAC < SS; ice application – ND
Magnusson et al (1996c)	Single application	SS, CR	PKE, torque measurement	CR < SS
Handel et al (1997)	8 weeks	CR	PKE, AKE	CR < baseline (PKE, not AKE)
Gribble et al (1999)	6 weeks	SS, CR	AKE	CR = SS < baseline
Schmitt et al (1999)	10 days	ACR	Sit and reach	ACR < baseline; different contraction durations – ND
Burke et al (2001)	5 days	ACR	Active SLR	ACR < baseline; hot/cold – ND
Feland et al (2001a)	Single application	SS, CR	PKE	SS = CR < control CR < SS (males < 65 yrs)
Spernoga et al (2001)	Single application	CR	AKE	CR < baseline
Ferber et al (2002a)	Single application	SS, CR, ACR	PKE	ACR < CR = SS ACR = CR = SS (untrained 65–75 yrs)
Ferber et al (2002b)	Single application	SS, CR, ACR	PKE	ACR < CR = SS
Mehta & Hatton (2002)	Single application	CR	PKE	CR < baseline; different contraction durations – ND
Stopka et al (2002)	Single application	SS, CR	Sit and reach	CR < SS < baseline
Ballantyne et al (2003)	Single application		PKE, torque measurement	
Funk et al (2003)	Single application	SS, CR, ± exercise	AKE	CR = SS; CR + exercise < CR
Rowlands et al (2003)	6 weeks	CRAC + SS	Passive SLR	CRAC < control; 10-sec contract < 5-sec contract
Feland & Marin (2004)	5 days	CR	PKE	CR < control; varied contract intensity – ND

CR = contract–relax, ACR = agonist contract–relax, CRAC = contract–relax agonist contract, SS = static stretch, PKE = passive knee extension, AKE = active knee extension, SLR = straight leg raise. ND = no difference

Feland et al (2001a) examined the hamstring extensibility of senior athletes (age range 55–79 years) after allocation to either a CR (*n* = 40), static stretch (*n* = 38) or control group (*n* = 19). The CR treatment consisted of a hamstring stretch using a straight leg raise (SLR) to the point of discomfort, followed by a maximal contraction of the hamstring and hip extensor muscles for 6 seconds, relaxation and further stretching for 10 seconds, and the procedure was repeated once. The static stretch intervention was maintained for 32 seconds, the same period as for the duration of the CR technique. The researchers found that both treatments were significantly more effective than no treatment (CR produced 5° mean increased ROM), but there was no overall difference between the two treatments. Only in the male subjects and those aged less than 65 years did the CR appear to be more effective than stretching. Feland et al speculated that age-related changes to the muscles of subjects over 65 years, such as an increase in collagen, myofibril degeneration and neurophysiological changes, could hamper the effect of PNF techniques. These interesting findings require further investigation before any conclusions can be made about the suitability of MET in older populations.

CR techniques have also been shown to produce immediate improvements in flexibility in subjects with mild–moderate intellectual disabilities. Stopka et al (2002) examined the ability of 18 Special Olympic athletes to perform sit-and-reach position after undergoing an application of static stretching and CR. The stretch was performed in the sit-and-reach position with a towel placed around the soles of their feet and used a 10-second stretch, followed by 10 seconds of relaxation. The CR was performed in the same position and used a 10-second plantar flexion isometric contraction, followed by 10 seconds of relaxation. Only one application of CR was used. The order of stretching was reversed (from stretch/CR to CR/stretch) in a trial 3–4 weeks later. Both static stretching and CR were effective in increasing ROM in the first trial (stretch/CR), but when the order was reversed (CR/stretch) only CR was effective, with an actual decrease in stretching performance following the static stretch. The researchers concluded that CR was more effective because it increased ROM regardless of the order of stretching.

Long-term effects of contract–relax techniques

Researchers have also established that contract–relax stretching programmes over a longer time period produce increased joint ROM and hamstring muscle extensibility compared with pre-stretching baseline measures, as well as to static stretching. Sady et al (1982) examined whether a programme of ballistic stretching, static stretching or CR was more effective in increasing the passive SLR measurement. Subjects ($n = 43$) engaged in a 3-day per week, 6-week flexibility programme where those in the ballistic group performed the stretch rapidly 20 times, and those in the static

group held the stretch for 6 seconds, relaxed and repeated the sequence twice. For those in the CR group, a partner stretched the leg to the limit of motion, followed by an isometric contraction of the hamstrings and hip extensors for 6 seconds, and relaxation and further stretching, all repeated two more times. The CR group achieved significantly greater ROM than the control group (10.6° and 3.4°, respectively), whereas the ballistic and static stretching groups were not significantly different from the control.

Wallin et al (1985) examined the effect of CR, ballistic stretching, and of frequency of stretching on hamstring, ankle plantar flexor and adductor muscle extensibility in 47 subjects. Subjects underwent a stretching programme (CR or ballistic stretching) three times a week for 30 days, and then CR once/twice/five times a week for the next 30 days. The CR technique involved five repetitions of stretching the muscle almost to its full range, a maximal isometric contraction for 7–8 seconds, 2–5 seconds of relaxation, and then fully stretched for 7–8 seconds. An equal time period was used for the ballistic stretching group. Hamstring extensibility was measured with a compass goniometer and PKE performed to the point of knee buckling. At 30 days, the CR group had significantly increased PKE (approximately 6°) compared with baseline, and significantly different from the ballistic stretching group, which only achieved approximately 2° change. After the 30-day period, those performing CR only once a week maintained their increased flexibility, whereas those that performed CR twice or five times a week gained further significant increases.

Handel et al (1997) also found that a CR stretching regimen produced significant increases in hamstring extensibility. Sixteen male athletes underwent a 10-minute CR stretching programme three times a week for 8 weeks. Knee flexors and extensors were stretched using eight cycles of a 10-second strong contraction, 1–2 seconds of relaxation, followed by 10–15 seconds of passive stretching. Seated PKE (but not seated AKE) was significantly increased at 4 and 8 weeks (5.6°), as well as active and passive knee flexion. Gribble et al (1999), however, found that while both CR and static stretching over a 6-week period increased hamstring extensibility (14° and 9° of AKE, respectively), the treatments were not significantly different from each other. In this study, the hamstrings of subjects in the CR group were stretched for 8 seconds in a straight leg raise (SLR) position, followed by a 7-second isometric contraction of the hamstrings, a 5-second rest, and a 10-second stretch, and was performed four times. Subjects in the stretching group underwent four 30-second stretches, with 30-second rests between each stretch. The relatively small numbers of volunteers in each group (16, 12, and 14) may have led to insufficient power to detect a significant difference between treatment effects.

There is little research on the effect of CR on muscles and joints other than the hamstrings and knee. In the only study found, Klein et al (2002) examined the effect of a 10-week flexibility programme (including warm-ups, CR and cool-down exercises, twice a week) on various muscles in 11 assisted-living older adults (73–94 years). The researchers found that the subjects gained significant improvements in ankle flexion and shoulder flexion ROM, in isometric strength, and in balance and mobility for sit-to-stand.

Agonist contract–relax versus contract–relax

Agonist contract–relax (ACR) is another PNF stretching technique commonly referred to in the research literature. In ACR, the agonist muscle group (e.g. quadriceps femoris muscle, when attempting to stretch the hamstrings) is contracted to actively move the limb or joint into increased ROM, in contrast to CR where the muscle undergoing the stretch produces an isometric contraction. Several researchers have compared the effectiveness of the two techniques and found that ACR produces more ROM gain than CR, although some have noted that it appeared to be less comfortable for the subjects, and it may not be effective in older untrained adults.

Osternig et al (1990) found that ACR produced 9–13% more knee joint ROM than CR and static stretching. These researchers examined the impact of the three techniques in 10 endurance athletes (distance runners), 10 high-intensity athletes (volleyball players and sprinters), and 10 control subjects (not involved in competitive sports). Those subjects in the CR group performed a trial

of 5-second maximal contraction of the hamstring, followed by a 5-second stretch, and the procedure was repeated to conclude one trial, with five trials performed. Those in the ACR group received a similar procedure except that the quadriceps musculature was contracted to extend the knee. Subjects in the static stretch group received an 80-second stretch. The ACR technique produced significantly greater ROM (approximately 20°) than the CR and static stretch groups. The subgroup of endurance athletes attained less ROM following ACR and CR than the high-intensity athletes and non-athletes. The researchers postulated that high-intensity short-term activity training might involve greater joint excursions than long-term endurance training, and necessitate less hamstring resistance.

ACR techniques have also been found more effective for increasing hamstring extensibility in older adults. Ferber et al (2002b) examined the effects of ACR, CR and static stretching of the hamstrings on PKE in adults aged 50–75 years. For subjects in the CR group, the hamstrings were passively stretched, followed by a 5-second maximal isometric contraction, and further stretching for 5 seconds, all performed eight times. The procedure for the ACR was the same except that the quadriceps muscle group, rather than the hamstring group, was contracted. Subjects undergoing static stretching had their hamstrings held in a position of stretch and gradually increased for 80 seconds. The mean change produced by the ACR was 15.7°, and was significantly greater than the CR (12.1°) and static stretch (11.7°). It is interesting to note that 77% of subjects found the ACR to be the most uncomfortable procedure. In another investigation of PNF stretching in older adults, Ferber et al (2002a) found that ACR produced 4–6° more knee ROM than CR and static stretch in trained subjects (master level endurance runners) aged 45–75 years and in untrained subjects aged 45–50 years, but not in untrained adults aged 65–75 years. The researchers suggested the lack of effect in this older untrained group was possibly due to a lack of neuromuscular control or strength.

Etnyre & Abraham (1986a) have found that a variation of ACR was more effective than CR to increase the range of ankle dorsiflexion. Twelve subjects performed contract–relax antagonist contract (CRAC, a combination of CR and ACR methods), CR and static stretching on separate days. The CRAC technique consisted of passive hamstring stretching followed by isometric contraction of the hamstrings against operator resistance, relaxation and additional passive stretching, and then contraction of the quadriceps muscles to further increase range of motion. The CRAC produced significantly greater increases in ROM than the CR, which was significantly better than static stretching. Godges et al (2003) applied a combination of soft tissue mobilisation (sustained pressure to the subscapularis muscle) and CRAC to subjects with limited shoulder external rotation and overhead reach. These researchers found that a single treatment intervention produced an immediate significant increase in external rotation (16.4°), compared with less than 1° in the control group.

Duration of contraction

Various authors and researchers have suggested different durations for the muscular contraction for MET and similar techniques, but this has received little attention in previous research. Many authors in the field of MET have advocated the use of 3–7 seconds of resisted contraction for adequate therapeutic effect (Mitchell & Mitchell 1995, Greenman 1996), whereas other authors and researchers have used 5-second (Ballantyne et al 2003), 5- and 20-second (Mehta & Hatton 2002), 6- and 12-second (Schmitt et al 1999), and 20-second (Ferber et al 2002b) contraction durations. The value of longer isometric contraction durations is uncertain, because conflicting results appear in the few studies that have examined this variable.

Schmitt et al (1999) examined the relationship between durations of sub-maximal isometric contraction on hamstring flexibility, and compared the effects of 6- and 12-second isometric contraction phases in 10 subjects, using an ACR technique. Both groups produced significant increases in ROM, measured by an active sit-and-reach test, but showed no significant differences between each other. Subjects in the 12-second contraction group achieved greater ROM than the 6-second group, and given the small numbers in each group ($n = 5$), this study may have lacked sufficient power

to detect differences between the contraction durations. Mehta & Hatton (2002) treated the hamstring muscles of asymptomatic subjects with CR using a 5-second sub-maximal contraction, and, after a 14-day washout period, treated them again using a 20-second contraction MET. The authors found a significant increase in the passive range of motion following both the 5-second and 20-second contractions, but no significant difference between the two treatments.

Nelson & Cornelius (1991) examined the effect of a 3-second, 6-second, and 10-second maximal contraction phase in a CRAC stretching procedure on the range of internal rotation of the shoulder joint in 60 subjects. The shoulders of subjects were passively internally rotated just short of end-range, followed by a maximal external rotation isometric effort, an internal rotation isometric effort (3, 6, or 10 seconds), and then relaxation and passive stretching for an unspecified duration. The isometric stretching procedures were performed three times. The researchers found all treatments produced significantly greater ROM than baseline measures, but there were no differences in the effect of varying the contraction duration. Similarly, Fryer & Ruszkowski (2004) examined the effect of both a 5-second and 20-second contraction phase in MET applied to the atlanto-axial joint of the upper cervical spine on active range of atlanto-axial rotation. They found that both techniques increased the range of rotation, but were not significantly different from one another, although the 5-second contraction appeared to be more effective (larger mean gain and effect size) than the 20-second contraction MET.

In contrast to these studies, Rowlands et al (2003) has reported that longer contraction times in CRAC resulted in greater increases in hamstring flexibility. Forty-three women were assigned to either a 5- or 10-second isometric contraction group, or a no-treatment control group, and ROM was measured by passive SLR to pain tolerance. The treatment groups followed a stretching programme twice a week for 6 weeks, which involved a 5-minute warm-up, 5-minute static stretching, and two CRAC techniques (supine and sitting). The hamstrings were passively stretched and the subject was asked to perform maximal contraction of the hamstrings for 5 or 10 seconds, followed by 5 seconds of relaxation, contraction of the agonist (quadriceps), and a passive stretch and hold for 10 seconds. Both treatment groups made significant increases over the control group, while the 10-second group made significantly greater gains than the 5-second group at both 3 weeks (20 and 16°) and 6 weeks (33 and 28°, respectively).

Force of contraction

The research literature has not yet adequately addressed the question of the optimal contraction force in isometric contraction used in MET for the purpose of producing greater muscle extensibility. Most researchers who have examined isometric stretching have used protocols with either moderate or maximal contraction intensities, but because of the different treatment and ROM measurement methodologies employed, it is impossible to make comparisons between these studies. Only two studies were found that have examined the effect of varying the force of contraction in isometric stretching, and the results of these two studies are conflicting.

Schmitt et al (1999) found that progressively increasing the intensity of isometric contraction over a 10-day stretching programme was more effective than maintaining a standard intensity. The standard programme used 6-second standard intensity (50% maximal back muscle contraction, 75% maximal hamstring contraction, measured by a FlexAbility machine), whereas the progressive programme prescribed 30% maximal contraction for days 1 and 2, 40% for days 3 and 4, 50% for days 5 and 6, 60% for days 7 and 8, and 70% for days 9 and 10. Those subjects in the progressive programme achieved significantly greater ROM than the standard group (12 cm compared with 4 cm, as measured by the sit-and-reach test). However, due to lack of examiner blinding and the small number of subjects in each group ($n = 5$), caution must be used in interpreting these results. In contrast to these findings, Feland & Marin (2004) found no difference by varying the intensity of isometric contraction. These researchers assigned 72 volunteers with tight hamstrings to a control or one of three CR treatment groups using 20%, 60% or 100% maximal voluntary isometric contraction. Subjects in the CR intervention groups performed a session of stretching once a day for 5 days consisting of three 6-second isometric contractions with a 10-second rest between contractions. Feland & Marin measured hamstring extensibility using PKE, and found that all CR groups achieved greater flexibility than the control, but there was no difference between these groups. Further research is warranted to determine the effect of isometric contraction intensity in MET.

Number of contraction/relaxation phases

There is little evidence available to guide the practitioner in deciding on the number of contraction–relaxation phases to use for optimal ROM gain. Osternig et al (1990) found that 64–84% of the ROM gain was produced in the first phase (one 5-second contraction, followed by 5-second relaxation and stretch) of each trial for passive stretching, CR and ACR. Magnusson et al (1996c) achieved a large hamstring ROM gain (33°) following only one 6-second CR isometric contraction phase. This suggests that there may be little benefit in many repetitions of isometric contraction, but this variable also warrants further investigation.

Duration of post-contraction stretch

Authors and researchers in the field of MET have used and advocated various durations for the passive stretch which follows the contraction phase in MET. Many American authors (Mitchell et al 1979, Greenman 1996, Goodridge 1997) have recommended only enough time to allow patient relaxation and to 'take up the tissue slack' to the new barrier, whereas other authors have recommended a stretching duration of up to 60 seconds (Chaitow 1997).

Little evidence exists to inform practitioners of the ideal duration for post-contraction stretching. Although a number of studies have used different durations of post-contraction stretching, these studies are not directly comparable because of different subject groups, treatment and measurement procedures. Bandy and Irion (1994) and Bandy et al (1997) have determined that 30 seconds of passive stretching was more effective than 15 seconds for increasing the extensibility of the hamstrings muscles, and that 60 seconds was no more effective than 30 seconds of stretching.

In contrast, Feland et al (2001b) found that a 60-second passive stretch was more effective for increasing hamstring length than shorter stretching durations, in an elderly population (older than 65 years). Feland et al speculated that a longer duration of stretch was more effective in elderly subjects because of the age-related changes in the muscles of these subjects.

The relevance of these studies to MET is uncertain. It may be possible to infer that each isometric contraction should be followed by 30 seconds of passive stretch for maximum benefit. However, Bandy et al (1997) reported that no increase in flexibility occurred when the application of 30-second stretch was increased from once a day to three times a day. Fryer (2000) suggested that the length of passive stretching might not be important, provided that the entire procedure (three repetitions of contraction, relaxation and stretching) is of at least 30 seconds duration, because the muscle would be relatively stretched throughout the duration of the technique. This important aspect of MET requires investigation.

Other factors

The frequency of MET stretching, such as the optimal number of treatment periods per week, has received little investigation by researchers. Wallin et al (1985) found that following a 30-day stretching programme (three sessions of CR or ballistic stretching per week), volunteers who performed CR once a week only maintained their improved flexibility, but those who stretched with CR twice or five times a week gained further increases in ROM. The effect of frequency of isometric stretching deserves further investigation.

CR has been demonstrated to be more effective immediately following exercise for producing increased hamstring extensibility. Funk et al (2003) examined hamstring extensibility using AKE of 40 elite college-aged athletes following either passive stretching or CR, and additionally for each of these groups either without exercise or immediately following a 60-minute cycling and upper body conditioning programme. The CR technique consisted of a maximal contraction of the hamstrings for 30 seconds, followed by relaxation and

passive stretching for an unspecified duration, all of which was repeated for a 5-minute period. The researchers found no significant differences between the two treatment groups but a significant increase in the CR group following exercise compared with baseline and CR pre-exercise (approximately mean $4°$ increase).

It has been suggested that the application of cold (cryotherapy) may facilitate PNF stretching because cold would increase the threshold stimulus of the muscle spindles and attenuate the stretch reflex, which may result in a more relaxed muscle and increase in ROM. However, Cornelius et al (1992) examined the effect of cold (ice cubes in a plastic bag placed on the posterior thigh for 10 minutes) or no cold on the hamstring extensibility of 120 male subjects immediately prior to the application of either passive stretch, CR, ACR, or CRAC techniques and found that the cold application did not influence the effectiveness of the techniques. The researchers did report that all PNF techniques produced significantly greater increases in ROM than the passive stretching. Similarly, Burke et al (2001) investigated the effect of 10 minutes of either hot- or cold-water immersion in addition to ACR over a 5-day stretching period. These researchers found that all ACR groups (ACR + heat, ACR + cold, ACR alone) produced significant increases in hamstring length compared with baseline as measured by active SLR, but neither application of hot or cold influenced post-treatment flexibility.

The effect of isometric techniques on muscle pain and tenderness has largely escaped the attention of researchers. In one of the few studies found, Lewit & Simons (1984) performed postisometric techniques on 244 patients who complained of pain and were found to have pain points within the muscle as well as increased tension on stretching. The problematic muscle was passively stretched to a point just short of pain, and the patient instructed to perform a gentle isometric contraction for 10 seconds, followed by relaxation and further stretching. This CR procedure was performed three to five times. The authors reported that treatment resulted in immediate pain relief in 94% of patients, and lasting relief in 63%. Lewit and Simons used palpation for tenderness to determine pain relief but due to lack of examiner blinding and the unknown reliability of this method of assessment, caution is needed when interpreting these findings.

MET applied to the spine

Few researchers have investigated effects of MET applied to the spine, despite the fact that many authors in the field of MET (Bourdillon et al 1992, Mitchell & Mitchell 1995, Greenman 1996, Goodridge & Kuchera 1997) have focused on its application for spinal dysfunction. Only a few studies have examined the effect of MET on spinal ROM, and, although more research is needed, these studies support the effectiveness of MET for increasing ROM. Very few clinical trials examining the effect of MET on spinal pain exist in the peer-reviewed literature and this is clearly an area that deserves further research.

Effect on range of motion

A small number of studies have reported that MET produces increased ROM in the cervical, thoracic and lumbar spine (Table 4.3). Schenk et al (1994) investigated the effect of MET treatment over a 4–week period on cervical ROM. Eighteen asymptomatic subjects with limitations (10° or more) of active motion in one or more planes (rotation, side-bending, flexion or extension) were randomly assigned to either a treatment or control group. Subjects in the treatment group underwent seven treatment sessions over a 4-week period where the joint was positioned against the restrictive barrier and using three repetitions of light 5-second isometric contractions. Pre and post ROM was measured using the cervical ROM device, and the post-test range was measured one day after the last treatment session. Those subjects in the MET group achieved significant gains in rotation (approximately 8°), and smaller non-significant gains in all other planes. The control group demonstrated little change.

MET has been demonstrated to produce increases in ROM when applied to a single motion segment. Fryer & Ruszkowski (2004) examined the effect of a single application of MET directed at the rotational restriction of the atlanto-axial (AA) articulation in the cervical spine. The AA segment was chosen because, using leverages of cervical flexion and rotation, it is possible to isolate ROM to this joint. Fifty-two asymptomatic volunteers who displayed at least 4° of asymmetry in active AA rotation (rotation with the cervical spine in approximately 45° of flexion to 'lock' the lower segments) were randomly allocated to either an MET (with either a 5- or 20-second isometric contraction phase) or sham 'functional technique' treatment (control). Those in the experimental group received a single application of MET which consisted of rotating the segment to the restrictive barrier, a light isometric

Table 4.3 Overview of studies that have investigated MET for increasing spinal range of motion

Study	Treatment duration	Technique	Measurement	Findings
Schenk et al (1994)	4 weeks	MET (CR)	Cervical rotation, SB, flexion, extension	MET < baseline rotation; non-significant increases in other ranges
			Cervical ROM device (goniometer)	MET < control
Schenk et al (1997)	4 weeks	MET (CR)	Lumbar extension	MET < baseline
			Bubble goniometer	MET < control
Lenehan et al (2003)	Single application	MET (CR)	Seated trunk rotation	MET < baseline
			ARMDno3 goniometer	MET < control
Fryer & Ruszkowski (2004)	Single application	MET (CR) (5 & 20 sec duration)	Cervical (AA) rotation Compass goniometer	MET 5 sec < MET 20 sec < sham control

contraction (5 or 20 seconds) away from the barrier, relaxation and repositioning to the new barrier, performed three times. Subjects were remeasured for active AA rotation using a compass goniometer by an examiner who was blinded to the group allocation. Fryer and Ruszkowski found that MET using a 5-second contraction phase produced a significantly greater increase in the restricted direction, but not the unrestricted range, than the control group. The increase in ROM was not made at the expense of the unrestricted direction, which also made small mean increases. The 20-second isometric contraction phase MET also produced increased ROM, but appeared to be less effective than the group treated with 5-second contractions.

Schenk et al (1997), in a study design similar to their investigation of cervical ROM, examined 26 asymptomatic subjects who presented with limited active lumbar extension (less than 25°), as measured with a bubble goniometer. Those subjects assigned to the treatment group received treatment twice a week for 4 weeks, which consisted of four repetitions of a light 5-second isometric contraction, with the joint positioned against the restrictive barriers in extension, rotation, and side-bending. Those in the MET group achieved significantly increased lumbar extension (7°), whereas there was no increase in the control group. It should be noted that in both studies by Schenk et al (1994, 1997) the examiner was not blinded to the group designation of subjects, and there exists the possibility of some examiner bias.

Lenehan et al (2003) examined the immediate effect of a single application of MET to active seated trunk rotation in asymptomatic subjects. Fifty-nine subjects were randomly assigned to either the MET or control group, and blinded pre- and post-intervention measurement of trunk rotation was performed using a custom made goniometer. Subjects in the treatment group were seated and positioned with their thoracolumbar spine rotated towards the barrier of restricted rotation, and received MET consisting of four applications of 5-second isometric contraction away from the barrier, followed by a 7-second period of relaxation and repositioning to the new barrier. The MET group achieved significantly greater trunk rotation (10.7°), but not to the non-restricted side or to either side in the untreated control group.

Effect on spinal pain

Very few researchers have examined the effect of MET on spinal pain, but the few existing studies support the effectiveness of this technique. MET has been reported to be effective for reducing pain intensity and disability in subjects suffering with low-back pain (LBP). Wilson et al (2003) examined 19 patients with acute LBP (less than 12 weeks duration) who were diagnosed with a segmental lumbar flexion restriction (extended, ipsilaterally rotated and side-bent – ERS dysfunction – according to the Fryette osteopathic model) using the methods advocated by Greenman (1996), and supported by observation of restricted active flexion, extension and side-bending. Patients were excluded if they had radiating pain, paraesthesia or numbness into their buttocks or lower extremities, motor weakness, diminished or absent reflexes, previous back surgery, or chronic pain of more than 12 weeks duration. Patients assigned into the MET group received a specific MET for their lumbar dysfunction and were given a home exercise programme that included an MET self-treatment component, abdominal 'drawing in', and progressive strengthening exercises. Those patients assigned to the control group (matched for age, gender and initial Oswestry Disability scores) received a sham treatment (side-lying passive ROM) by the same practitioner who performed the MET, and the home exercise programme without the MET self-treatment component. All patients were asked to perform these exercises once a day, and were seen twice a week for 4 weeks. At each subsequent visit, patients were re-examined and the MET was performed only if the flexion restriction was present. All patients then performed a strengthening exercise programme supervised by an instructor who was blinded to the treatment allocation. Those patients treated with MET showed a significantly higher change in Oswestry Disability Index scores than the matched control patients (mean change of 83% compared with 65% for the control), and every patient treated with MET had a greater improvement than those in the control group.

In a study by Brodin (1982), a physiotherapist treated 41 LBP patients for nine sessions over 3 weeks (if required), but no details of the techniques used in the MET sessions were reported. Reduction of more than two steps in a nine-point pain scale was achieved for 17 of the MET group ($n = 21$), but for only four subjects of the control group ($n = 20$). However, the author did not offer any statistical analysis to support his conclusion that MET was effective for LBP.

Cassidy et al (1992b) compared the immediate effect of a single application of manipulation (high-velocity thrust) or MET in 100 subjects with unilateral neck pain. The MET techniques consisted of five 5-second isometric contractions with increasing rotation or side-bending of the neck. Both groups experienced small increases in ROM, but these were not significant. The manipulated group displayed a significant decrease in pain scores, whereas the MET group did not, and the authors concluded that manipulation appeared more effective than MET for pain relief. Osteopathic authors claim that MET applied to the spine requires skill and substantial experience in localising motion barriers, and it was not stated whether the chiropractors in this study were experienced in the use of this technique.

These studies support the use of MET to increase spinal ROM and improve clinical indicators of pain and disability, but further investigation of the duration of these effects and the clinical benefit to symptomatic individuals is needed.

Research into the mechanisms of therapeutic effect

Myofascial extensibility

The physiological mechanisms behind the changes in muscle extensibility produced by MET – as well as those produced by passive stretching – remain controversial. Of the three most studied mechanisms that have been proposed to account for the short- and medium-term changes in muscle extensibility – reflex relaxation, viscoelastic or muscle property change, and changes to stretch tolerance – a change to tolerance to stretching is most supported by the scientific literature.

Reflex muscle relaxation

Many authors have proposed that MET and PNF techniques facilitate stretching by producing neurological reflex muscle relaxation following isometric muscle contraction (Osternig et al 1987, Kuchera & Kuchera 1992, Mitchell & Mitchell 1995, Greenman 1996). Muscle relaxation following contraction has been proposed to occur by activation of the golgi tendon organs and their inhibitory influence on the a-motor neuron pool, or due to reciprocal inhibition produced by contraction of a muscle antagonist (Kuchera & Kuchera 1992). Although it is accepted that these reflex pathways exist, their role in postisometric relaxation has not been established.

Several studies have lent support for the concept of neurological muscle relaxation in MET by providing evidence of a strong, brief neuromuscular inhibition following isometric muscle contraction. Moore & Kukulka (1991) examined H-reflexes (an indicator of a-motor neuron pool excitability) of the soleus muscle in 16 subjects who performed isometric (65–75% maximal) plantar flexion contractions. Monitoring of the tibialis anterior muscle EMG activity revealed minimal activity, consistent with rest, to exclude the possibility of reciprocal inhibition. The researchers found that a strong brief depression of the soleus H-reflex occurred in all subjects and lasted for about 10 seconds, with maximal depression between 0.1 and 1 second post contraction, which was attributed to pre-synaptic inhibition.

Similarly, Etnyre and Abraham (1986b) found that static stretching of the soleus muscle reduced the H-reflex only slightly, whereas CR and CRAC produced profound inhibition of the reflex. The H-reflex in the CR group increased to values similar to those of the stretching group 2 seconds post contraction, but there was only a slight increase towards baseline after 2 seconds following the CRAC technique. Carter et al (2000) found that three repetitions of 7-second CR produced decreased biceps femoris EMG activity in response to a sudden stretch, compared with a control group.

Gandevia et al (1999) used transmastoid electrical stimulation to assess motor neuron activity before and after a maximal isometric contraction of the elbow flexor muscles. The researchers found an immediate reduction to approximately half of the pre-contraction value that lasted for about 2 minutes, and occurred regardless of whether the isometric contraction was performed for the duration of 5 seconds or 2 minutes. The responses to transmastoid stimulation showed no depression when the muscle and motor neurons were activated by stimulation of the peripheral nerve, which indicated that the depressed responses were likely to involve corticospinal axons and their actions on the motor neuron synapse.

These studies support the proposition that MET may produce reflex inhibition to the a-motor neuron pool, and is consistent with many protocols which recommend 5–10 seconds of stretching following isometric contraction. While these studies suggest that MET may have the potential to produce reflex relaxation, evidence of a decrease in EMG activity following the use of MET is needed before accepting neurological inhibition as a likely mechanism.

In order for the proposal that MET produces increased muscle length by reflex muscle relaxation to be plausible, it should also be established that low-level motor activity plays a role in limiting the passive stretch of a muscle. Many studies have demonstrated, however, that active motor activity appears to have little role in producing resistance to stretch when relaxed muscles are passively stretched. The hamstring muscles have been shown to demonstrate a low-level EMG response when undergoing static stretch (Magnusson et al 1995, 1996b, 1996d), which has been described as having an amplitude of below 1% (when peak torque was 23% of maximal voluntary contraction), and therefore it is unlikely that muscle activity contributes significantly to passive peak torque (passive resistance to stretch) (Magnusson et al 1996b). Furthermore, several studies have demonstrated that increases in muscle length following 90 seconds of passive stretching occur without any change to the low-level EMG activity of that muscle (Magnusson et al 1996b, 1996d). Additionally, one study found that the decline in resistance to stretch and lack of EMG activity were similar in subjects with spinal cord injury (with loss of motor control in their lower extremities) and normal controls (Magnusson et al 1996d).

Given that neurological motor activity appears not to play a role in passive resistance to stretch, it is not surprising that researchers have found that MET and PNF techniques do not decrease the low-level EMG activity associated with muscle stretching. Magnusson et al (1995) found that the low-level EMG response of the hamstrings was unchanged within 60 seconds after 40 maximal-effort, repetitive hamstring contractions (concentric or eccentric) prior to the second stretch. In a later study, Magnusson et al (1996c) compared the effects of passive stretching (80 seconds) and a 6-second forceful isometric contraction of the hamstrings (in a position of stretch, followed by 80 seconds of stretch) on ROM and hamstring EMG. They found that the low-level EMG activity was unchanged after both stretching procedures.

Osternig et al (1987) examined the effect of static stretching, CR and ACR on hamstring extensibility and EMG activity in 10 subjects. Five trials of both CR (5-second maximal contraction followed by stretching, performed three times) and ACR (5-second maximal quadriceps contraction followed by stretching, performed three times) were used, and the passive stretching treatment was performed for 80 seconds. Static stretching produced a small decrease (11%) in hamstring EMG response between the first and second application, whereas CR and ACR produced *increases* in hamstring EMG activity. In the final trial for each technique, passive stretching produced a mean EMG activity of 10 mV, CR produced 15 mV, and ACR produced 25 mV, all recorded during the stretch (relaxation) phase of the respective techniques.

In a later study, Osternig et al (1990) found the same pattern of EMG activity in different athlete populations, with ACR producing greater ROM and greater hamstring EMG activity than either CR or static stretching (89% and 110% greater EMG activity, respectively). Similarly, Ferber et al (2002b) examined the effects of static hamstring stretching, CR and ACR in a population of older adults (50–75 years). The authors found that ACR produced greater ROM as well as greater hamstring EMG activity than the CR and stretching groups (65% and 119%, respectively). The authors of both these studies concluded that factors other than muscle relaxation were responsible for the greater muscle extensibility and ROM that resulted from PNF techniques.

It appears clear from the evidence that neurological EMG activity in the hamstring muscles does not contribute to resistance to passive stretching, and although MET techniques produce greater ROM changes than static stretching, they paradoxically produce greater EMG activity in the muscle undergoing the stretch. It seems reasonable to conclude that increased extensibility must occur due to other factors, such as viscoelastic change or increase to stretch tolerance.

Viscoelastic or muscle property change

Connective tissues display mechanical properties relating to their fluid or gel components (viscous) and their elastic properties, called viscoelasticity. Connective tissue elongation is time and history dependent, and if a constant stretching force is loaded on a tissue, the tissue will respond with slow elongation or 'creep'. The tissue creep results in loss of energy (hysteresis), and repetition of loading before the tissue has recovered will result in greater deformation (Norkin & Levangie 1992). Additional loading may cause more permanent 'plastic' change, which is caused by microtearing of collagen fibres (which would cause an immediate change in the stiffness of the tissue) and subsequent remodelling of fibres to a longer length (Lederman 1997).

Isometric muscle contraction has been found to produce similar reductions in tissue tension as produced by passive stretching. Taylor et al (1997) measured the tensile load changes in the tibialis anterior muscles of eight rabbits by measuring passive tension at neutral length, and using a silk suture implanted from the muscle origin to the dorsum of the foot to measure muscle length. One hind limb of each rabbit was randomly assigned to a repeated muscular contraction group, and the other limb to a repeated passive stretching group. These researchers found that both muscle contraction and muscle stretching resulted in passive tension reductions of similar magnitude, indicating viscoelastic stress relaxation of the muscle–tendon unit. Taylor et al reasoned that for a muscle to stay the same length during an isometric contraction, the connective tissues must undergo lengthening to compensate for contractile element shortening. They suggested that a combination of

contractions and stretches (as used in MET) might be more effective for producing viscoelastic change than passive stretching alone, because the greater forces could produce increased viscoelastic change and passive extensibility.

Lederman (1997) noted that myofascial structures have two distinct connective tissue arrangements: elastic 'parallel' fibres, arranged parallel to the muscle fibres, and the stiffer 'in series' fibres that lie perpendicular to muscle fibres and found mainly at the tendinous junctions. Lederman proposed that passive stretching would elongate the parallel fibres but have little effect on the 'in series' fibres; however, the addition of an isometric contraction would place loading on these fibres to produce viscoelastic or plastic change above and beyond that achieved by passive stretching alone (Figs 4.1 and 4.2).

Stretch and isometric contraction of connective tissues may affect the water content and produce

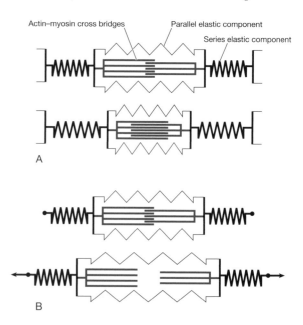

Figure 4.1 Changes in the connective tissue element of the muscle during muscle contraction and passive stretching. **A** During contraction, the series elastic components are under tension and elongate, whilst the tension in the parallel elastic components is reduced. **B** During passive stretching, both the parallel and elastic components are under tension. However, the less stiff parallel fibres will elongate more than the series component. (The separation between the actin and myosin has been exaggerated.)

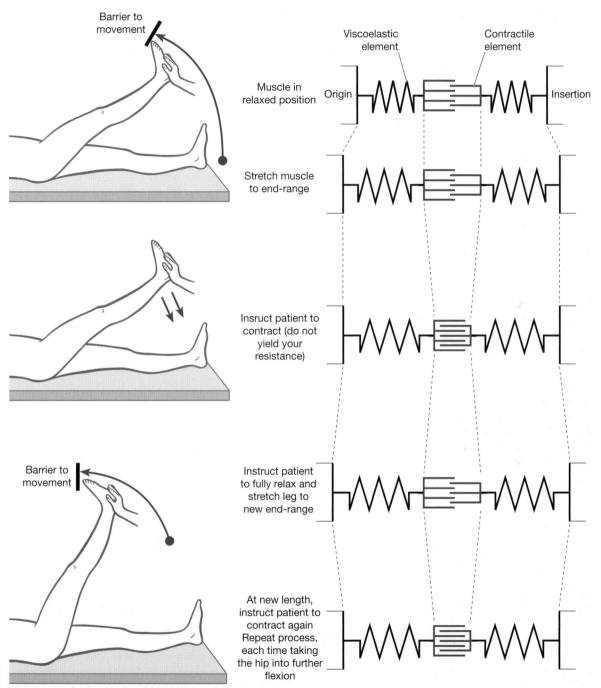

Figure 4.2   Sequence of active muscle stretching.

subsequent alteration to the length and stiffness of the tissue. Lanir et al (1988) investigated the mechanism of viscoelastic change in rat collagen fibre bundles following stretch. Under high-strain loads, the researchers found that there was an initial reduction in fibre diameter due to loss of water and glycosaminoglycan molecules (GAG), followed by a swelling of the fibre beyond its initial diameter. Similarly, Yahia et al (1993) examined the viscoelastic properties of human lumbodorsal fascia and found tissue stiffness increased after successive stretching (initial, 30 minutes and 1 hour later), and that greater loads were required to deform (lengthen) the tissue on subsequent stretch applications. Schleip et al (2004) extended this work and found a 'sponge' effect following stretch, where water was squeezed out of the fascia during stretching, but recovered in a few minutes. If the stretch was strong enough and a rest period long enough, water continued to soak into the ground substance to swell the fibre and increase its elastic stiffness. An increase in the water content of a ligament has been demonstrated to increase pre-stress (tension when only slightly loaded) and decrease (shorten) the functional length of the ligament (Thornton et al 2001). The clinical implications of these findings are unclear. Schleip et al (2004) proposed that this hydration effect might have a role in the therapeutic action of stretching and connective tissue manipulation by increasing the tissue water content to alter the stiffness and mechanical property of the tissue. Lanir et al (1988), however, suggested that the fibre swelling was a result of weakening of the structural elements of the isolated fibre in vitro, and that this might not occur in living tissue because the collagen fibres are tightly packed and isolated by the membranic epitenon. The 'sponge effect' is an interesting phenomenon, which may have a role in tissue texture change following MET or connective tissue manipulation, and warrants further research.

Most researchers who have reported ROM gains following passive stretching of the hamstring muscles have monitored hamstring length using PKE and have not measured the passive torque (force applied to produce the stretch) applied to the muscles (Bandy & Irion 1994, Bandy et al 1997, Feland et al 2001b). Similarly, most researchers who have reported ROM gains following CR or AKE have used methods such as AKE (Gribble et al 1999, Spernoga et al 2001), sit-and-reach (Stopka et al 2002), PKE (Wallin et al 1985, Handel et al 1997, Ferber et al 2002b), and SLR (Burke et al 2001) without measurement of passive torque. Measurement of ROM without passive torque provides no indication of a change in muscle property (change

in the biomechanical structure of the muscle) because there is no way of determining whether the same amount of torque (force used to passively stretch the muscle) was used in pre- and post-measurements. For example, when using PKE to the point of discomfort or knee buckling, there is no way to be certain that the force used to stretch and measure the hamstrings was the same as before the treatment intervention. Similarly, when using AKE, there is no certainty that the subject did not use greater active muscle effort during the post-treatment measure. Only with a measurement of torque can passive stretching force be kept consistent pre and post intervention, and information gained about any change to the property of muscle tissue.

Evidence of lasting viscoelastic change, however, has been hard to demonstrate in human muscle. Researchers who have investigated the effect of passive stretching on hamstring extensibility using torque-controlled PKE have found little evidence of any lasting change to tissue property. Magnusson et al (1996a) examined the effect of five consecutive 90-second static stretches on stiffness and energy of the hamstring muscle, measuring passive torque, velocity and ROM in a seated PKE. They found that stiffness, energy and passive torque all significantly declined between the first and fifth passive stretch, indicating viscoelastic stress relaxation, but these variables returned to baseline when tested 1 hour later. Similarly, Magnusson et al (2000) tested the effect of three consecutive 45-second stretches separated by 30 seconds – a realistic stretching protocol – on viscoelastic stress relaxation of the hamstrings unit. They found that although each of the 45-second stretches produced some viscoelastic change, each stretch did not affect the resistance of the subsequent stretch 30 seconds later. In other words, viscoelastic stress relaxation was so transient that the energy loss was recovered in the 30-second rest period between the stretches. Other studies have confirmed the lack of viscoelastic stress relaxation following stretching protocols (Magnusson et al 1996b, 1998).

Similarly, it appears that MET produces little immediate viscoelastic change in the hamstring muscles. Magnusson et al (1996c) and Ballantyne et al (2003) both measured PKE and passive torque following an MET contraction to the hamstrings and found little evidence of viscoelastic change. Both studies did find that MET produced significant ROM gains, but only when the passive torque was increased to stretch the hamstrings to the point of discomfort, which indicated that this increase was not due to a change in muscle property.

It seems possible that both passive stretching and MET may produce tissue property change in certain groups of people using certain protocols. An example of this might be ballet dancers or gymnasts, who often appear to have muscle and joint flexibility well in excess of normal ranges. It could be that relentless stretching, particularly in a growing teenager, might achieve greater and lasting ROM increases than when performed less vigorously by a mature adult. This is speculative, but research into the training and joint flexibility of these elite groups of athletes may shed light on what is required to produce permanent increases in joint flexibility and muscle extensibility. Research into the effect of MET on the recovery of injured muscles may also reveal evidence of tissue property change, because it is feasible that MET may help realign maturing connective tissue along lines of force, and break poorly aligned cross-linkages. Hopefully we may see research in these fields in the future.

Stretch tolerance

Despite the lack of evidence of viscoelastic change in human muscle following either passive stretching or MET, many studies have reported ROM gains. The majority of studies that have found increased ROM following passive hamstring stretching have not measured the passive torque used to extend the muscle, and so have not provided evidence of a change in the physical property of the muscle (Bandy & Irion 1994, Bandy et al 1997, Feland et al 2001b). If viscoelastic change is not responsible for the increased muscle extensibility, what could be the cause? PKE (when passive torque is not measured) and AKE are usually performed to the point of hamstring tension or pain. Magnusson et al (1996b, 1998) measured the passive torque of the hamstring muscle during PKE before and after the muscle was stretched (90 seconds) to the point of pain, and

they found that both ROM and passive torque were increased following the stretch. In other words, no change to the physical property of the muscle occurred, but subjects were able to tolerate a stronger stretch.

Ballantyne et al (2003) similarly found that MET (5-second moderate force contraction, 3-second stretch and relaxation, performed four times) applied to the hamstrings produced no evidence of viscoelastic change, but when the PKE was taken to pain tolerance (pre and post MET), a greater passive torque was tolerated post MET that allowed a subsequent increase in ROM. Magnusson et al (1996c) compared the effect of a 90-second passive stretch and stretching with the addition of a 6-second CR contraction and found no change in EMG activity or viscoelastic property. They did find that both ROM and passive torque increased – indicating an increase in stretch tolerance – and that the CR produced significantly more ROM and passive torque than the passive stretch.

The results of the study by Magnusson et al (1996c), and the fact that many studies have found that MET produced greater ROM gain than passive stretching, strongly suggest that MET methods produce a greater change in stretch tolerance than passive stretching. The application of MET would appear to decrease an individual's perception of muscle pain and is greater than that which occurs with passive stretching. Stretching and isometric contraction stimulate muscle and joint mechanoreceptors and proprioceptors, and it is possible that this may attenuate the sensation of pain. According to Melzack and Wall's 'gate control theory' (1965), stimulation of large-diameter mechanoreceptors produces inhibition of the incoming messages of pain at the dorsal horn of the spinal cord. MET and stretching appear to produce lasting changes in stretch tolerance, and so the mechanism is likely to be more complex than just gating at the spinal cord, and may also involve changes in the higher centres of the CNS.

The fact that it appears that MET does not have an obvious effect on the viscoelastic property of muscle tissue does not mean that it has no clinical relevance for enhancing stretching and performance. A change in stretch tolerance may help condition and prepare the muscle in preparation for athletic activity. It is also possible that if MET can alter neurological pain mechanisms more strongly than passive stretching, it may also have a role in improving joint and muscle proprioception for improved coordination and performance. Hopefully we will see studies in the future that examine the effect of MET on sporting performance and injury prevention.

Spinal dysfunction

Increase in range of motion

A small number of studies have demonstrated that MET can produce increased ROM in the cervical, thoracic and lumbar spine (Schenk et al 1994, Schenk et al 1997, Lenehan et al 2003, Fryer & Ruszkowski 2004). All these studies examined the effect of MET on active ROM where no measure of passive torque could be made, and so little can be concluded regarding the possible mechanism behind the increased range of motion. Changes to the viscoelasticity of segmental muscles or periarticular tissues are unlikely given the evidence relating to stretching and hamstring extensibility. The lighter loads applied to spinal tissues (most authors of MET recommend positioning the spinal segment at the 'first' or 'featheredge' restrictive barrier) would mean there is little loading on tissues to produce viscoelastic or plastic change. The theory of reflex muscle relaxation following MET applied to muscles is not supported by evidence (discussed above), and no study has examined changes to paraspinal muscle EMG activity or reflex relaxation following spinal MET. Given that only active spinal ROM has been reported to increase, it seems likely that a change in stretch tolerance (as appears to be the case when stretching muscles) may be responsible for spinal ROM gains.

Decrease in pain

The few studies that have examined the effect of MET on spinal pain (Brodin 1982, Cassidy et al 1992b; Wilson et al 2003) offer support for the hypoalgesic effects of this technique. This research is consistent with the evidence of mechanisms behind MET for increasing muscle extensibility, where it appears that MET reduces the pain sensitivity (stretch tolerance) of treated muscles.

How might MET reduce pain? There is growing evidence of the hypoalgesic effect of a number of manual therapy techniques. Fryer et al (2004a) demonstrated that both spinal manipulation and mobilisation decreased thoracic pain sensitivity to pressure, with mobilising appearing to be more effective. Studies by Sterling et al (2001) and Vicenzino et al (1998) have shown increases in pain thresholds in both symptomatic and asymptomatic subjects following posterior–anterior mobilisation applied to the cervical spine. Vicenzino et al (1996) also confirmed increases in pain thresholds occurring at sites remote from the application of mobilisation. These researchers found that mobilisation at the level of C5/6 in subjects with lateral epicondylitis produced a resultant increase in pressure pain thresholds of up to 25% at the head of the radius. A number of studies have reported cervical manipulation to be effective for pain relief (Cassidy et al 1992a, 1992b, van Schalkwyk & Parkin-Smith 2000), with one study finding pain reduction in as many as 85% of subjects (Cassidy et al 1992b).

The exact mechanism of pain relief from manual techniques is unclear, but it has been suggested that pain is modulated at either the spinal cord or in the higher centres of the central nervous system (Wright 1995, Shacklock 1999). Manipulation has been proposed to affect pain processing at the spinal cord level via the gate control theory (Melzack & Wall 1965). According to this theory, passive joint mobilisation and manipulation would stimulate joint and muscle mechanoreceptors, which would modulate and inhibit the incoming pain information at the dorsal horn of the spinal cord and potentially provide pain relief (Melzack & Wall 1965). Descending inhibition of pain from higher centres in the CNS, particularly from the dorsal periaqueductal grey region (dPAG), may also play a role in manipulation-induced hypoalgesia. Stimulation of the dPAG produces a profound and selective analgesia (Kandel et al 2000), and because manipulation has been shown to produce concurrent sympathetic stimulation (another function of the dPAG), it has been proposed that spinal manipulative therapy may exert its initial effects by activating this region (Wright 1995, Vincenzino et al 1998).

It is quite plausible that MET may exert a strong effect on pain perception. This may be true of its use in muscle stretching as well as when applied to spinal dysfunction in subjects with spinal pain. Once again, more research is needed to determine the effects of MET on patients with spinal and non-spinal sites of pain.

Other possible effects

Many osteopathic authors have described detailed and specific MET to address intervertebral dysfunction (also known as somatic dysfunction or segmental dysfunction) (Mitchell & Mitchell 1995, Greenman 1996, DiGiovanna & Schiowitz 1997). Somatic dysfunction has been defined by the Educational Council on Osteopathic Principles (1981) as: 'Impaired or altered function of related components of the somatic (body framework) system: skeletal, arthrodial, and myofascial structures, and related vascular, lymphatic, and neural elements' (p 1138).

Authors in the field of osteopathy claim that intervertebral dysfunction can be detected by manual palpation and corrected with skilled manipulation (Greenman 1996, DiGiovanna & Schiowitz 1997, Kappler 1997, Kuchera et al 1997). The diagnostic indicators of segmental dysfunction are said to be segmental asymmetry of bony landmarks, range of motion abnormality (increased, decreased or a change in quality), and tissue texture changes (Kuchera & Kuchera 1992, Greenman 1996). Some authors also include tenderness (DiGiovanna & Schiowitz 1997, Kuchera et al 1997). The acronym 'TART' is sometimes used as a memory aid for the features of tissue texture, asymmetry, range of motion abnormality and tenderness.

Part of the problem in assessing the evidence of the therapeutic action of MET in the spine is that the nature and pathophysiology of intervertebral dysfunction is unknown (Fryer 2003). Intervertebral dysfunction may not necessarily produce obvious spinal pain or restrict gross ROM. Unfortunately the reliability for the detection of intervertebral dysfunction has not been established. Many studies have demonstrated the poor reliability for motion palpation (Harrison et al 1998), palpation of static asymmetry (Freburger &

Riddle 1999, O'Haire & Gibbons 2000, Spring et al 2001), and for where to manipulate (French et al 2000, Hestboek & Leboeuf 2000). Palpation for tenderness and examination for symptomatic joints using pain provocation appear to be the most reliable clinical methods (Jull et al 1988, 1997, Boline et al 1993, Hubka & Phelan 1994, Phillips & Twomey 1996). It is not possible to examine the effectiveness of treating intervertebral dysfunction with techniques like MET until there are objective characteristics of its pathophysiology or reliable methods to detect it. Measures such as pain sensitivity and ROM are likely, but unproven, indicators of dysfunction.

It is possible that intervertebral dysfunction may produce disturbances in proprioception and motor control that may potentially be improved by manual techniques such as MET. It has been proposed that intervertebral dysfunction could be initiated by minor trauma to the intervertebral joint complex and injury to the zygapophysial joint, the annulus fibrosis and periarticular soft tissues, creating signs of somatic dysfunction such as tissue texture changes (periarticular inflammation) and ROM changes (synovial effusion of the zygapophysial joint). Minor injury would trigger nociceptor (pain receptor) activity, and in addition to tenderness and possible awareness of pain, nociception may create a regional proprioceptive deficit and changes in segmental motor control (Fryer 2003).

There is growing evidence that pain interferes with normal proprioception. Researchers have demonstrated that patients suffering with pain display decreased awareness of direction of lumbar motion and position (Gill & Callaghan 1998, Taimela et al 1999, Leinonen et al 2002), and cutaneous touch perception (Voerman et al 2000, Stohler et al 2001). It has been proposed that intervertebral sprains that activate nociceptors in any spinal structure would activate nociceptive pathways and may lead to a reduction in the proprioceptive input from that segment (Fryer 2003). In addition, spinal pain appears to produce changes in paraspinal muscle activity, by inhibiting the deeper 'stabilising' paraspinal musculature, while changing the control of the more superficial spinal muscles to overreact to stimuli at times when the muscles should be relatively silent (Fryer et al 2004b, 2004c). The resulting loss of regional proprioception and altered motor control is likely to affect segmental stability and predispose the segment to further strain following trivial trauma.

It is possible that improvements in proprioception and motor control may underlie both short- and long-term benefits for patients receiving manual therapy. MET applied to the spine involves applying specific leverages and localisation to spinal articulations, and carefully controlled, purposeful isometric muscle contraction from the patient. This has been proposed to stimulate joint proprioceptors, highlight a different pattern of afferent activity in the proprioceptive-impaired region, and allow the CNS to normalise the proprioceptive and motor coordination from that segment (Fryer 2000, 2003). Patients often volunteer feelings of being more 'balanced', with the painful region 'back in place' and 'part of the body again', following treatment. Such comments could be attributed to a placebo response, but also suggest an improvement in proprioception and motor control.

There is limited evidence to suggest that manual treatment can produce improvements in proprioception and control, but no study has yet investigated the effect of MET in this area. Cervical manipulation (high-velocity thrust) has been reported to improve head repositioning after active displacement in patients with chronic neck pain (Rogers 1997), and patients with vertigo and dizziness (Heikkila et al 2000). Cervical mobilisation has been demonstrated to improve body sway in patients with whiplash trauma (Karlberg et al 1991), and decrease superficial neck muscle recruitment during staged cervical flexion (Sterling et al 2001). It would be interesting to see comparisons between MET and these more passive techniques (manipulation and mobilisation) because it is feasible that the active participation of the patient may produce greater changes in proprioceptive feedback, motor control and motor learning.

MET has been proposed to be useful for promoting fluid drainage and relieving tissue congestion (Mitchell & Mitchell 1995, Greenman 1996, Goodridge & Kuchera 1997). Minor injury to the intervertebral joint complex may produce tissue damage and inflammation, resulting in fluid congestion in the periarticular tissues which could present as palpable tissue texture change and alteration of joint end-feel. Active muscle contraction and relaxation has a strong effect on lymphatic and venous drainage (Lederman 1997), and MET may act to relieve periarticular congestion to improve tissue texture and joint mobility. Although this proposal appears reasonable, it is likely to remain speculative because of the difficulty in examining changes to deep paraspinal fluid drainage.

Directions for research

Myofascial extensibility

MET and similar isometric stretching techniques appear to be more effective for producing greater muscle extensibility than passive stretching, but the most efficacious type of application remains uncertain. CRAC and ACR appear to be more effective than CR methods for this purpose, but the optimal passive torque for stretching, the force and duration of isometric contraction, and number of repetitions all need to be determined. The length of treatment effect and influence on sporting injuries also requires study. Additionally, it would be useful to examine whether any particular stretching programme, or the application of a programme in a younger age group, is able to produce change to the muscle property (viscoelastic or plastic change), rather than just a change in tolerance to stretch.

Application to spinal dysfunction

More research is required to evaluate the clinical usefulness of MET in treating spinal dysfunction and pain. There is growing evidence that MET can increase spinal ROM in individuals with restricted ROM, but most of these studies have examined asymptomatic subjects, and the relevance of asymmetrical ROM to clinical problems is presently only speculative. There is a need to examine the effectiveness of MET in treating symptomatic subjects, and comparing the efficacy of this technique to other manual interventions. Researchers could examine the effect of MET on pain using either technical means (pressure algometry) or self-reported pain and disability, and compare this method to other manual and conventional treatments. The possibility of MET improving proprioception, stability and motor control is an avenue that may yield promising results.

Mechanisms of therapeutic effect

The mechanisms behind the therapeutic effect of MET warrant investigation, although the first concern to researchers and practitioners alike should be to establish clinical efficacy. Passive torque could be examined to establish whether increased ROM following MET is a result of increased stretch tolerance (as appears to be the case in muscle stretching) or whether there is evidence of biomechanical change. Examination of MET applied to a painful spinal segment using pressure algometry may establish whether the hypoalgesic effects are localised to the treated site (suggesting a spinal cord reflex) or more general (suggesting descending inhibition of pain).

MET is a manual technique that is being widely adopted because it appears safe and gentle and is believed to be effective. If the research base that supports this technique can be broadened and evidence of its efficacy in patients with a variety of symptoms can be established, the popularity of MET will justifiably increase for the benefit of practitioners and patients alike.

References

Ballantyne F, Fryer G, McLaughlin P 2003 The effect of muscle energy technique on hamstring extensibility: the mechanism of altered flexibility. Journal of Osteopathic Medicine 6(2): 59–63

Bandy W D, Irion J M 1994 The effect of time on static stretch on the flexibility of the hamstring muscles. Physical Therapy 74(9): 845–850

Bandy W D, Irion J M, Briggler M 1997 The effect of time and frequency of static stretching on flexibility of the hamstring muscles. Physical Therapy 77: 1090–1096

Boline P D, Haas M, Meyer J J et al 1993 Interexaminer reliability of eight evaluative dimensions of lumbar segmental abnormality: Part 2. Journal of Manipulative and Physiological Therapeutics 16: 363–374

Bourdillon J F, Day E A, Bookhout M R 1992 Spinal manipulation, 5th edn. Butterworth-Heinemann, Oxford

Brodin H 1982 Lumbar treatment using the muscle energy technique. Osteopathic Annals 10(12): 23–24

Burke D G, Holt L E, Rasmussen R et al 2001 Effects of hot or cold water immersion and modified proprioceptive neuromuscular facilitation flexibility exercise on hamstring length. Journal of Athletic Training 36(1): 16–19

Carter A et al 2000 Proprioceptive neuromuscular facilitation decreases muscle activity during the stretch reflex in selected posterior thigh muscles. Journal of Sport Rehabilitation 9: 269–278

Cassidy D J, Quon J A, Lafrance L J et al 1992a The effect of manipulation on pain and range of motion in the cervical spine: a pilot study. Journal of Manipulative and Physiological Therapeutics 15: 495–500

Cassidy D J, Lopes A A, Yong-Hing K 1992b The immediate effect of manipulation versus mobilization on pain and range of motion in the cervical spine: a randomized controlled trial. Journal of Manipulative and Physiological Therapeutics 15: 570–575

Chaitow L 1997 Muscle energy techniques. Churchill Livingstone, Edinburgh

Cornelius W L, Ebrahim K, Watson J et al 1992 The effects of cold application and modified PNF stretching techniques on hip joint flexibility in college males. Research Quarterly in Exercise and Sport 63(3): 311–314

DiGiovanna E L, Schiowitz S 1997 An osteopathic approach to diagnosis and treatment, 2nd edn. Lippincott, Philadelphia

DiGiovanna E L, Schiowitz S, Dowling D J 2005 An Osteopathic Approach to Diagnosis & Treatment, 3rd ed. Philadelphia: Lippincott William & Wilkins

Educational Council on Osteopathic Principles of the American Association of Colleges of Osteopathic Medicine 1981 Glossary of osteopathic terminology. In: Ward R C (ed.) 1997 Foundations for osteopathic medicine. Williams & Wilkins, Baltimore, p 1138

Etnyre B R, Abraham L D 1986a Gains in range of ankle dorsiflexion using three popular stretching techniques. American Journal of Physical Medicine 65(4): 189–196

Etnyre B R, Abraham L D 1986b H-reflex changes during static stretching and two variations of proprioceptive neuromuscular facilitation techniques. Electroencephalography and Clinical Neurophysiology 63(2): 174–179

Feland J B, Marin H N 2004 Effect of submaximal contraction intensity in contract–relax proprioceptive neuromuscular facilitation stretching. British Journal of Sports Medicine 38(4): E18

Feland J B, Myrer J W, Merrill R M 2001a Acute changes in hamstring flexibility: PNF versus static stretch in senior athletes. Physical Therapy in Sport 2(4): 186–193

Feland J B, Myrer J W, Schulthies S S et al 2001b The effect of duration of stretching of the hamstring muscle group for increasing range of motion in people aged 65 years or older. Physical Therapy 81: 1100–1117

Ferber R, Gravelle D C, Osternig L R 2002a Effect of proprioceptive neuromuscular facilitation stretch techniques on trained and untrained older adults. Journal of Aging and Physical Activity 10: 132–142

Ferber R, Osternig L R, Gravelle D C 2002b Effect of PNF stretch techniques on knee flexor muscle EMG activity in older adults. Journal of Electromyography and Kinesiology 12: 391–397

Freburger J K, Riddle D L 1999 Measurement of sacroiliac dysfunction: a multicenter intertester reliability study. Physical Therapy 79(12): 1134–1141

French S D, Green S, Forbes A 2000 Reliability of chiropractic methods commonly used to detect manipulable lesions in patients with chronic low-back pain. Journal of Manipulative and Physiological Therapeutics 23(4): 231–238

Fryer G 2000 Muscle energy concepts – a need for change. Journal of Osteopathic Medicine 3(2): 54–59

Fryer G 2003 Intervertebral dysfunction: a discussion of the manipulable spinal lesion. Journal of Osteopathic Medicine 6(2): 64–73

Fryer G, Ruszkowski W 2004 The influence of contraction duration in muscle energy technique applied to the atlanto-axial joint. Journal of Osteopathic Medicine 7(2): 79–84

Fryer G, Carub J, McIver S 2004a The effect of manipulation and mobilisation on pressure pain thresholds in the thoracic spine. Journal of Osteopathic Medicine 7(1): 8–14

Fryer G, Morris T, Gibbons P 2004b Paraspinal muscles and intervertebral dysfunction, Part 1. Journal of Manipulative and Physiological Therapeutics 27(4): 267–274

Fryer G, Morris T, Gibbons P 2004c Paraspinal muscles and intervertebral dysfunction, Part 2. Journal of Manipulative and Physiological Therapeutics 27(5): 348–357

Funk D C, Swank A M, Mikla B M et al 2003 Impact of prior exercise on hamstring flexibility: a comparison of proprioceptive neuromuscular facilitation and static stretching. Journal of Strength and Conditioning Research 17(3): 489–492

Gandevia S C, Peterson N, Butler J E, Taylor J L 1999 Impaired response of human motorneurones to corticospinal stimulation after voluntary exercise. Journal of Physiology 521(3): 749–759

Gibbons P, Tehan P 1998 Muscle energy concepts and coupled motion of the spine. Manual Therapy 3(2): 95–101

Gill K P, Callaghan M J 1998 The measurement of lumbar proprioception in individuals with and without low back pain. Spine 23(3): 371–377

Godges J J, Mattson-Bell M, Thorpe D et al 2003 The immediate effects of soft tissue mobilisation with proprioceptive neuromuscular facilitation on glenohumeral external rotation and overhead reach. Journal of Orthopaedic and Sports Physical Therapy 33: 713–718

Goodridge J P 1997 Muscle energy technique procedures. In: Ward R C (ed) Foundations for osteopathic medicine. Williams & Wilkins, Baltimore, pp 691–696

Goodridge J P, Kuchera W A 1997 Muscle energy treatment techniques for specific areas. In: Ward R C (ed) Foundations for osteopathic medicine. Williams & Wilkins, Baltimore, pp 697–761

Greenman P E 1996 Principles of manual medicine, 2nd edn. Williams & Wilkins, Baltimore

Greenman P E 2003 Principles of Manual Medicine, 3rd ed. Philadelphia: Lippincott William & Wilkins

Gribble P A, Guskiewicz K M, Prentice W E et al 1999 Effects of static and hold-relax stretching on hamstring range of motion using the FlexAbility LE1000. Journal of Sport Rehabilitation 8: 195–208

Handel M, Horstmann T, Dickhuth H H et al 1997 Effects of contract-relax stretching training on muscle performance in athletes. European Journal Applied Physiology 76(5): 400–408

Harrison D E, Harrison D D, Troyanovich S J 1998 Motion palpation: it's time to accept the evidence (Commentary). Journal of Manipulative and Physiological Therapeutics 21(8): 568–571

Heikkila H, Johansson M, Wenngren B I 2000 Effects of acupuncture, cervical manipulation and NSAID therapy on dizziness and impaired head positioning of suspected cervical origin: a pilot study. Manual Therapy 5(3): 151–157

Hestboek L, Leboeuf-Y de C 2000 Are chiropractic tests for the lumbo-pelvic spine reliable and valid? A systematic critical literature review. Journal of Manipulative and Physiological Therapeutics 23(4): 258–275

Hubka M J, Phelan S P 1994 Interexaminer reliability of palpation for cervical spine tenderness. Journal of Manipulative and Physiological Therapeutics 17: 591–594

Jull G A, Bogduk N, Marsland A 1988 The accuracy of manual diagnosis for cervical zygapophysial joint pain syndromes. Medical Journal of Australia 148: 233–236

Jull G A, Zito G, Trott P et al 1997 Inter-examiner reliability to detect painful upper cervical joint dysfunction. Australian Journal of Physiotherapy 43(2): 125–129

Kandel E R, Schwartz J H, Jessell T M 2000 Principles of neural science, 4th edn. McGraw-Hill, New York

Kappler R E 1997 Palpatory skills. In: Ward R C (ed) Foundations for osteopathic medicine. Williams & Wilkins, Baltimore, pp 473–477

Karlberg M, Magnusson M, Malmstrom E M et al 1991 Postural and symptomatic improvement after physiotherapy in patients with dizziness of suspected cervical origin. Archives Physical Medicine and Rehabilitation 72: 288–291

Klein D A, Stone W J, Phillips W T et al 2002 PNF training and physical function in assisted-living older adults. Journal of Aging and Physical Activity 10: 476–488

Kuchera M L, Jones J M, Kappler R E et al 1997 Musculoskeletal examination for somatic dysfunction. In: Ward R C (ed) Foundations for osteopathic medicine. Williams & Wilkins, Baltimore

Kuchera W A, Kuchera M L 1992 Osteopathic principles in practice. Kirksville College of Osteopathic Medicine Press, Missouri

Lanir Y, Salant E L, Foux A 1988 Physio-chemical and microstructural changes in collagen fibre bundles following stretching in-vitro. Biorheology 25: 591–603

Lederman E 1997 Fundamentals of manual therapy. Churchill Livingstone, London

Lederman E 2005 The Science and Practice of Manual Therapy, 2nd ed. Edinburgh: Elsevier Churchill Livingstone

Leinonen V, Maatta S, Taimela S et al 2002 Impaired lumbar movement perception in association with postural stability and motor- and somatosensory-evoked potentials in lumbar spinal stenosis. Spine 27(9): 975–983

Lenehan K L, Fryer G, McLaughlin P 2003 The effect of muscle energy technique on gross trunk range of motion. Journal of Osteopathic Medicine 6(1): 13–18

Lewit K, Simons D G 1984 Myofascial pain: relief by post-isometric relaxation. Archives of Physical Medicine and Rehabilitation 65: 452–456

Magnusson M, Simonsen E B, Aagaard P et al 1995 Contraction specific changes in passive torque in human skeletal muscle. Acta Physiologica Scandinavica 155(4): 377–386

Magnusson M, Simonsen E B, Aagaard P et al 1996a Biomechanical responses to repeated stretches in human hamstring muscle in vivo. American Journal of Sports Medicine 24(5): 622–628

Magnusson M, Simonsen E B, Aagaard P et al 1996b A mechanism for altered flexibility in human skeletal muscle. Journal of Physiology 497(Part 1): 293–298

Magnusson S P, Simonsen E B, Aagaard P et al 1996c Mechanical and physiological responses to stretching with and without preisometric contraction in human skeletal muscle. Archives of Physical Medicine and Rehabilitation 77: 373–377

Magnusson M, Simonsen E B, Dyhre-Poulsen P et al 1996d Viscoelastic stress relaxation during static stretch in human skeletal muscle in the absence of EMG activity. Scandinavian Journal of Medicine and Science in Sport 6(6): 323–328

Magnusson M, Aagaard P, Simonsen E B et al 1998 A biomechanical evaluation of cyclic and static stretch in human skeletal muscle. International Journal of Sports Medicine 19: 310–316

Magnusson M, Aagaard P, Nielson J J 2000 Passive energy return after repeated stretches of the hamstring muscle-tendon unit. Medicine and Science in Sports and Exercise 32(6): 1160–1164

Mehta M, Hatton P 2002 The relationship between the duretion of sub-maximal isometric contraction (MET) and improvement in the range of passive knee extension (abstract). In: Abstracts from 3rd International Conference for the Advancement of Osteopathic Research, Melbourne, 2002. Journal of Osteopathic Medicine 5(1): 40

Melzack R, Wall P D 1965 Pain mechanisms: a new theory. Science 150: 971–979

Mitchell F L Jnr, Mitchell P K G 1995 The muscle energy manual, vol 1. MET Press, Michigan

Mitchell F L Jnr, Moran P S, Pruzzo N A 1979 An evaluation and treatment manual of osteopathic muscle energy procedures. Mitchell, Moran and Pruzzo Associates, Missouri

Moore M, Kukulka C 1991 Depression of Hoffman reflexes following voluntary contraction and implications for proprioceptive neuromuscular facilitation therapy. Physical Therapy 71(4): 321–329

Nelson K C, Cornelius W L 1991 The relationship between isometric contraction durations and improvement in shoulder joint range of motion. Journal of Sports Medicine and Physical Fitness 31(3): 385–388

Norkin C C, Levangie P K 1992 Joint structure and function. A comprehensive analysis, 2nd edn. F A Davis, Philadelphia

O'Haire C, Gibbons P 2000 Inter-examiner and intra-examiner agreement for assessing sacroiliac anatomy using palpation and observation: pilot study. Manual Therapy 5: 13–20

Osternig L R, Robertson R, Troxel R K et al 1987 Muscle activation during proprioceptive neuromuscular facilitation (PNF) stretching techniques. American Journal of Physical Medicine 66(5): 298–307

Osternig L R, Robertson R N, Troxel R K et al 1990 Differential responses to proprioceptive neuromuscular facilitation (PNF) stretch techniques. Medicine and Science in Sports Exercise 22(1): 106–111

Peace S, Fryer G 2004 Methods used by members of the Australian osteopathic profession to assess the sacroiliac joint. Journal of Osteopathic Medicine 7(1): 26–33

Phillips D R, Twomey L T 1996 A comparison of manual diagnosis with a diagnosis established by a uni-level lumbar spinal block procedure. Manual Therapy 2: 82–87

Rogers R G 1997 The effects of spinal manipulation on cervical kinesthesia in patients with chronic neck pain: a pilot study. Journal of Manipulative and Physiological Therapeutics 20(2): 80–85

Rowlands A V, Marginson V F, Lee J 2003 Chronic flexibility gains: effect of isometric contraction duration during proprioceptive neuromuscular facilitation stretching techniques. Research Quarterly Exercise and Sport 74(1): 47–51

Sady S P, Wortman M, Blanke D 1982 Flexibility training: ballistic, static or proprioceptive neuromuscular facilitation? Archives of Physical Medicine and Rehabilitation 63(6): 261–263

Schenk R J, Adelman K, Rousselle J 1994 The effects of muscle energy technique on cervical range of motion. Journal of Manual and Manipulative Therapy 2(4): 149–155

Schenk R J, MacDiarmid, Rousselle J 1997 The effects of muscle energy technique on lumbar range of motion. Journal of Manual and Manipulative Therapy 5(4): 179–183

Schleip R, Klingler W, Lehman-Horn F 2004 Active contraction of the thoracolumbar fascia (abstract). 5th Interdisciplinary World Congress on Low Back and Pelvic Pain, Melbourne

Schmitt G D, Pelham T W, Holt L E 1999 From the field. A comparison of selected protocols during proprioceptive neuromuscular facilitation stretching. Clinical Kinesiology 53(1): 16–21

Shacklock M O 1999 Central pain mechanisms: A new horizon in manual therapy. Australian Journal of Physiotherapy 45: 83–92

Spernoga S G, Uhl T L, Arnold B L et al 2001 Duration of maintained hamstring flexibility after a one-time, modified hold-relax stretching protocol. Journal of Athletic Training 36(1): 44–48

Spring F, Gibbons P, Tehan P 2001 Intra-examiner and inter-examiner reliability of a positional diagnostic screen for the lumbar spine. Journal of Osteopathic Medicine 4(2): 47–55

Sterling M, Jull G A, Wright A 2001 Cervical mobilisation: concurrent effects on pain, sympathetic nervous system activity and motor activity. Manual Therapy 6(2): 72–81

Stohler C S, Kowalski C J, Lund J P 2001 Muscle pain inhibits cutaneous touch perception. Pain 92: 327–333

Stopka C, Morley K, Siders R et al 2002 Stretching techniques to improve flexibility in special olympics athletes and their coaches. Journal of Sport Rehabilitation 11: 22–34

Taimela S, Kankaanpaa M, Luoto S 1999 The effect of lumbar fatigue on the ability to sense a change in lumbar position. Spine 24(13): 1322–1327

Taylor D C, Brooks D E, Ryan J B 1997 Visco-elastic characteristics of muscle: passive stretching versus muscular contractions. Medicine and Science in Sports and Exercise 29(12): 1619–1624

Thornton G M, Shrive N G, Frank C B 2001 Altering ligament water content affects ligament pre-stress and creep behaviour. Journal of Orthopaedic Research 19: 845–851

van Schalkwyk R, Parkin-Smith G F 2000 A clinical trial investigating the possible effect of the supine cervical rotatory manipulation and the supine lateral break manipulation in the treatment of mechanical neck pain: A pilot study. Journal of Manipulative and Physiological Therapeutics 23(5): 324–331

Vincenzino B, Collins D, Benson H et al 1998 An investigation of the interrelationship between manipulative therapy-induced hypoalgesia and sympathoexcitation. Journal of Manipulative and Physiological Therapeutics 21(7): 448–453

Vincenzino B, Collins D, Wright A 1996 The initial effects of a cervical spine manipulative physiotherapy treatment on the pain and dysfunction of lateral epicondylalgia. Pain 68: 69–74

Voerman V F, Van Egmond J, Crul B J P 2000 Elevated detection thresholds for mechanical stimuli in chronic pain patients: support for a central mechanism. Archives of Physical Medicine and Rehabilitation 81(April): 430–435

Wallin D, Ekblam B, Grahn R et al 1985 Improvement of muscle flexibility. A comparison between two techniques. American Journal of Sports Medicine 13(4): 263–268

Wilson E, Payton O, Donegan-Shoaf L et al 2003 Muscle energy technique in patients with acute low back pain: a pilot clinical trial. Journal of Orthopaedic and Sports Physical Therapy 33: 502–512

Wright A 1995 Hypoalgesia post-manipulative therapy: a review of a potential neurophysiological mechanism. Manual Therapy 1(1): 11–16

Yahia L H, Pigeon P, DesRosiers E A 1993 Viscoelastic properties of the human lumbodorsal fascia. Journal of Biomedical Engineering 15: 425–429

Sequential assessment and MET treatment of main postural muscles

5

CHAPTER CONTENTS

Clinical research evidence **133**
MET results in treatment of myofascial pain 134
MET results in treatment of fibromyalgia 134
Objectives of manual treatment **135**
Evaluating muscle shortness **136**
Important notes on assessments and use
of MET **137**
Stretching – what is happening? 139
MET for joints, and post-treatment discomfort 140
Postural muscle assessment sequence checklist 140
Sequential assessment and MET treatment
of postural muscles **140**
1. Assessment of tight gastrocnemius (01)²
and soleus (02) 141
2. Assessing for shortness in medial hamstrings
(03) (semi-membranosus, semi-tendinosus as
well as gracilis) and short adductors (04)
(pectineus, adductors brevis, magnus and longus) 143
3. Assessment and treatment of hip flexors – rectus
femoris (05), Iliopsoas (06) 145
4. Assessment and treatment of hamstrings (07) 154

5. Assessment and treatment of tensor fascia lata
(TFL) (08) 158
6. Assessment and treatment of piriformis (09) 162
7. Assessment and treatment of quadratus
lumborum (10) 166
8. Assessment and treatment of pectoralis
major (11) and latissimus dorsi (12) 170
9. Assessment and treatment of upper
trapezius (13) 176
10. Assessment and treatment of scalenes (14) 180
11. Assessment for shortness of
sternocleidomastoid (15) 183
12. Assessment and treatment of levator
scapulae (16) 185
13. Assessment and treatment of shortness
in infraspinatus (17) 187
14. Assessment and treatment of subscapularis (18) 189
15. Assessment for shortness of supraspinatus (19) 190
16. Assessment and treatment of flexors
of the arm (2) 191
17. Assessment and treatment of paravertebral
muscles (21) 193
References **197**

Clinical research evidence

As outlined in Ch. 4, research into the mechanisms associated with, and efficacy of MET usage, is growing, but remains – as with many aspects of manual therapy – partial. Numerous studies show the benefits in enhanced muscle flexibility follow-ing use of MET-type stretching. The variables – including length of contraction, number of repetitions, etc., remain open to debate (Bandy et al 1997, Shrier & Gossal 2000, Feland et al 2001).

Two examples of the value of MET in common clinical settings associated with myofascial pain and fibromyalgia are described below.

MET results in treatment of myofascial pain (Lewit & Simons 1984)

David Simons, co-researcher with Janet Travell into trigger points, and Karel Lewit, the Czech developer of gentler MET, have fairly demonstrated the efficiency of MET in a study involving assessment and treatment of severe muscular pain using MET. The study involved 244 patients with pain diagnosed as musculoskeletal in nature. These patients were examined and found to have between them 351 muscle groups requiring attention, based on their having:

1. Trigger points in the muscle and/or its insertion
2. Increased muscular tension during stretch
3. Muscular tension shortening which was not secondary to movement restriction caused by joint dysfunction.

These were muscular/soft tissue restrictions and not joint problems.

The method used in treating these muscles involved Lewit's postisometric relaxation approach (as described in Chs 2 and 3) in which mild isometric contractions against resistance were carried out for 10 seconds before releasing. Following complete 'letting go' by the patient, and on a subsequent exhalation, any additional slack was taken up and the muscle moved to its new barrier ('stretch was stopped at the slightest resistance').

From the new position, the process was repeated, although if no release was apparent, contractions, which remained mild, were extended for up to 30 seconds. The authors noted that it was only after the second or third contraction that a release was obtained, and three to five repetitions were usually able to provide as much progress as was likely at one session.

When release was achieved the operator was careful not to move too quickly: 'At this time the operator was careful not to interfere with the process and waited until the muscle relaxed completely. When the muscle reached a full range of motion the tension and the tender (trigger) points in the muscle were gone.'

The results were impressive, with 330 (94%) of the 351 muscles or muscle groups treated demonstrating immediate relief of pain and/or tenderness.

The technique was required to be precise concerning the direction of forces, which needed to be aligned to stretch the fibres demonstrating greatest tension. The patient's effort therefore needed to involve contraction in the direction which precisely affected these fibres. This was most important in triangular muscles such as pectoralis major and trapezius.

At a 3-month follow-up, lasting relief of pain was found to have been achieved in 63% of cases (referring to the pain originally complained of) and lasting relief of tenderness (relating to relief of tenderness in the treated muscles) in a further 23% of muscles. Among the muscles treated in this study, those which were found to respond most successfully are given in Table 5.1.

Lewit & Simons point out that: 'The technique not only abolished trigger points in muscles, but also relieved painful ligaments and periosteum in the region of attachment. The fact that increasing the length of shortened muscles relieved tenderness and pain, supports a muscular origin of the pain.'

The authors further point out that those patients achieving the greatest degree of long-term relief were those who carried out home treatment using MET stretches under instruction.

MET results in treatment of fibromyalgia

Drs Stotz and Kappler (1992) of the Chicago College of Osteopathic Medicine report having treated patients with fibromyalgia utilising a variety of osteopathic approaches including MET. The results given below were achieved by incorporating MET alongside positional release methods, together with a limited degree of more active manipulation (personal communication 1994).

Fibromyalgia is notoriously unresponsive to standard methods of treatment and continues to be treated, in the main, by resort to mild antidepressant medication, despite many of the primary researchers' insistence that in most instances depression is a result, rather than a cause of the condition (Block 1993, Duna & Wilke 1993).

The Chicago physicians measured the effects of osteopathic manipulative therapy (OMT – which included MET as a major element) on the intensity of pain reported from tender points in 18

Table 5.1 Results of use of MET in myofascial pain study

Muscle	Number treated	Pain relief	Tenderness relief	No relief
Upper trapezius	7	7		
Wrist and finger flexors	5	5		
Lateral epicondyle of arm involving spinator, wrist and finger extensors and/or biceps brachii	20	19	1	
Suboccipital	23	21	2	
Soleus (Achilles tendon)	6	5	1	
Sternomastoid	9	7	2	
Hamstrings	8	5	2	1
Pelvic muscles/ligaments	29	22	4	3
Gluteus maximus (coccyx attachment)	27	15	9	3
Levator scapulae	19	10	7	2
Piriformis	21	11	6	4
Erector spinae	28	13	12	3
Deep paraspinal	15	7	5	3
Upper pectorals	22	10	5	7
Biceps femoris (fibula head)	18	8	6	4
Biceps femoris (long head)	7	2	0	5

patients, who met all the criteria for fibromyalgia syndrome (FMS) (Goldenberg 1993).

Each patient had six visits/treatments and it was found over a 1-year period that 12 of the patients responded well in that their tender points became less sensitive (14% reduction against a 34% increase in the six patients who did not respond well). Activities of daily living were significantly improved and general pain symptoms decreased.

In another study, 19 patients with all the criteria of FMS were treated once a week for 4 weeks at Kirksville, Missouri, College of Osteopathic Medicine, using OMT which included MET as a major component: 84.2% showed improved sleep patterns, 94.7% reported less pain, and most patients had fewer tender points on palpation (Rubin et al 1990).

In these fibromyalgia examples, MET is seen to have been used as part of a wider range of soft tissue modalities, and this model is the recommendation of the lead author of this text. Before describing protocols for the use of MET in treating specific muscular dysfunction (such as shortness, tightness, weakness) the broader objectives of manual therapy deserve brief attention.

Objectives of manual treatment

What are the focuses and objectives of manual treatment in general, and manipulation in particular?

- Lewit (1985a) summarises what he believes manipulation is concerned with in the phrase 'restricted mobility', with or without pain.

- Evjenth (1984) is equally succinct, and states that what is needed to become proficient in treating patients with symptoms of pain or 'constrained movement' is 'experience gained by thoroughly examining every patient'. The only real measure of successful treatment is, he states, 'restoration of muscle's normal pattern of movement with freedom from pain'.

- Janda (1988) seems mainly to be concerned with 'imbalances' and the implications of dysfunctional patterns in which some muscles become weaker (inhibited) and others progressively tighter.

- Greenman (1996) reports on the conclusion of a 1983 workshop in which manual experts from around the world considered the question of the 'goal of manipulation'. The conclusion was: 'To restore maximal pain-free movement of the musculoskeletal system in postural balance'.

Previous chapters have discussed concepts relating to 'tight–loose', 'ease–bind' and particular muscle groups – however they are categorised – being subject, as part of their adaptation to the stresses of life, to shortening, while others are subject to weakening and/or lengthening. It is in the context of such adaptation, compensation and decompensation that soft tissue and articular changes can be identified by means of diligent palpation and assessment. Hopefully attention will also be paid to any habits of use that have contributed to the dysfunctional pattern being treated.

Restoration of a more normal function demands the availability of therapeutic tools by means of which change can be engineered. Biomechanical (manipulation, exercise, etc.) solutions and strategies that retard the chances of recurrence may focus on key muscles that require strengthening, or on enhancing posture or breathing function.

Re-education strategies depend for success, at least partly, on correction or improvement of the structural and functional imbalances which are present at the outset. As these imbalances are modified they allow change towards improved posture, fuller breathing, etc. No one with restricted and shortened accessory breathing/upper fixator muscles can learn to breathe correctly until these have, to an extent, been normalised; no one with short lumbar erector spinae and weak abdominal muscles can learn to use their spine in a posturally correct manner until these muscular imbalances have, to an extent, been normalised.

The structure–function continuum demands that therapeutic attention be paid to both aspects. Function cannot change until structure allows it to do so, and structure will continue to modify and adapt at the expense of optimal function until dysfunctional patterns of use are altered for the better.

Part of a solution is offered by the methods used in MET, in which the short and tight structures are identified and lengthened, while the weak and inhibited muscles are encouraged

towards enhanced tone, strength and stamina. Rehabilitation and re-education methods can then work in a relatively unhindered environment as new habits of use are learned.

Greenman (1996) offers a summary of this clinical approach: 'After short tight muscles are stretched, muscles that are inhibited can undergo retraining ... as in all manual medicine procedures, after assessment, stretching, and strengthening, reevaluation of faulty movement patterns ... is done.'

Dommerholt (2000) discussing enhancement of posture and function in musicians, has summarised an important concept:

In general, assessment and treatment of individual muscles must precede restoration of normal posture and normal patterns of movement. Claims that muscle imbalances would dissolve following lessons in Alexander technique are not substantiated in the scientific literature (Rosenthal 1987). Instead, muscle imbalances must be corrected through very specific strengthening and flexibility exercises ... myofascial trigger points must be inactivated ... [and] ... associated joint dysfunction ... must be corrected with joint mobilisation. Once the musculoskeletal conditions of 'good posture' have been met, postural retraining can proceed.

Evaluating muscle shortness

Many of the problems of the musculoskeletal system seem to involve pain or restriction related to aspects of muscle shortening (Lewit 1999). For example, simple dysfunctional patterns such as restricted hip extension can be shown to directly relate to shortness of hip flexors (Tyler et al 1996).

Where weakness (or lack of tone) is found to be a major element, it will often be noted that antagonists to these muscles are hypertonic and/or shortened, reciprocally inhibiting their tone. As discussed in Chs 2 and 3, many experts hold that prior to any effort to strengthen weak muscles, shortened ones should be dealt with by appropriate means, after which spontaneous toning usually occurs in the previously 'weakened' muscles. If muscle tone remains inadequate, then, and only then, should exercise and/or isotonic procedures be initiated. This is, however, not a universally accepted model, with many clinicians preferring to work on weak structures first, so reducing tone in their (usually) hypertonic antagonists. Attention to weak structures as a primary therapeutic effort may usefully reduce hypertonicity in antagonists; however, such treatment methods cannot reverse fibrotic states present in many chronically shortened structures, and until this is achieved the author contends that enhancing the strength of previously weak phasic (stabiliser, see Ch. 2) muscles is unlikely in itself to restore functional balance.

Janda (1983) tells us that short, tight muscles usually maintain their strength; however, in extreme cases of tightness some decrease in strength occurs. In such cases stretching (MET) of the tight muscle usually leads to a rapid recovery of strength (as well as toning of the antagonists via removal of reciprocal inhibition). As noted in Ch. 3, weakened postural muscles benefit from slowly applied isotonic eccentric methods (Norris 1999).

It is therefore important that short, tight muscles are assessed in a systematic, standardised manner. Janda (1983) suggests that, in order to obtain a reliable evaluation of muscle shortness:

- The starting position, method of fixation and direction of movement must be observed carefully.

- The prime mover must not be exposed to external pressure.

- If possible, the force exerted on the tested muscle must not work over two joints.

- The examiner should perform, at an even speed, a slow movement that brakes slowly at the end of the range.

- To keep the stretch and the muscle irritability about equal, the movement must not be jerky.

- Pressure or pull must always act in the required direction of movement.

- Muscle shortening can only be correctly evaluated if the joint range is not decreased, as might be the case should an osseous limitation or joint blockage exist.

It is also in shortened muscles that local reflex dysfunction is most commonly noted (Scudds 1995, Gerwin & Dommerholt 2002) – variously called trigger points (Simons et al 1999), tender points, zones of irritability, hyperalgesic zones (Lewit 1999), neurovascular and neurolymphatic reflexes, etc. (Chaitow 1991). Localising these areas of altered function is usually possible via normal palpatory methods. Identification and treatment of tight muscles may also be systematically carried out using the methods described later in this chapter.[1]

Important notes on assessments and use of MET

1. When the term 'restriction barrier' is used in relation to soft tissue structures, it is meant to indicate the place where the first signs of resistance are noted (as palpated by sense of 'bind', or sense of effort required to move the area, or by visual or other palpable evidence), and not the greatest possible range of pain-free movement obtainable. (Refer to the ease–bind palpation exercise involving the adductors in Ch. 3 and to Fig. 3.1A, B.)

2. In all treatment descriptions involving MET (apart from the first set of assessment tests involving gastrocnemius and soleus) it will be assumed that the 'shorthand' reference to 'acute' and 'chronic' will be adequate to alert the reader to the variations in methodology which these variants call for, as discussed in Ch. 3, where appropriate barriers for use in acute and chronic situations were summarised (see also Box 5.1).

3. Assistance from the patient is valuable as movement is made to, or through, a barrier, provided that the patient can be educated to gentle cooperation and can learn not to use excessive effort.

---

[1] Note that the assessment methods presented are not themselves diagnostic but provide strong indications of probable shortness of the muscles being tested.

4. In most MET treatment guidelines in this chapter the method described will involve isometric contraction of the agonist(s) – i.e. the muscle(s) which require stretching. It is assumed that the reader is now familiar with the possibility of using the antagonists to achieve reciprocal inhibition (RI) before initiating stretch or movement to a new barrier, and will use this alternative when appropriate (for example, if there is pain on use of agonist, or if there has been prior trauma to the agonist, or in an attempt to see if more release can be made available after the initial use of the agonist isometrically). See Ch. 4 for discussion of the current degree of research evidence relative to choice of RI or PIR in MET usage. Recall also that, as discussed in Ch. 1, there exists some controversy relating to the use of the words 'antagonist' and 'agonist' in some MET-like methods.

Box 5.1 'Acute' and 'chronic'

The words 'acute' and 'chronic' should alert the reader to the differences in methodology which these variants call for in applying MET, especially in terms of the starting position for contractions and whether or not stretching should take place after the contraction.

In acute conditions the isometric contraction starts at the barrier, whereas in chronic conditions the contraction starts short of the barrier (Janda 1983, Liebenson 1996, Lewit 1999). After the contraction the practitioner takes the area to the new barrier in acute conditions, or through the previous resistance barrier into slight sustained stretch in chronic conditions.

The term 'acute' may be applied to strain or injury which has occurred within the past 3 weeks, or where the symptoms such as pain are acute, or where active inflammation is present.

Use of the antagonists to the affected muscle(s) offers an alternative to activation of an isometric contraction in such muscles if this proves painful or difficult for the patient to perform.

A further alternative is to use Ruddy's repetitive pulsing contractions, rather than a sustained contraction, if the latter is painful or difficult for the patient to perform (see Ch. 3).

---

5. Isolytic methods (rapidly stretched eccentric isotonic contractions) will be suggested in a few instances, most notably in treating tensor fascia lata (TFL), but these are not generally recommended for application in sensitive patients or in potentially 'fragile' areas such as the muscles associated with the cervical spine.

6. Careful reading of Chs 1 and 3 in particular is urged before commencing practice of the methods listed below.

7. There should be no pain experienced during application of MET, although mild discomfort (stretching) is acceptable.

8. The methods of assessment and treatment of postural muscles given here are far from comprehensive or definitive. There are many other assessment approaches, and numerous treatment/stretch approaches, using variations on the theme of MET, as evidenced by the excellent texts by Janda, Basmajian, Lewit, Liebenson, Greenman, Grieve, Mattes, Hartman, Evjenth and Dvorak, among others. The methods recommended below provide a sound basis for the application of MET to specific muscles and areas, as do the methods suggested for spinal, pelvic, neck and shoulder regions in Chs 6 and 8. By developing the skills with which to apply the methods, as described, a repertoire of techniques can be acquired, offering a wide base of choices that will be appropriate in numerous clinical settings.

9. Some of the discussion of particular muscles will include notes containing information unrelated to the main objective, which is to outline assessment and MET treatment possibilities. These notes are included where the particular information they carry is likely to be useful clinically.

10. Breathing cooperation can, and should, be used as part of the methodology of MET. This, however, will not be repeated as an instruction in each example of MET use below. Basically, if appropriate (that is, if the patient is cooperative and capable of

following instructions), the patient should be given the instructions outlined in Box 5.2. A note which gives the instruction to 'use appropriate breathing', or some variation on it, will be found in the text describing various MET applications, and this refers to the guidelines outlined in Box 5.2.

11. Various eye movements are sometimes advocated during contractions and stretches, particularly by Lewit (1999) who uses these methods to great effect. The only specific recommendations for use of visual synkinesis in this chapter will be found in regard to muscles such as the scalenes and sternomastoid, where the use of eye movements is particularly valuable in terms of the gentleness of the contractions they induce.

12. 'Pulsed muscle energy technique' is based on Ruddy's work (see Ch. 3). It can be substituted for any of the methods described in the text below for treating shortened soft tissue structures, or for increasing the range of motion in joints (Ruddy 1962).

13. There are times when 'co-contraction' seems to be clinically useful, involving contraction of both the agonist and the antagonist. Studies have shown that this approach is particularly useful in treatment of the

hamstrings, when both these and the quadriceps are isometrically contracted prior to stretch (Moore at al 1980).

14. It is seldom necessary to treat all the shortened muscles that are identified via the methods described below.

For example, Lewit and Simons (1984) mention that postisometric relaxation of the suboccipital muscles will also relax the sternocleidomastoid muscles; treatment of the thoracolumbar muscles induces relaxation of iliopsoas, and vice versa; treatment (MET) of the sternocleidomastoid and scalene muscles relaxes the pectorals. These interactions are worthy of greater study.

Stretching – what is happening?

As previously discussed, when muscles and other soft tissues are placed at stretch following an isometric contraction, it has been widely assumed that subsequent benefits, for example involving enhanced extensibility, derive from reflex muscular neurological influences, such as postisometric relaxation (PIR), and/or reciprocal inhibition (RI) (Mitchell et al 1979, Kuchera & Kuchera 1992, Greenman 1996). It has also been hypothesised that stretching, if maintained, results in visco-elastic deformation of connective tissue, resulting in increased ranges of motion and extensibility (Taylor et al 1990, 1997).

These beliefs and concepts are both questioned and are examined in some depth in Ch. 4, along with the current favoured explanation for muscle extensibility, following isometric contraction, the phenomenon of increased stretch tolerance. How strong a contraction should be, and how long a stretch is appropriate to achieve optimal benefit, along with other MET variables, are also examined in Ch. 4.

The degree of force requested of the patient in application of isometric contractions will vary depending on the nature of the dysfunction and the age and status of the patient. However, in general it is the recommendation of the lead author that when treating *soft tissue problems* only moderate degrees of force (under 35%) should be employed, at most, and that very light contractions are frequently all that is needed, particularly in acute

---

Box 5.2 Notes on respiratory synkinesis during MET (Lewit 1999)

Patients who are cooperative and capable of following instructions should be asked to:

- Inhale as they slowly build up an isometric contraction
- Hold the breath during the 7–10 second contraction, and
- Release the breath as they slowly cease the contraction
- Inhale and exhale fully once more, following cessation of all effort, as they are asked to 'let go completely'.

During this second exhalation the tissues are taken to their new barrier in an acute condition, or the barrier is passed as the muscle is stretched in a chronic condition (with patient assistance if possible).

settings. It is also the lead author's clinical opinion based on clinical experience that in treating chronic *soft tissue problems*, contractions should be held for 7–10 seconds, and that ideally stretches should be held for 30 seconds or more, to allow a slow lengthening process to begin.

Experience suggests that a second stretch be introduced, and sometimes a third, although clinical experience points to very little additional gain being likely if the first two stretches have been adequately performed, always following an isometric contraction. See below for Greenman's (1996) suggestions regarding the number of contraction repetitions when treating joints.

MET for joints, and post-treatment discomfort

When treating restricted joints using MET (see Ch. 6) *no stretching* should be introduced following isometric contractions. The MET approach suggested is precisely that indicated (see Chs 2 and 3) for acute soft tissue problems. The barrier should be engaged and, following an isometric contraction, movement should be made passively to a new barrier, without force or stretching.

Unlike the period required to hold soft tissues at stretch, in order to achieve increased extensibility, no such feature is part of the protocol for treatment of joints, when using MET. Once a new barrier is reached, having taken out available slack without force after the isometric contraction, the subsequent contraction is called for and the process is repeated.

The lead author has found that a variety of directions of resisted effort are useful (or put differently, a range of different muscles should be contracted isometrically) when attempting to achieve release and mobilisation of a restricted joint, including those where there is no specific muscular control over the joint, such as the sacroiliac, sternoclavicular and acromioclavicular joints.

Patient-directed isometric efforts towards the restriction barrier, as well as away from it, and using a combination of forces, often of a 'spiral' nature, should be experimented with, if a joint does not release using the most obvious directions of contraction (see notes in Ch. 6 on MET treat-

ment of iliosacral and shoulder joints in particular). Additionally the author highly recommends the use of Ruddy's pulsed MET approaches as variations on the theme of MET, when attempting to release blocked joints.

Greenman (1996) advocates three to five repetitions of contractions when treating joints with MET (each lasting just 3–4 seconds), and warns that discomfort should be anticipated for 12–36 hours after the treatment. He explains why this occurs:

> [MET] *muscle contractions influence the surrounding fascia, connective tissue ground substance, and interstitial fluids, and alter muscle physiology by reflex mechanisms. Fascial length and tone is altered by muscle contraction. Alteration in fascia influences not only its biomechanical function but also the biochemical and immunological functions. The patient's muscle effort requires energy and the metabolic process of muscle contraction results in carbon dioxide, lactic acid, and other metabolic waste products that must be transported and metabolized.*

Effleurage, applied to the tissues following MET, appears to assist in reducing the degree of discomfort which Greenman suggests is likely.

Postural muscle assessment sequence checklist

The checklist in Box 5.3 can be used to follow (and record results of) the simple sequence of postural muscle assessment as described in detail later in this chapter.

Sequential assessment and MET treatment of postural muscles

The assessment and treatment recommendations that follow represent a synthesis of information derived from personal clinical experience, as well as from the numerous sources cited, or are based on the work of named researchers, clinicians and therapists (Fryette 1954, Cailliet 1962, Mennell 1964, Williams 1965, Basmajian 1974, Rolf 1977, Janda 1983, Dvorak & Dvorak 1984, Greenman 1989, 1996, Lewit 1992, 1999).

Box 5.3 Postural muscle assessment sequence

NAME _____

E = Equal (circle both if both are short)

L or R are circled if left or right are short

Spinal abbreviations indicate low-lumbar, lumbodorsal junction, low-thoracic, mid-thoracic and upper thoracic areas (of flatness and therefore reduced ability to flex – short erector spinae)
01. Gastrocnemius E L R
02. Soleus E L R
03. Medial hamstrings E L R
04. Short adductors E L R
05. Rectus femoris E L R
06. Psoas E L R
07. Hamstrings
    a) upper fibres E L R
    b) lower fibres E L R
08. Tensor fascia lata E L R
09. Piriformis E L R
10. Quadratus lumborum E L R
11. Pectoralis major E L R
12. Latissimus dorsi E L R
13. Upper trapezius E L R
14. Scalenes E L R
15. Sternocleidomastoid E L R
16. Levator scapulae E L R
17. Infraspinatus E L R
18. Subscapularis E L R
19. Supraspinatus E L R
20. Flexors of the arm E L R
21. Spinal flattening:
    a) seated legs straight LL LDJ LT MT UT
    b) seated legs flexed LL LDJ LT MT UT
22. Cervical spine extensors short? Yes No

1. Assessment of tight gastrocnemius (01)[2] and soleus (02) (Fig. 5.1A, B)

- The patient lies supine with feet extending over the edge of the table.

- For right leg examination the practitioner's left hand cradles the Achilles tendon just above the heel, avoiding pressure on the tendon.

_____

[2] The 'code' number assigned to each listed muscle links it to the postural muscle assessment sequence checklist in Box 5.3.

- The heel lies in the palm of the hand, fingers curving round it.

- The practitioner's right hand is placed so that the fingers rest on the dorsum of the foot (these are not active and do not apply any pulling stretch), with the thumb on the sole, lying along the medial margin. (This position is important for adequate control – it is a mistake to place the thumb too near the centre of the sole of the foot.)

- Stretch is introduced by means of a pull on the heel with the left hand, taking out the slack of the muscle, while at the same time the right hand maintains light cephalad pressure on the sole of the foot, via the thumb (along its entire length). This directs the foot towards an upright position without force (Fig. 5.1A).

- The leg should remain resting on the table throughout the assessment. The arm and hand controlling the removal of slack via the hold on the heel should be placed so that it is an extension of the leg, not allowing an upward (towards the ceiling) pull when stretch is introduced.

- If the muscles being assessed are in a normal state, a range of movement should be achieved which takes the sole of the foot to a 90° angle to the leg without any force being applied.

- If this is not possible (i.e. if force is required to achieve the 90° angle between the sole of the foot and the leg), there is shortness in gastrocnemius and/or soleus. Further screening is then required to identify precisely which muscle is involved (see soleus assessment below).

Assessment of tight soleus (02)

The method described above assesses both gastrocnemius and soleus. To assess only the soleus, precisely the same procedure is adopted, with the knee passively flexed (over a cushion, for example) (Fig.5.1B).

- If the sole of the foot fails to easily come to a 90° angle with the leg, without force, once slack has been taken out of the tissues via

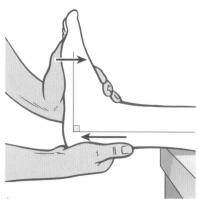

A

Figure 5.1A Assessment or treatment of gastrocnemius and soleus. During assessment the sole of the foot should achieve a vertical position without effort once slack is taken out via traction on the heel. Treatment would involve taking the tissues to or through (acute/chronic) the identified barrier following an isometric contraction.

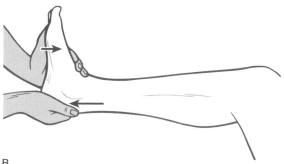

B

Figure 5.1B With the knee flexed, the same assessment is evaluating the status of soleus alone. Treatment would involve taking the tissues to or through (acute/chronic) the identified barrier following an isometric contraction.

traction through the long axis of the calf from the heel, soleus is considered short.

- If the previous test (in which the leg was straight) indicated shortness of gastrocnemius *or* soleus, and this test (in which the knee is flexed) is normal, then gastrocnemius alone is short.

Squat test

A further screening test for soleus involves the patient being asked to squat, with the trunk in slight flexion, feet placed shoulder width apart, so

that the buttocks rest between the legs (which face forwards rather than outwards). If the soleus muscles are normal then it should be possible to go fully into this position with the heels remaining flat on the floor. If not, and the heels rise from the floor as the squat is performed, the soleus muscles are probably shortened.

MET treatment of shortened gastrocnemius and soleus (Fig. 5.1A, B)

Precisely the same position is adopted for treatment as for testing, with the knee flexed over a rolled towel or cushion if soleus is being treated, and with the knee straight if gastrocnemius is being treated.

- If the condition is acute (defined as a dysfunction/injury of less than 3 weeks' duration) the area is treated with the foot dorsiflexed to the restriction barrier.

- If it is a chronic problem (longer duration than 3 weeks) the barrier is assessed and the muscle treated in a position of ease, slightly towards the mid-range, away from the restriction barrier.

- Starting from the appropriate position, at the restriction barrier or just short of it, based on the degree of acuteness or chronicity, the patient is asked to exert a small effort (no more than 20% of available strength) towards plantarflexion, against unyielding resistance, with appropriate breathing (see Box 5.2).

- This effort isometrically contracts either gastrocnemius or soleus (depending on whether the knee is unflexed or flexed).

- This contraction is held for 7–10 seconds.

- On slow release, on an exhalation, the foot/ankle is dorsiflexed (be sure to flex the whole foot and not just the toes) to its new restriction barrier if acute, or slightly and painlessly beyond the new barrier if chronic, *with the patient's assistance.*

- If chronic, the tissues should be held in slight stretch for up to 30 seconds, to allow a slow lengthening of tissues (see notes on 'creep' and viscoelasticity in Ch. 2).

- This pattern is repeated until no further gain is achieved (backing off to mid-range for the next contraction, if chronic, and commencing the next contraction from the new resistance barrier if acute).

- Alternatively, if there is undue discomfort when contracting the agonists (the muscles being treated), the antagonists to the shortened muscles can be used, by introducing resisted dorsiflexion with the muscle at its barrier or just short of it, followed by a painless move to the new barrier (if acute) or beyond it (if chronic), ideally during an exhalation.

- Use of antagonists in this way is less effective than use of the agonist, but may be a useful strategy if trauma has taken place.

NOTE: Figure 5.2 illustrates an alternative treatment position for gastrocnemius which can also be used for assessment. Flexion of the knee would allow this position to be used for treating soleus.

2. Assessing for shortness in medial hamstrings (03) (semi-membranosus, semi-tendinosus as well as gracilis) and short adductors (04) (pectineus, adductors brevis, magnus and longus)

Test A

- The patient lies so that the non-tested leg is abducted slightly, heel over the end of the table.

- The leg to be tested should be close to the edge of the table, and the practitioner ensures that the tested leg is in its anatomically correct position, knee in full extension and with no external rotation of the leg, which would negate the test.

- The practitioner should effectively stand between patient's leg and the table so that all control of the tested leg is achieved with his lateral (non-table-side) arm/hand, while the table-side hand can rest on, and palpate, the inner thigh muscles for sensations of bind as the leg is taken into abduction.

- Abduction of the tested leg is introduced passively until the first sign of resistance is

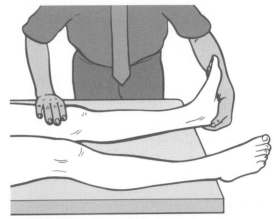

Figure 5.2 MET treatment position for gastrocnemius. If knee were flexed the same position would focus on treatment of soleus only.

noted (see Fig. 5.3). There are effectively three indicators of this resistance:
- A sense of increased effort should be noted by the hand carrying the leg at the moment that the first resistance barrier is passed.
- The sense of bind should be noted by the palpating hand at this same moment.
- A visual sign, movement of the pelvis as a whole, laterally towards the tested side, should be observed as this barrier is passed.

- If abduction produces an angle with the midline of 45° or more before a resistance barrier is reached, then no further test is needed, the degree of abduction is normal, and there is probably no shortness in the short or long adductors (medial hamstrings or, more correctly, gracilis and biceps femoris).

- If, however, abduction ceases before a 45° angle is easily achieved (without effort, or a sense of bind in the tissues), then restriction exists in either the medial hamstrings or the short adductors of the thigh.

Screening short adductors (04) from medial hamstrings (03)

As in the tests for gastrocnemius and soleus, it is necessary to differentiate between shortness of the one and two joint muscles (in this case the short adductors and the medial hamstrings).

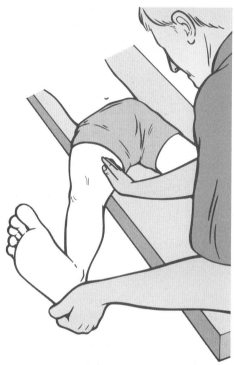

Figure 5.3 Assessment and treatment position for medial hamstrings. Adductor shortness may be evaluated and treated in the same relative position but with the knee of the leg to be treated in flexion.

- This is achieved by abducting the leg to its easy barrier and then introducing flexion of the knee, allowing the lower leg to hang down freely.

- If (after knee flexion has been introduced) further abduction is now easily achieved to 45° when previously it was restricted, this indicates that any previous limitation into abduction was the result of medial hamstring shortness.

- If, however, restriction remains, as evidenced by continued 'bind', or obvious restriction in movement towards a 45° excursion, once knee flexion has been introduced to the abducted leg, then the short adductors are continuing to prevent movement, and are short.

Test B

- The patient lies at the very end of table (coccyx close to edge), non-tested leg fully flexed at the hip and knee, and held towards the chest

by the patient (or the sole of the patient's foot may rest against the practitioner's lateral chest wall) to stabilise the pelvis in full rotation, so that the lumbar spine is not in extension.

- The tested leg is grasped both above and below the knee and taken into abduction to the first sign of resistance. The practitioner has two free hands in this position, one of which can usefully palpate the inner thigh for bind during the assessment.

- If abduction reaches 45°, then the test has revealed no shortness.

- If a restriction/resistance barrier is noted before 45°, then the knee should be flexed to screen the short adductors from the medial hamstrings as in method A, above.

- In all other ways the findings are interpreted as above.

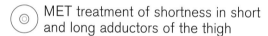 MET treatment of shortness in short and long adductors of the thigh

Precisely the same positions may be adopted for treatment as for testing, whether test A or test B was used.

- If the short adductors (pectineus, adductors brevis, magnus and longus) are being treated, then the leg, *with knee flexed*, is held at the barrier (for an acute condition) or a little short of the barrier (if chronic).

- An isometric contraction is introduced by the patient using around 20–30% of available strength employing the agonists (the patient pushes away from the barrier of resistance) or the antagonists (the patient pushes towards the barrier of resistance) for 7–10 seconds.

- Appropriate breathing instructions should be given (see notes on breathing in Box 5.2).

- After the contraction ceases and the patient has relaxed, the leg is eased to its new barrier (if acute) or painlessly (assisted by the patient) beyond the new barrier and into stretch (if chronic), where it is held for not less than 30 seconds (longer if possible), in order to stretch shortened tissue.

- The process is repeated at least once more.

If the medial hamstrings (semi-membranosus, semi-tendinosus, as well as gracilis) are being treated, all elements are the same, except that the *knee should be held in extension* (see Fig. 5.4). Whichever position is used, the subsequent movement, on an exhalation, is to (if acute), or through (if chronic) the barrier, to commence normalisation of the shortened muscles.

NOTE: Either approach (knee straight or flexed) can be performed with the patient side-lying as in Fig. 5.5 – see description below.

Caution and alternative treatment position (Fig. 5.5)

A major error made in treating these particular muscles, using MET, relates to allowing a pivoting of the pelvis and a spinal side-bending to occur. Maintenance of the pelvis in a stable position is important, and this can most easily be achieved via suitable straps when supine or, during treatment, by having the patient side-lying with the affected side uppermost.

- Patient is side-lying.
- Practitioner stands behind and uses the caudad arm and hand to control the leg and to palpate for bind, with the treated leg flexed or straight as appropriate.

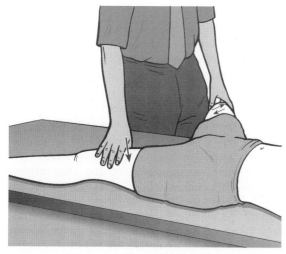

Figure 5.4 Position for treatment of shortness in adductors of the thigh.

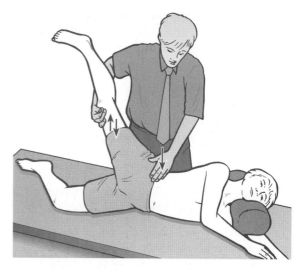

Figure 5.5 Side-lying position for treatment of two-joint adductors of the thigh.

- The cephalad hand maintains a firm downwards pressure on the lateral pelvis to ensure stability during stretching.
- All other elements of treatment are identical to those described for supine treatment above.

3. Assessment and treatment of hip flexors – rectus femoris (05), Iliopsoas (06) (see also Box 5.4 and Fig. 5.6A)

- The patient lies supine with buttocks (coccyx) as close to the end of the table as possible, the non-tested leg in flexion at both hip and knee, held by the patient, or with the sole of the foot of the non-tested side placed against the lateral chest wall of the practitioner.
- Full flexion of the hip helps to maintain the pelvis in full rotation with the lumbar spine flat. This is essential if the test is to be meaningful and stress on the spine avoided.
- If the thigh of the tested leg lies in a horizontal position in which it is parallel to the floor/table (Fig. 5.6A), then the indication is that iliopsoas is not short.
- If, however, the thigh rises above the horizontal (Fig. 5.6B) then iliopsoas is probably short.

- Even if the thigh is able to lie parallel to the floor, a slight degree (±10°) of hip extension should be possible in this position in response to a gentle push downwards on the thigh by the practitioner, with no knee extension occurring as this is done.

- If effort is required to achieve 10° of hip extension, this suggests iliopsoas shortening on that side.

- If the knee straightens when the thigh is eased towards the floor, this suggests rectus femoris (or possibly tensor fascia lata) shortening on that side.

- Rectus femoris shortness can be confirmed by seeing whether or not the heel on the tested side can easily flex to touch the buttock when the patient is prone. If rectus femoris is short the heel will not easily reach the buttock (Fig. 5.7B).

- In the supine testing position, if the lower leg of the tested side fails to hang down to an almost 90° angle with the thigh, vertical to the floor, then shortness of rectus femoris is indicated (see Fig. 5.6B).

- If this is not clearly observed, as suggested above, application of light pressure towards the floor on the lower third of the thigh will produce a compensatory extension of the lower leg only, when rectus femoris is short.

- If both iliopsoas and rectus femoris are short, passive flexion of the knee will result in compensatory lumbar lordosis and increased hip flexion. (See also functional assessment method for psoas in Ch. 8 and notes on psoas in Box 5.4.)

- If both psoas and rectus are short, rectus should be treated first.

- If the line of the suspended thigh lies below a parallel (with the floor) position, this indicates a degree of laxity in iliopsoas (see Fig. 5.6C).

- If TFL structure is short (a further test proves it, see Test 5, later in this chapter) then there should be an obvious groove apparent on the lateral thigh, and sometimes the whole lower leg will deviate laterally.

Mitchell's strength test

Before using MET methods to normalise a short psoas, Mitchell recommended that the patient should lie at the end of the table, both legs hanging down, with feet turned in so that they can rest on your lateral calf areas, as you stand facing the patient. The patient should press firmly against your calves with her feet as you rest your hands on her thighs and she attempts to lift you from the floor. In this way you can assess the relative strength of one leg's effort, as against the other.

Judge which psoas is weaker or stronger than the other. If a psoas has tested short (as in the test described above) and also tests strong in this test, then it is suitable for MET treatment, according to Mitchell's guidelines (Mitchell et al 1979). If it tests both short and weak, then other factors such as tight erector spinae muscles, or of trigger points in the low-back muscles (multifidus, iliocostalis) or in psoas should be treated first until psoas tests strong and short, at which time MET should be applied to start the lengthening process (Simons et al 1999).

It has been found to be clinically useful to suggest that before treating a shortened psoas, any shortness in rectus femoris on that side should first be treated.

What if one psoas is inhibited and the other tight?

Schamberger (2002) discusses an imbalance ('malalignment syndrome') in which the psoas on one side is inhibited while the other is tight. As one might expect a pelvic tilt is a likely, but not certain outcome, with elevation on the short, tight, side. However, Schamberger reports the work of Maffetone (1999) who suggests that the reverse might also be true, with psoas inhibition being located on the side of pelvic elevation.

Testing for length and for weakness (as above) would lead to revelation of the true picture, whatever the underlying cause(s) (see Fig. 5.7).

Psoas strength test and toning exercise (Fig. 2.13) (Norris 1999)

A different test for psoas weakness/inhibition can become a toning exercise when repeated regularly:

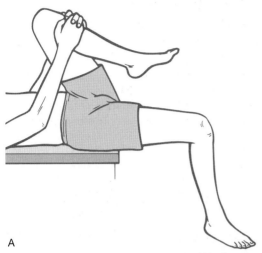

A

Figure 5.6A   Test position for shortness of hip flexors. Note that the hip on the non-tested side must be fully flexed to produce full pelvic rotation. The position shown is normal.

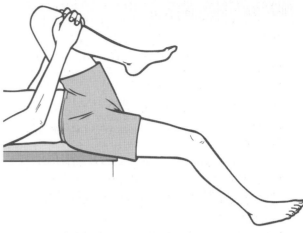

C **Figure 5.6C**   The fall of the thigh below the horizontal indicates hypotonic psoas status. Rectus femoris is once again seen to be short, while the relative external rotation of the lower leg (see angle of foot) hints at probable shortened TFL involvement.

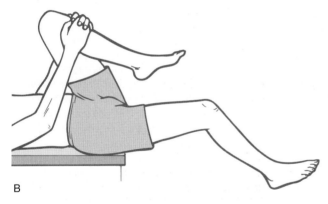

B

Figure 5.6B   In the test position, if the thigh is elevated (i.e. not parallel to the table) probable psoas shortness is indicated. The inability of the lower leg to hang more or less vertically towards the floor indicates probable rectus femoris shortness (TFL shortness can produce a similar effect).

- Patient sits on an upright chair, with spine in neutral and with the knee flexed at 90°.

- The leg on the side to be tested, or on which psoas is to be toned (right in this example), should be raised about 5 cm from the floor.

- If psoas is strong it should be possible to hold this raised leg for 10 seconds before lowering and repeating the raise and hold nine more times.

During this test, if psoas is strong, there should be:

1. No loss of the upright, neutral, spinal position, or

2. No quiver or twitch of the anterior thigh muscles, and

3. It should be possible to perform the 10 repetitions of 10-second holds without distress.

Box 5.4 Notes on psoas

- Lewit (1985b) mentions that in many ways the psoas behaves as if it were an internal organ. Tension in the psoas may be secondary to kidney disease, and one of its frequent clinical manifestations, when in spasm, is that it reproduces the pain of gall-bladder disease (often after the organ has been removed).

- The definitive signs of psoas problems are not difficult to note, according to Fryette (1954). He maintains that the distortions produced in inflammation and/or spasm in the psoas are characteristic and cannot be produced by other dysfunction. The origin of the psoas is from 12th thoracic to (and including) the 4th lumbar, but not the 5th lumbar. The insertion is into the lesser trochanter of the femur, and thus, when psoas spasm exists unilaterally, the patient is drawn forwards and side-bent to the involved side. The ilium on the side will rotate backwards on the sacrum, and the thigh will be everted. When both muscles are involved the patient is drawn forward, with the lumbar curve locked in flexion. This is the characteristic reversed lumbar spine. Chronic bilateral psoas contraction creates either a reversed lumbar curve if the erector spinae of the low back are weak, or an increased lordosis if they are hypertonic.

- Lewit (1999) says, 'Psoas spasm causes abdominal pain, flexion of the hip and typical antalgesic (stooped) posture. Problems in psoas can profoundly influence thoraco-lumbar stability.'

- The 5th lumbar is not involved directly with psoas, but great mechanical stress is placed upon it when the other lumbar vertebrae are fixed in either a kyphotic or an increased lordotic state. In unilateral psoas spasms, a rotary stress is noted at the level of 5th lumbar. The main mechanical involvement is, however, usually at the lumbodorsal junction. Attempts to treat the resulting pain (frequently located in the region of the 5th lumbar and sacroiliac) by attention to these areas will be of little use. Attention to the muscular component should be a primary focus, ideally using MET.

- Bogduk (Bogduk et al 1992, Bogduk 1997) provides evidence that psoas plays only a small role in the action of the spine, and states that it 'uses the lumbar spine as a base from which to act on the hip'. He goes on to discuss just how much pressure derives from psoas compression on discs: 'Psoas potentially exerts massive compression loads on the lower lumbar discs ... upon maximum contraction, in an activity such as sit-ups, the two psoas muscles can be expected to exert a compression on the L5–S1 disc equal to about 100 kg of weight.'

- There exists in all muscles a vital reciprocal agonist–antagonist relationship that is of primary importance in determining their tone and healthy function. Psoas–rectus abdominis have such a relationship and this has important postural implications (see notes on lower crossed syndrome in Ch. 2).

- Observation of the abdomen 'falling back' rather than mounding when the patient flexes indicates normal psoas function. Similarly, if the patient, when lying supine, flexes knees and 'drags' the heels towards the buttocks (keeping them together), the abdomen should remain flat or fall back. If the abdomen mounds or the small of the back arches, psoas is incompetent (Liebenson 1996).

- If the supine patient raises both legs into the air and the belly mounds it shows that the recti and psoas are out of balance. Psoas should be able to raise the legs to at least 30° without any help from the abdominal muscles.

- Psoas fibres merge with (become 'consolidated' with) the diaphragm and it therefore influences respiratory function directly (as does quadratus lumborum).

- Basmajian (1974) informs us that the psoas is the most important of all postural muscles. If it is hypertonic and the abdominals are weak and exercise is prescribed to tone these weak abdominals (such as curl-ups with the dorsum of the foot stabilised), then a disastrous negative effect will ensue in which, far from toning the abdominals, increase of tone in psoas will result, due to the sequence created by the dorsum of the foot being used as a point of support. When this occurs (dorsiflexion), the gait cycle is mimicked and there is a sequence of activation of tibialis anticus, rectus femoris and psoas. If, on the other hand, the feet could be plantarflexed during curl-up exercises, then the opposite chain is activated (triceps surae, hamstrings and gluteals) inhibiting psoas and allowing toning of the abdominals.

- When treating, it is sometimes useful to assess changes in psoas length by periodic comparison of apparent arm length. Patient lies supine, arms extended above head, palms together so that length can be compared. A shortness will commonly be observed in the arm on the side of the shortened psoas, and this should normalise after successful treatment (there may of course be other reasons for apparent difference in arm length, and this method provides an indication only of changes in psoas length).

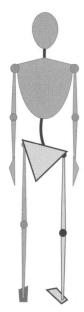

Figure 5.7 Static postural assessment of malalignment caused by psoas inhibition on the right, leading to medial rotation of the ipsilateral foot, with excessive pronation. The lumbar spine is shown to be convex on the left, involving a tight psoas. As noted by Maffetone (1996), the pelvis may be higher or lower on the side of the inhibited psoas. (Redrawn from Schamberger 2002, p 90, figure 3.2A.)

Psoas toning exercise:

- Precisely the same procedure as the test should be performed once or twice daily, until 10 repetitions of 10 seconds are possible without strain.

If shortness is still evident, once tone and strength are restored, MET should be applied.

NOTE: It is worth recalling Norris's (1999) advice that a slowly performed isotonic eccentric exercise will normally strengthen a weak postural muscle. As discussed in Ch. 2, psoas is classified as postural, and a mobiliser, depending on the descriptive model being used.

Richardson et al (1999) describe psoas as 'an exception' to their deep/superficial rule (see Ch. 2) since, 'it is designed to act exclusively on the hip'.

There is therefore virtually universal agreement that psoas will shorten in response to stress.

◎ MET treatment for shortness of rectus femoris

- The patient lies prone, ideally with a cushion under the abdomen to help avoid hyperlordosis.

- The practitioner stands on the side of the table of the affected leg so that he can stabilise the patient's pelvis (hand covering the sacral area or ischial tuberosity) during the treatment, using the cephalad hand.

- The affected leg is flexed at hip and knee.

- The practitioner can either hold the lower leg at the ankle (as in Fig. 5.8), or the upper leg can be cradled so that the hand curls under the lower thigh and is able to palpate for bind, just above the knee, with the practitioner's upper arm offering resistance to the lower leg.

- Either of these holds allows flexion of the knee to the barrier, perceived either as increasing effort, or as palpated bind.

- If rectus femoris is short, then the patient's heel will not easily be able to touch the buttock (Fig. 5.8).

- Once the restriction barrier has been established (how close can the heel get to the buttock before the barrier is noted?) the decision will have been made as to whether to treat this as an acute problem (commencing the contraction from the barrier), or as a chronic problem (commencing the contraction from short of the barrier).

- Appropriate degrees of resisted isometric effort are then introduced. For an acute problem a mild 15% of MVC (maximum voluntary contraction). For a chronic problem, a longer, stronger (up to 25% of MVC) effort is used, as the patient tries to both straighten the leg and take the thigh towards the table (this activates both ends of rectus femoris).

- Appropriate breathing instructions should be given (see notes on breathing in Box 5.2).

- The contraction is followed, on an exhalation, by taking of the muscle to, or stretching through, the new barrier, by taking the heel towards the buttock with the patient's help.

- The stretch should be held for 30 seconds or more.

- Remember to increase slight hip extension before the next contraction (using a cushion to support the thigh) as this removes slack from the cephalad end of rectus femoris.

- Repeat once or twice using agonists or antagonists.

Once a reasonable degree of increased range has been gained in rectus femoris it is appropriate to treat psoas, if this has tested as short.

Alternative rectus femoris MET treatment, using slow eccentric isotonic stretching (SEIS) of the hamstrings

- The patient lies prone, as in the previous description.

- The heel is eased towards the buttock to establish the first sign of resistance (bind).

- The heel should be held towards the buttock by the patients own effort.

- The practitioner then slowly eases (forces) the leg towards a straightened position, the patient having been given the instruction that, 'I am going to try to straighten your leg. You should resist this but not totally, so that you allow me to slowly overcome your effort.'

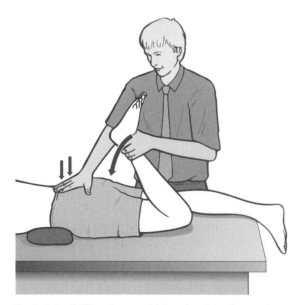

Figure 5.8   MET treatment of left rectus femoris muscle. Note that the practitioner's right hand stabilises the sacrum and pelvis to prevent undue stress during the stretching phase of the treatment.

- This slow eccentric stretch of the hamstrings tones these, and inhibits quadriceps/rectus femoris – or (see Ch. 4) increases tolerance to the stretch that follows.

- After the SEIS procedure the knee is flexed again and the heel eased towards the buttock to stretch rectus femoris as in the previous exercise.

MET treatment of psoas

Method A (Fig. 5.9A and B)   Psoas can also be treated in the prone position described for rectus femoris above. The stretch follows the patient's isometric effort to bring the thigh to the table against resistance (see Fig. 5.9A).

- The patient is prone with a pillow under the abdomen to reduce the lumbar curve (or the contralateral leg can be placed so that the foot touches the floor, neutralising the lumbar curve) and offering a stable pelvis from which to apply the subsequent stretch (see Fig. 5.9B).

- The practitioner stands contralateral to the side of psoas to be treated, with the table-side hand supporting the thigh.

- The non-table-side hand is placed so that the heel of that hand is on the sacrum, applying pressure towards the floor, to maintain pelvic stability.

- The fingers of that hand can be placed so that the middle, ring and small fingers are on one side of L2/3 segment and the index finger on the other. This allows these fingers to sense a forward (anteriorly directed) 'tug' of the vertebrae when psoas is stretched past its barrier as the thigh is elevated from the table.

- An alternative hand position is offered by Greenman (1996) who suggests that the stabilising contact on the pelvis should apply pressure towards the table, on the ischial tuberosity, as thigh extension is introduced (see Fig. 5.9A and B). The author agrees that this is a more comfortable contact than the sacrum. However, it fails to allow access to palpation of the lumbar spine during the procedure.

- The practitioner eases the thigh (knee is flexed) off the table surface and senses for ease of movement into extension of the hip. If there is a strong sense of resistance there should be an almost simultaneous awareness of the palpated vertebral segment moving anteriorly.

- It should be possible – if psoas is normal – to achieve approximately 10° of hip extension before that barrier is reached, without force. Greenman (1996) suggests that 'Normally the knee can be lifted 6 inches [15 cm] off the table. If less, tightness and shortness of psoas is present.'

- Having identified the barrier, the practitioner either works from this (in an acute setting) or short of it (in a chronic setting) as the patient is asked to bring the thigh towards the table against resistance, using 15–25% of their maximal voluntary contraction potential, for 7–10 seconds.

- Following release of the effort the thigh is eased to its new barrier if acute, or past that barrier, into stretch, with the patient's assistance ('gently push your foot towards the ceiling').

- If stretch is introduced, this is held for up to 30 seconds.

- It is important that as stretch is introduced no hyperextension occurs of the lumbar spine. Pressure from the heel of hand on the sacrum or ischial tuberosity usually ensures that spinal stability is maintained.

- The process is then repeated.

  Method B (Fig. 5.10A) Grieve's method involves using the supine test position, in which the patient lies with the buttocks at the very end of the table, with the non-treated leg fully flexed at the hip and knee, and either held in that state by the patient, or by placement of the patient's foot against the practitioner's lateral chest wall (Fig. 5.10A).

- The leg on the affected side is allowed to hang freely with the medio-plantar aspect resting on the practitioner's knee or shin.

- The practitioner stands sideways on to the patient, at the foot of the table, with both

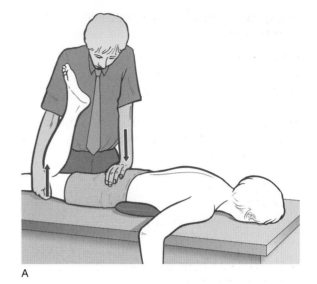

A

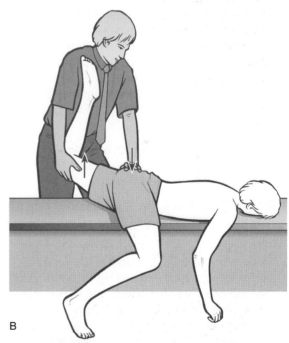

B

Figure 5.9 MET treatment of psoas with stabilising contact on ischial tuberosity as described by Greenman (1996).

hands holding the thigh of the extended leg. The practitioner's far leg should be flexed slightly at the knee so that the patient's foot can rest as described.

- This is used as a contact which, with the hands, resists the attempt of the patient to *externally rotate the leg* and, at the same time, *flex the hip* for 7–10 seconds. This combination of forces focuses the contraction effort into psoas very precisely.

- The practitioner resists both efforts, and an isometric contraction of the psoas and associated muscles therefore takes place.

- Appropriate breathing instructions should be given (see notes on breathing, Box 5.2).

- If the condition is acute, the treatment commences from the restriction barrier, whereas if the condition is chronic, the leg is elevated into a somewhat more flexed hip position.

- After the isometric contraction, using an appropriate degree of effort the thigh should, on an exhalation, either be taken to the new restriction barrier, without force (if acute), or through that barrier with slight, painless pressure towards the floor on the anterior aspect of the thigh (if chronic), and held there for 30 seconds (see Fig 5.10A and also a variation, Fig. 5.10B).

- Repeat until no further gain is achieved.[3]

MET treatment of psoas:

Method C (Fig. 5.11A, B) This method is appropriate for chronic psoas problems only.

- The supine test position is used in which the patient lies with the buttocks at the very end of the table, the non-treated leg fully flexed at the hip and knee, and either held in that state by the patient (Fig 5.11A), or by the practitioner's hand (Fig 5.11B), or by placement of the patient's foot against the practitioner's lateral chest wall.

- The leg on the affected side is allowed to hang freely.

---

[3] Direct inhibitory pressure techniques applied to the vertebral attachments of psoas through the mid-line is an effective alternative approach, especially in acute psoas conditions. This is not usually applicable in overweight individuals.

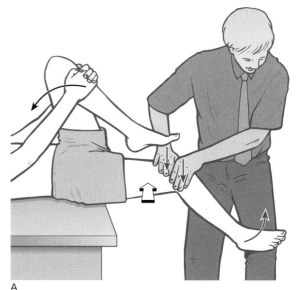

A

Figure 5.10A MET treatment of psoas using Grieve's method, in which there is placement of the patient's foot, inverted, against the practitioner's thigh. This allows a more precise focus of contraction into psoas when the hip is flexed against resistance.

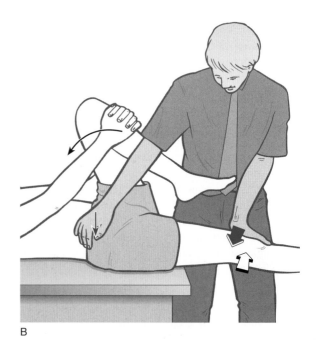

B

Figure 5.10B Psoas treatment variation, with the leg held straight and the pelvis stabilised.

- The practitioner resists a light attempt by the patient to flex the hip for 7–10 seconds.

- Appropriate breathing instructions should be given (see notes on breathing, Box 5.2).

- After the isometric contraction, using an appropriate degree of effort, on an exhalation the thigh should be taken slightly beyond the restriction barrier, with a light degree of painless pressure towards the floor, and held there for 30 seconds (Fig. 5.11B).

- Repeat until no further gain is achieved (see footnote 3).

Self-treatment of psoas

Method A

- Lewit suggests self-treatment in a position as above in which the patient lies close to the end of a bed as shown in Fig. 5.6B, with one leg fully flexed at the hip and knee and held in this position throughout, while the other leg is allowed to reach the limit of its stretch, as gravity pulls it towards the floor.

- The patient then lifts this leg slightly (say a further 2 cm) to contract psoas, holding this for 7–10 seconds, before slowly allowing the leg to ease towards the floor.

- This stretch position is held for a further 30 seconds, and the process is repeated three to five times.

- The counterpressure in this effort is achieved by gravity.

Method B (Fig. 5.12)

- The patient stands facing a chair or stool onto which is placed the non-treated-side foot.

- The flexed knee should be above hip height.

- The treated-side leg is placed behind the trunk so that all hip flexion is eliminated, until a sense of light stretching is noted on the anterior thigh, but not in the low back.

- The patient places both hands on hips and ensures that no hyperextension of the lumbar spine is occurring.

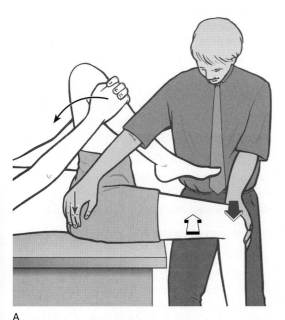

A

Figure 5.11A MET treatment involves the patient's effort to flex the hip against resistance.

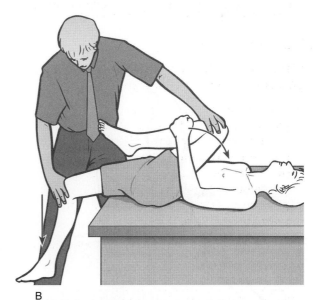

B

Figure 5.11B Stretch of psoas, which follows the isometric contraction (Fig. 5.10A) and is achieved by means of gravity plus additional practitioner effort.

- The patient is instructed to ease the trunk anteriorly, without any spinal flexion or extension, until a sense of additional stretch is noted on the anterior thigh.

- This is held for 30 seconds before a further movement anteriorly, of the patient's trunk, reproduces the sense of stretching in the anterior thigh.

- This again is held for 30 seconds.

4. Assessment and treatment of hamstrings (07) (Fig. 5.13A and B)

Should obviously tight hamstrings always be treated? Van Wingerden (1997), reporting on the earlier work of Vleeming (Vleeming et al 1989), states that both intrinsic and extrinsic support for the sacroiliac joint derives in part from hamstring (biceps femoris) status. Intrinsically the influence is via the close anatomical and physiological relationship between biceps femoris and the sacrotuberous ligament (they frequently attach via a strong tendinous link): 'Force from the biceps femoris muscle can lead to increased tension of the sacrotuberous ligament in various ways. Since increased tension of the sacrotuberous ligament diminishes the range of sacroiliac joint motion, the

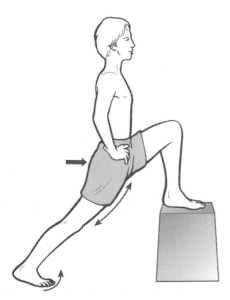

Figure 5.12   Psoas self-stretch.

biceps femoris can play a role in stabilisation of the SIJ.'

Van Wingerden also notes that in low-back patients, forward flexion is often painful as the load on the spine increases. This happens whether flexion occurs in the spine or via the hip joints (tilting of the pelvis). If the hamstrings are tight and short they effectively prevent pelvic tilting: 'In this respect, an increase in hamstring tension might well be part of a defensive arthrokinematic reflex mechanism of the body to diminish spinal load.' If such a state of affairs is longstanding, the hamstrings (biceps femoris) will shorten, possibly influencing sacroiliac and lumbar spine dysfunction.

The decision to treat tight ('tethered') hamstrings should therefore take account of *why they are tight*, and consider that, in some circumstances, they might be offering beneficial support to the SIJ, or be reducing low-back stress.

Methodology

If the hip flexors (psoas, etc.) have previously tested as short, then the test position for the hamstrings needs to commence with the non-tested leg flexed at both knee and hip, foot resting flat on the treatment surface to ensure full pelvic rotation into neutral (as in Fig 5.13B). If no hip flexor shortness was observed, then the non-tested leg should lie flat on the surface of the table.

Hamstring test A

- The patient lies supine with non-tested leg either flexed or straight, depending on previous test results for hip flexors.

- The tested leg is taken into a straight-leg-raised (SLR) position, no flexion of the knee being allowed, with minimal force employed.

- The first sign of resistance (or palpated bind) is assessed as the barrier of restriction.

- If straight leg raising to 80° is not easily possible, then there exists some shortening of the hamstrings and the muscles can be treated in the straight leg position (see below).

Hamstring test B (Fig. 5.14)   Whether or not an 80° elevation is easily achieved, a variation in

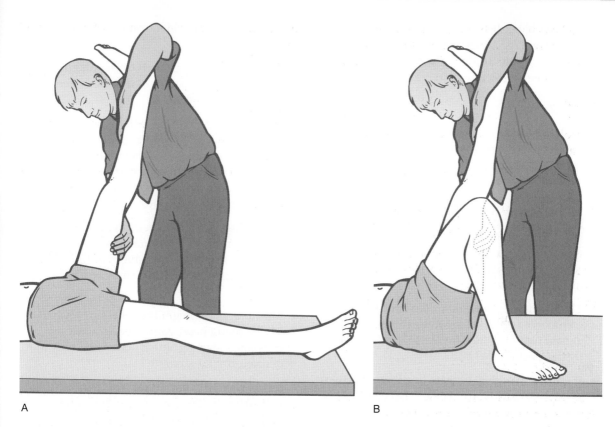

A

B

Figure 5.13A Assessment for shortness in hamstring muscles. The practitioner's right hand palpates for bind/the first sign of resistance, while the left hand maintains the patient's knee in extension.

Figure 5.13B MET treatment of shortened hamstrings. Following an isometric contraction, the leg is taken to or through the resistance barrier (depending on whether the problem is acute or chronic).

testing is also needed to evaluate the lower hamstring fibres.

- To achieve this assessment the tested leg is taken into *full* hip flexion (helped by patient holding upper thigh with both hands (see Fig. 5.14). The knee is then straightened until resistance is felt, or bind is noted by palpation of the lower hamstrings.

- If the knee cannot straighten with the hip flexed, this indicates shortness in the lower hamstring fibres, and the patient will report a degree of pull behind the knee and lower thigh. MET treatment of this is carried out in the test position.

- If, however, the knee is capable of being straightened with the hip flexed, having

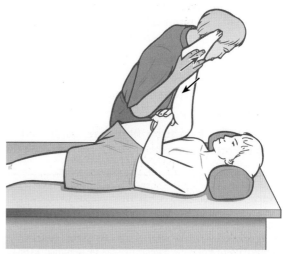

Figure 5.14 Assessment and treatment position for lower hamstring fibres.

previously not been capable of achieving an 80° straight leg raise, then the lower fibres are not responsible for the restriction, and it is the upper fibres of hamstrings that require attention using MET, working from the SLR test position.

Hamstring test C   Lewit (1999) describes a functional test which helps to screen for overactivity in the erector spinae and/or hamstrings, while also indicating weakness of gluteus maximus.

- The patient is prone and the practitioner places palpating hands on the lower buttock/upper thigh (gluteal/hamstring contact) and the low-back (erector spinae contact) as the patient is asked to extend the hip, leg kept straight.

- The normal sequence is for the hamstrings to commence the elevation of the thigh with almost instant gluteal involvement, followed by the erectors.

- If gluteus maximus is weak (see lower crossed syndrome notes in Ch. 2) there may still be strong extension of the thigh, but with the hamstrings and erectors doing most of the work.

- This is an indication of overactivity (i.e. stress) in these postural muscles and therefore suggests shortness.

- In extreme cases the movement of thigh/hip extension is initiated by the erector spinae themselves, and these are then almost certainly short.[4]

Method A. MET for shortness of lower hamstrings

If the lower hamstring fibres are implicated as being short (see hamstring test B above), then the

---

[4] Extension of the hip is a normal part of the gait cycle and therefore a movement which is usually made thousands of times daily. It is easy to imagine the degree of overuse stress (and therefore ultimately shortness) in hamstrings which is compensating for the weakness in the gluteal muscles. If this pattern exists the hamstrings can be assumed to be short and out of balance with their synergists and likely to benefit from MET.

treatment position is identical to the test position (see Fig. 5.14).

- The non-treated leg needs to be either flexed (if hip flexors are short, as described above) or straight on the table.

- The treated leg should be flexed at both the hip and knee, and then straightened by the practitioner until the restriction barrier is identified (one hand should palpate the tissues behind the knee for sensations of bind as the lower leg is straightened).

- Depending upon whether it is an acute or a chronic problem, the isometric contraction against resistance is introduced at this 'bind' barrier (if acute) or a little short of it (if chronic).

- The instruction might be something such as 'try to gently bend your knee, against my resistance, starting slowly and using only a quarter of your strength'.

- It is particularly important with the hamstrings to take care regarding cramp, and so it is suggested that no more than 25% of patients' strength should ever be used during isometric contractions in this region.

- Following the 7–10 seconds of contraction (for notes on respiratory synkinesis see Box 5.2) followed by complete relaxation, the leg should, on an exhalation, be straightened at the knee towards its new barrier (in acute problems) and through that barrier, with a degree of stretch (if chronic), with the patient's assistance.

- This slight stretch should be held for up to 30 seconds.

- Repeat the process until no further gain is possible (usually one or two repetitions achieve the maximum degree of lengthening available at any one session).

Antagonist muscles can also be used isometrically by having the patient try to extend the knee during the contraction, rather than bending it, followed by the stretching procedure described above.

Method B. MET treatment of lower hamstrings (Fig. 5.14)

- The supine patient fully flexes the hip on the affected side.

- The flexed knee is extended by the practitioner to the point of resistance (identifying the barrier).

- The calf of the treated leg is placed on the shoulder of the practitioner, who stands facing the head of the table on the side of the treated leg.

- If the right leg of the patient is being treated, the calf will rest on the practitioner's right shoulder, and the practitioner's right hand stabilises the patient's extended unaffected leg against the table.

- The practitioner's left hand holds the treated leg thigh to both maintain stability and to palpate for bind when the barrier is being assessed.

- The patient is asked to attempt to *straighten* the lower leg (i.e. extend the knee) utilising the antagonists to the hamstrings, employing 20% of the strength in the quadriceps.

- This is resisted by the practitioner for 7–10 seconds.

- Appropriate breathing instructions should be given (see notes in Box 5.2).

- The leg is then extended at the knee to its new hamstring limit if the problem is acute (or stretched slightly if chronic) after relaxation and the procedure is then repeated.

Method C. Co-contraction MET method of hamstring treatment

- Starting from the same position, a combined contraction may be introduced (Moore et al 1980).

- The instruction to the patient would be to pull the thigh towards her face (i.e. to flex the hip) and to push the lower leg downward onto the practitioner's shoulder (i.e. flexing the knee).

- This effectively contracts both the quadriceps and the hamstrings, facilitating subsequent easing to, or stretching through, the restriction barrier of the tight as described above.

Method D. Simultaneous toning of hamstring antagonists (quadriceps) and preparation for stretch of shortened hamstrings using SEIS

As discussed in Ch. 3 a slow eccentric isotonic stretch (SEIS) of a muscle tones this, while simultaneously preparing the antagonist for subsequent stretching.

- The patient is supine with hip and knee of the leg to be treated, flexed.

- The practitioner extends the flexed knee to its first barrier of resistance, palpating the tissues proximal to the knee crease for first sign of 'bind'.

- The patient is asked to resist, using a little more than half available strength, an attempt by the practitioner to slowly flex the knee fully (stretching the contracting quadriceps, toning these).

- An instruction should be given which makes clear the objective, 'I am going to slowly bend your knee, and I want you to partially resist this, but to let it slowly happen'.

- After performing the slow isotonic stretch of the quadriceps the hamstring should be retested for length and ease of straight-leg raising, and if necessary, the hamstrings should be taken into a stretched position and held for 30 seconds before repeating the procedure.

MET for shortness of upper hamstrings

- If the upper fibres are involved (i.e. hamstring test A, above), then treatment is performed in the SLR position, with the knee maintained in extension at all times.

- The non-treated leg should be flexed at hip and knee or straight, depending on the hip flexor findings as explained above.

- In all other details the procedures are the same as for treatment of lower hamstring fibres except that the leg is kept straight.

5. Assessment and treatment of tensor fascia lata (TFL) (08) (see also Box 5.5)

- The test recommended is a modified form of Ober's test (see Fig. 5.15).

- The patient is side-lying with back close to the edge of the table.

- The practitioner stands behind the patient, whose lower leg is flexed at hip and knee and held in this position, by the patient, for stability.

- The tested leg is supported by the practitioner, who must ensure that there is *no hip flexion*, which would nullify the test.

- The leg is extended to the position where the iliotibial band lies over the greater trochanter.

- The tested leg is held by the practitioner at ankle and knee, with the whole leg in its anatomical position, neither abducted nor adducted, and not forward or backward of the trunk.

- The practitioner carefully introduces flexion at the knee to 90°, *without allowing the hip to flex*, and then, while supporting the limb at the ankle, allows the knee to fall towards the table.

- If the TFL is normal, the thigh and knee will fall easily, with the knee usually contacting the table surface (unless there is unusual hip width, or a short thigh length prevents this).

- If the upper leg remains aloft, with little sign of 'falling' towards the table, then either the patient is not letting go, or the TFL is short and does not allow it to fall.

- As a rule the band will palpate as tender under such conditions.

Lewit's (1999) TFL palpation

See also the functional assessment method in Ch. 8.

- The patient is side-lying and the practitioner stands facing the patient's front, at hip level.

- The patient's non-tested leg is slightly flexed to provide stability, and there should be a vertical line to the table between one anterior superior iliac spine (ASIS) and the other (i.e. no forwards or backwards 'roll' of the pelvis).

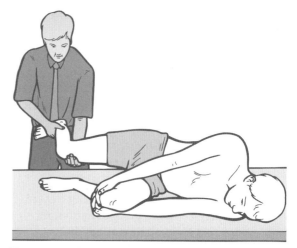

Figure 5.15 Assessment for shortness of TFL – modified Ober's test. When the hand supporting the flexed knee is removed the thigh should fall to the table if TFL is not short.

- The practitioner's cephalad hand rests over the ASIS so that it can also palpate over the trochanter, with the fingers resting on the TFL and the thumb on gluteus medius.

- The caudad hand rests on the mid-thigh to apply slight resistance to the patient's effort to abduct the leg.

- The patient abducts the upper leg (which should be extended at the knee and slightly hyperextended at the hip) and the practitioner should feel the trochanter 'slip away' as this is done.

- If, however, the whole pelvis is felt to move rather than just the trochanter, there is inappropriate muscular imbalance.

- In balanced abduction gluteus comes into action at the beginning of the movement, with TFL operating later in the pure abduction of the leg.

- If there is an overactivity (and therefore shortness) of TFL, then there will be pelvic movement on the abduction, and TFL will be felt to come into play before gluteus medius.

- The abduction of the thigh movement will have been modified to include external rotation and flexion of the thigh (Janda 1996).

Box 5.5 Notes on TFL

- Mennell (1964) and Liebenson (1996) say that TFL shortness can produce all the symptoms of acute and chronic sacroiliac problems.
- Pain from TFL shortness can be localised to the posterior superior iliac spine (PSIS), radiating to the groin or down any aspect of the thigh to the knee.
- Although the pain may arise in the sacroiliac (SI) joint, dysfunction in the joint may be caused and maintained by taut TFL structures.
- Pain from the band itself can be felt in the lateral thigh, with referral to hip or knee.
- TFL can be 'riddled' with sensitive fibrotic deposits and trigger point activity.
- There is commonly a posteriority of the ilium associated with short TFL.
- TFL's prime phasic activity (all postural structures also have some phasic function) is to assist the gluteals in abduction of the thigh.
- If TFL and psoas are short they may, according to Janda, 'dominate' the gluteals on abduction of the thigh, so that a degree of lateral rotation and flexion of the hip will be produced, rotating the pelvis backwards.
- Rolf (1977) points out that persistent exercise such as cycling will shorten and toughen the fascial iliotibial band 'until it becomes reminiscent of a steel cable'. This band crosses both hip and knee, and spatial compression allows it to squeeze and compress cartilaginous elements such as the menisci. Ultimately, it will no longer be able to compress, and rotational displacement at knee and hip will take place.

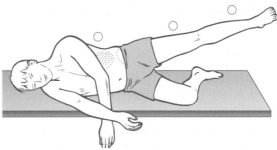

Figure 5.16 Hip abduction observation test.

- When quadratus is overactive it will often initiate the abduction along with TFL, thus producing a pelvic tilt.[5] (See also Fig. 5.11A and B.)

Observation assessment – hip abduction test (Fig. 5.16)

- The patient is side-lying, ideally with head on a cushion, with the upper leg straight and the lower leg flexed at hip and knee, for balance.
- The practitioner, who is observing not palpating, stands in front of the patient and towards the head end of the table.
- The patient is asked to slowly raise the leg into abduction.
- Normal is represented by pure hip abduction to 45°.
- Abnormal is represented by:
  - hip flexion during abduction, indicating TFL shortness
  - the leg externally rotating during abduction, indicating piriformis shortness
  - 'hip hiking', indicating quadratus lumborum shortness (and gluteus medius weakness)
  - posterior pelvic rotation, suggesting short antagonistic hip adductors.

- This indicates a stressed postural muscle (TFL), which implies shortness.
- It may be possible (depending on the practitioner's hand size and patient anatomical size) to increase the number of palpation elements involved by having the cephalad hand also palpate (with an extended small finger) quadratus lumborum during leg abduction.
- In a balanced muscular effort to lift the leg sideways, quadratus lumborum should not become active until the leg has been abducted to around 25–30°.

---

[5] Remember that a lateral 'corset' of muscles exists to stabilise the pelvic and low-back structures and that if TFL and quadratus (and/or psoas) shorten and tighten, the gluteal muscles will weaken. This test gives the proof of such imbalance existing. (See notes on lower crossed syndrome in Ch. 2.)

Method A. Supine MET treatment of shortened TFL (Fig. 5.17)

- The patient lies supine with the unaffected leg flexed at hip and knee.

- The practitioner stands facing the contralateral leg at approximately knee level.

- The affected-side leg is adducted to its barrier, requiring it to be brought under the contralateral leg/foot.

- Observing the guidelines previously discussed for acute and chronic problems, TFL will either be treated at, or short of, the barrier of resistance, using light to moderate degrees of effort involving isometric contractions of 7–10 seconds.

- The practitioner uses his trunk to stabilise the patient's pelvis by leaning against the flexed contralateral knee.

- The practitioner's caudad arm supports the affected leg so that the knee is stabilised by the hand. The other hand maintains a firm contact on the affected side ASIS.

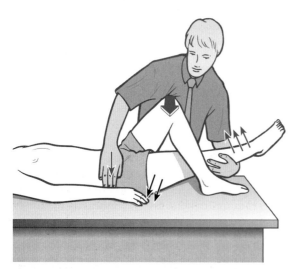

Figure 5.17   MET treatment of TFL (see Fig. 1.4 for description of isolytic variation). If a standard MET method is being used, the stretch will follow the isometric contraction in which the patient will attempt to move the right leg to the right against sustained resistance. It is important for the practitioner to maintain stability of the pelvis during the procedure.

- The patient is asked to abduct the leg against resistance using minimal force ('Using less than a quarter of your strength, slowly take your leg back towards the midline, against my resistance').

- After the contraction ceases, and the patient has relaxed, and on an exhalation, the leg should be taken to or through the new restriction barrier (into adduction past the barrier) to stretch the muscular fibres of TFL (the upper third of the structure).

- Care should be taken to ensure that the pelvis is not tilted during the stretch.

- Stability is achieved by the practitioner maintaining pressure against the flexed knee/thigh.

- The entire process should be repeated several times, or until no further gain is possible.

Method B. Greenman alternative supine MET treatment of shortened TFL (Fig. 5.18)

- The patient adopts the same position as for psoas assessment, lying at the end of the table with the non-treated-side leg in full hip flexion and held by the patient, with the tested leg hanging freely, knee flexed.

- For a right-sided TFL treatment the practitioner stands at the end of the table facing the patient so that his left lower leg can contact the patient's foot.

- The practitioner's left hand is placed on the patient's distal femur, and with this he introduces internal rotation of the thigh, while simultaneously introducing external rotation of the tibia, by means of light pressure on the distal foot from his lower leg.

- During this process the practitioner senses for resistance (the movements should be easy and 'springy' without any hard end-feel).

- If while maintaining these rotational holds a characteristic depression or groove can be observed on the lateral thigh, this strongly suggests shortness and tension involving TFL (Greenman 1996, p 464).

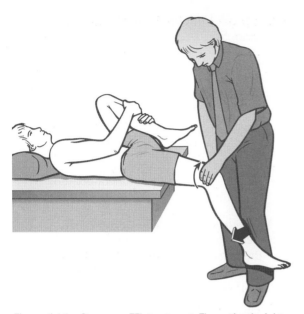

Figure 5.18 Greenman TFL treatment: The patient's right thigh is held at resistance barrier of internal rotation, together with external rotation of the tibia, as the patient introduces adduction of the femur and external rotation of the tibia aginst resistance. This is followed by the barriers being re-engaged and the stretch held for 30 seconds.

- Once the resistance barrier has been identified, the leg should be held just short of this for a chronic problem, as the patient is asked to *externally rotate the tibia*, and to *adduct the femur*, against resistance, for 7–10 seconds.

- Following this the practitioner eases the leg into a greater degree of internal hip rotation and external tibial rotation, and holds this stretch for up to 30 seconds.

Method C. Isolytic variation (Fig. 1.4)

If an isolytic contraction is introduced in order to actively stretch the interface between elastic and non-elastic tissues, then there is a need to stabilise the pelvis more efficiently, either by use of wide straps, or another pair of hands holding the ASIS to the table during the stretch.

- The procedure consists of the patient attempting to abduct the leg as the practitioner overcomes the muscular effort, forcing the leg into adduction.

- The contraction/stretch should be rapid (2–3 seconds at most to complete).

- Repeat several times.

Method D. Side-lying MET treatment of TFL

- The patient lies on the affected TFL side with the upper leg flexed at hip and knee and resting forward of the affected leg.

- The practitioner stands behind patient and uses caudad hand and arm to raise the affected leg (which is on the table) while stabilising the pelvis with the cephalad hand, or uses both hands to raise the affected leg into slight adduction (appropriate if strapping used to hold pelvis to table).

- The patient contracts the muscle against resistance by trying to take the leg into abduction (towards the table) using breathing assistance as appropriate (see notes on breathing, Box 5.2).

- After the effort, on an exhalation, the practitioner lifts the leg into adduction beyond the barrier to stretch the interface between elastic and non-elastic tissues.

- Repeat as appropriate or modify to use as an isolytic contraction (method C above) by stretching the structure past the barrier during the contraction.

Additional TFL methods

Mennell (1964) has described efficient soft tissue stretching techniques for releasing TFL. These involve a series of snapping actions applied by thumbs to the anterior fibres with patient side-lying, followed by a series of heel-of-hand thrusts across the long axis of the posterior TFL fibres.

Additional release of TFL contractions is possible by use of elbow or heel-of-hand 'stripping' of the structure, neuromuscular deep tissue approaches (using thumb or a rubber-tipped T-bar) applied to the upper fibres and those around the knee, and specific deep tissue release methods.

Most of these methods are distinctly uncomfortable and all require expert tuition.[6]

Self-treatment and maintenance

- The patient lies on her side, on a bed or table, with the affected leg uppermost and hanging over the edge (lower leg comfortably flexed).

- The patient may then introduce an isometric contraction by slightly lifting the hanging leg a few centimetres, and holding this position for 10 seconds, before slowly releasing and allowing gravity to take the leg towards the floor, so introducing a greater degree of stretch.

- This is held for up to 30 seconds and the process is then repeated several times in order to achieve the maximum available stretch in the tight soft tissues.

- The counterforce in this isometric exercise is gravity.

6. Assessment and treatment of piriformis (09) (see also Boxes 5.6 and 5.7)

◎ Test A. Piriformis stretch test

- When it is short, piriformis will usually cause the affected side leg of the supine patient to appear to be short and externally rotated.

- The supine patient's tested leg should be placed into flexion at the hip and knee so that the foot rests on the table lateral to the contralateral knee (the tested leg is crossed over the straight non-tested leg, as shown in Fig. 5.19).

- The angle of hip flexion should not exceed 60° (see notes on piriformis in Box 5.6).

- The non-tested side ASIS is stabilised to prevent pelvic motion during the test and the knee of the tested side is pushed into adduction, to place a stretch on piriformis.

- If piriformis is shortened the degree of adduction will be limited and the patient will report discomfort posterior to the trochanter.

◎ Test B. Piriformis palpation test (Fig. 5.20)

- The patient is side-lying, tested side uppermost.

- The practitioner stands at the level of the pelvis in front of and facing the patient, and, in order to contact the insertion of piriformis, draws imaginary lines between:
  - ASIS and the ischial tuberosity
  - PSIS and the most prominent point of trochanter.

- Where these reference lines cross, just posterior to the trochanter, is the insertion of the muscle, and digital pressure here will produce marked discomfort if the structure is short or irritated.

- To locate the most common trigger point site in the belly of the muscle, a line from the ASIS should be taken to the tip of the coccyx, rather than to the ischial tuberosity.

- The mid-point of the belly of piriformis, where triggers are common, is found where this line crosses the line from the PSIS to the trochanter. Light compression here that produces a painful

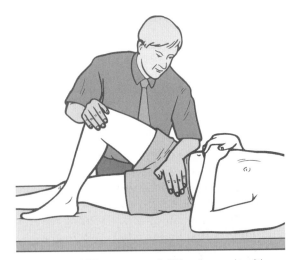

Figure 5.19 MET treatment of piriformis muscle with patient supine. The pelvis must be maintained in a stable position as the knee (right in this example) is adducted to stretch piriformis following an isometric contraction.

---

[6] These methods are fully described in Chaitow (2003).

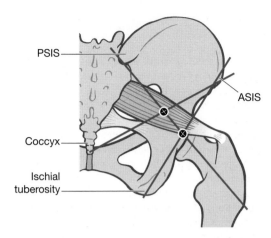

PSIS

ASIS

Coccyx

Ischial
tuberosity

Figure 5.20 Using bony landmarks as coordinates the commonest tender areas are located in piriformis, in the belly and at the attachment of the muscle.

response is indicative of a stressed muscle, and possibly an active myofascial trigger point.

Piriformis strength test

- The patient lies prone, both knees flexed to 90°, with the practitioner at the foot of the table grasping the lower legs at the limit of their separation.

- This internally rotates the hip and therefore allows comparison of the range of movement

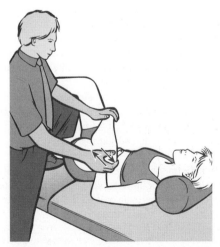

Figure 5.21 MET treatment of piriformis with hip fully flexed and externally rotated (see Box 5.6, first bullet point).

permitted by shortened external rotators such as the piriformis.

- The patient attempts to bring the ankles together as the practitioner assesses the relative strength of the two legs.

Mitchell et al (1979) suggest that if there is relative shortness (as evidenced by the lower leg not being able to travel as far from the mid-line as its pair in this position), and if that same side also tests strong, then MET is called for. However, if there is shortness as well as relative weakness, then the reasons for the weakness (trigger points for example) need to be dealt with prior to stretching using MET.

MET treatment of piriformis

Method A. Side-lying

- The patient should be side-lying, close to the edge of the table, affected side uppermost, both legs flexed at hip and knee.

- The practitioner stands facing the patient at hip level.

- The practitioner places his cephalad elbow tip gently over the point behind trochanter, where piriformis inserts.

- The patient should be close enough to the edge of the table for the practitioner to stabilise the pelvis against his trunk (see Fig. 5.22).

- At the same time, the practitioner's caudad hand grasps the patient's ankle and uses this to bring the upper leg/hip into internal rotation, taking out all the slack in piriformis.

- A degree of inhibitory pressure (sufficient to cause discomfort but not pain) is applied via the elbow for 5–7 seconds while the muscle is kept at a reasonable but not excessive degree of stretch.

- The practitioner maintains contact on the point, but eases pressure, and asks the patient to introduce an isometric contraction (25% of strength for 5–7 seconds) to piriformis, by bringing the lower leg towards the table against resistance.

Box 5.6 Notes on piriformis

- Piriformis paradox. The performance of external rotation of the hip by piriformis occurs when the angle of hip flexion is 60° or less. Once the angle of hip flexion is greater than 60° piriformis function changes, so that it becomes an internal rotator of the hip (Lehmkuhl & Smith 1983, Gluck & Liebenson 1997). The implications of this are illustrated in Figs 5.19 and 5.21.
- This postural muscle, like all others which have a predominence of type I fibres, will shorten if stressed. In the case of piriformis, the effect of shortening is to increase its diameter and because of its location this allows for direct pressure to be exerted on the sciatic nerve, which passes under it in 80% of people. In the other 20% the nerve passes through the muscle so that contraction will produce veritable strangulation of the sciatic nerve.
- In addition, the pudendal nerve and the blood vessels of the internal iliac artery, as well as common perineal nerves, posterior femoral cutaneous nerve and nerves of the hip rotators, can all be affected.
- If there is sciatic pain associated with piriformis shortness, then on straight leg raising, which reproduces the pain, external rotation of the hip should relieve it, since this slackens piriformis. (This clue may, however, only apply to any degree if the individual is one of those in whom the nerve actually passes through the muscle.)
- The effects can be circulatory, neurological and functional, inducing pain and paraesthesia of the affected limb as well as alterations to pelvic and lumbar function.
- Diagnosis usually hinges on the absence of spinal causative factors and the distributions of symptoms from the sacrum to the hip joint, over the gluteal region and down to the popliteal space. Palpation of the affected piriformis tendon, near the head of the trochanter, will elicit pain and the affected leg will probably be externally rotated.
- The piriformis muscle syndrome is frequently characterised by such bizarre symptoms that they may seem unrelated. One characteristic complaint is a persistent, severe, radiating low-back pain extending from the sacrum to the hip joint, over the gluteal region and the posterior portion of the upper leg, to the popliteal space. In the most severe cases the patient will be unable to lie or stand comfortably, and changes in position will not relieve the pain. Intense pain will occur when the patient sits or squats since this type of movement requires external rotation of the upper leg and flexion at the knee.
- Compression of the pudendal nerve and blood vessels which pass through the greater sciatic foramen and re-enter the pelvis via the lesser sciatic foramen is possible because of piriformis contracture. Any compression would result in impaired circulation to the genitalia in both sexes. Since external rotation of the hips is required for coitus by women, pain noted during this act could relate to impaired circulation induced by piriformis dysfunction. This could also be a basis for impotency in men. (See also Box 5.7.)
- Piriformis involvement often relates to a pattern of pain which includes:
- pain near the trochanter
- pain in the inguinal area
- local tenderness over the insertion behind trochanter
- SI joint pain on the opposite side
- externally rotated foot on the same side
- pain unrelieved by most positions with standing and walking being the easiest
- limitation of internal rotation of the leg which produces pain near the hip
- short leg on the affected side.
- The pain itself will be persistent and radiating, covering anywhere from the sacrum to the buttock, hip and leg including inguinal and perineal areas.
- Bourdillon (1982) suggests that piriformis syndrome and SI joint dysfunction are intimately connected and that recurrent SI problems will not stabilise until hypertonic piriformis is corrected.
- Janda (1996) points to the vast amount of pelvic organ dysfunction to which piriformis can contribute due to its relationship with circulation to the area.
- Mitchell et al (1979) suggest that (as in psoas example above) piriformis shortness should only be treated if it is tested to be short and stronger than its pair. If it is short and weak (see p 000 for strength test), then whatever is hypertonic and influencing it should be released and stretched first (Mitchell et al 1979). When it tests strong and short, piriformis should receive MET treatment.
- Since piriformis is an external rotator of the hip it can be inhibited (made to test weak) if an internal rotator such as TFL is hypertonic or if its pair is hypertonic, since one piriformis will inhibit the other.

Box 5.7 Working and resting muscles

Richard (1978) reminds us that a working muscle will mobilise up to 10 times the quantity of blood mobilised by a resting muscle. He points out the link between pelvic circulation and lumbar, ischiatic and gluteal arteries and the chance this allows to engineer the involvement of 2400 square metres of capillaries by using repetitive pumping of these muscles (including piriformis).

The therapeutic use of this knowledge involves the patient being asked to repetitively contract both piriformis muscles against resistance. The patient is supine, knees bent, feet on the table; the practitioner resists their effort to abduct their flexed knees, using a pulsed muscle energy approach (Ruddy's method) in which two isometrically resisted pulsation/contractions per second are introduced for as long as possible (a minute seems a long time doing this).

- The same acute and chronic rules as discussed previously are employed, together with cooperative breathing if appropriate (see Box 5.2).

- After the isometric contraction ceases, and the patient relaxes, the lower limb is taken to its new resistance barrier and elbow pressure is reapplied.

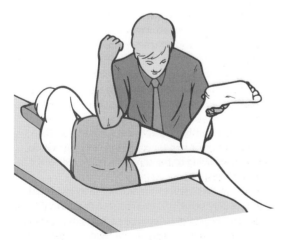

Figure 5.22 A combined ischaemic compression (elbow pressure) and MET side-lying treatment of piriformis. The pressure is alternated with isometric contractions/stretching of the muscle until no further gain is achieved.

- This process is repeated until no further gain is achieved.

Method B This method is a variation on the method described by TePoorten (1960) which calls for longer and heavier compression, and no intermediate isometric contractions.

- The patient lies on the non-affected side with knees flexed and hip joints flexed to 90°.

- The practitioner places his elbow on the piriformis musculotendinous junction, and a steady firm pressure is applied.

- With his other hand the practitioner abducts the foot in order to force an internal rotation of the hip.

- The leg is held in this position for up to 2 minutes with sustained compression by the elbow of the piriformis attachment area.

- The entire procedure is repeated two or three times.

- The patient is then placed in the supine position and piriformis is retested.

Method C This method is based on the test position (see Fig. 5.19) and is described by Lewit (1992).

- With the patient supine, the treated leg is placed into flexion at the hip and knee, so that the foot rests on the table lateral to the contralateral knee (the leg on the side to be treated is crossed over the other, straight, leg).

- The angle of hip flexion should not exceed 60° (see notes on piriformis, Box 5.6, for explanation).

- The practitioner places one hand on the contralateral ASIS to prevent pelvic motion, while the other hand is placed against the lateral flexed knee as this is pushed into resisted abduction to contract piriformis for 7–10 seconds.

- Following the contraction the practitioner eases the treated-side leg into adduction until a sense of resistance is noted; this is held for 10–30 seconds.

Method D

- The position illustrated in Fig. 5.21 is adopted (see explanatory notes in Box 5.6, first bullet point).

- The hip is flexed beyond 60° and the hip fully externally rotated to its barrier.

- The patient attempts – using minimal effort – to internally rotate the hip against resistance.

- Following this the hip is flexed further and externally rotated further and held for 30 seconds, before repeating the sequence.

7. Assessment and treatment of quadratus lumborum (10) (see also Box 5.8)

It is suggested that you review Lewit's functional palpation test described above under heading 5, 'Assessment and treatment of tensor fascia lata'.

Box 5.8 Notes on quadratus lumborum

Norris (2000) describes the divided roles in which quadratus is involved:

- The quadratus lumborum has been shown to be significant as a stabiliser in lumbar spine movements (McGill et al 1996), while tightening has also been described (Janda 1983). It seems likely that the muscle may act functionally differently in its medial and lateral portions, with the medial portion being more active as a stabiliser of the lumbar spine, and the lateral more active as a mobiliser (see stabiliser/mobiliser discussion Ch. 2). Such sub-division is seen in a number of other muscles, for example the gluteus medius, where the posterior fibres are more posturally involved (Jull 1994); the internal oblique, where the posterior fibres attaching to the lateral raphe are considered stabilisers (Bergmark 1989); the external oblique, where the lateral fibres work during flexion in parallel to the rectus abdominis (Kendall et al 1993).

- Janda (1983) observes that, when the patient is side-bending (as in method B) 'when the lumbar spine appears straight, with compensatory motion occurring only from the thoraco-lumbar region upwards, tightness of quadratus lumborum may be suspected'. This 'whole lumbar spine' involvement differs from a segmental restriction which would probably involve only a part of the lumbar spine.

- Quadratus fibres merge with the diaphragm (as do those of psoas), which makes involvement in respiratory dysfunction a possibility since it plays a role in exhalation, both via this merging and by its attachment to the 12th rib.

- Shortness of quadratus, or the presence of trigger points, can result in pain in the lower ribs and along the iliac crest if the lateral fibres are affected.

- Shortness of the medial fibres, or the presence of trigger points, can produce pain in the sacroiliac joint and the buttock.

- Bilateral contraction produces extension and unilateral contraction produces extension and side-bending to the same side.

- The important transition region, the lumbodorsal junction (LDJ), is the only one in the spine in which two mobile structures meet, and dysfunction results in alteration of the quality of motion between these structures (upper and lower trunk/dorsal and lumbar spines). In dysfunction there is often a degree of spasm or tightness in the muscles which stabilise the region, notably: psoas and erector spinae of the thoracolumbar region, as well as quadratus lumborum and rectus abdominis.

- Symptomatic differential diagnosis of muscle involvement at the LDJ is possible as follows:
  - psoas involvement usually triggers abdominal pain if severe and produces flexion of the hip and the typical antalgesic posture of lumbago
  - erector spinae involvement produces low-back pain at its caudad end of attachment and interscapular pain at its thoracic attachment (as far up as the mid-thoracic level)
  - quadratus lumborum involvement causes lumbar pain and pain at the attachment of the iliac crest and lower ribs
  - rectus abdominis contraction may mimic abdominal pain and result in pain at the attachments at the pubic symphysis and the xiphoid process, as well as forward-bending of the trunk and restricted ability to extend the spine.

- There is seldom pain at the site of the lesion in LDJ dysfunction. Lewit (1992) points out that even if a number of these muscles are implicated, it is seldom necessary, using PIR methods, to treat them all since, as the muscles most involved (discovered by tests for shortness, overactivity, sensitivity and direct palpation) are stretched and normalised, so will others begin automatically to normalise.

Quadratus lumborum test A (Fig. 5.23, also Fig. 5.11A, B)

- The patient is side-lying and is asked to take the upper arm over the head to grasp the top edge of the table, 'opening out' the lumbar area.

- The practitioner stands facing the back of the patient, and has easy access for palpation of quadratus lumborum's lateral border – a major trigger point site (Travell & Simons 1992) – with the cephalad hand.

- Activity of quadratus is tested (palpated for) with the cephalad hand as the leg is abducted, while also palpating gluteus medius (and TFL) with the caudad hand.

- If the muscles act simultaneously, or if quadratus fires first, then it is stressed, probably short, and will benefit from stretching.

- When the leg of the side-lying patient is abducted, and the practitioner's palpating hand senses that quadratus becomes actively involved in this process before the leg has reached at least 25° of elevation, then quadratus is probably overactive.

- If quadratus has been overactive for any length of time then it is almost certainly hypertonic and short, and a need for MET can be assumed.

Quadratus lumborum test B (Fig. 3.2A–C) (see CD-ROM of TFL assessment on p. 157 for observation of QL over activity)

- The patient stands, back towards crouching practitioner.

- Any leg length disparity (based on pelvic crest height) is equalised by using a book or pad under the short-leg-side heel.

- With the patient's feet shoulder-width apart, a pure side-bending is requested, so that the patient runs a hand down the lateral thigh/calf. (Normal level of side-bending excursion allows the fingertips to reach to just below the knee.)

- The side to which the fingertips travel furthest is assessed.

- If side-bending to one side is limited, then quadratus on the opposite side is probably short.

- Combined evidence from palpation (test A) and this side-bending test indicate whether or not it is necessary to treat quadratus.

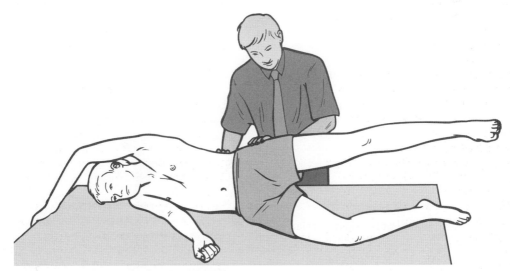

Figure 5.23 Palpation assessment for quadratus lumborum overactivity. The muscle is palpated, as is gluteus medius, during abduction of the leg. The correct firing sequence should be gluteus, followed at around 25° elevation by quadratus. If there is an immediate 'grabbing' action by quadratus it indicates overactivity, and therefore stress, so shortness can be assumed (see details of similar functional assessments in Ch. 5).

Method A. MET for shortness in quadratus lumborum ('banana') (Fig. 5.24)

- The patient lies supine with the feet crossed (the side to be treated crossed under the non-treated-side leg) at the ankle.

- The patient is arranged in a light side-bend, away from the side to be treated, so that the pelvis is towards that side, and the feet and head away from that side ('banana shaped').

- As this side-bend is being achieved the affected quadratus can be palpated for bind so that the barrier is correctly identified.

- The patient's heels are placed just off the side of the table, anchoring the lower extremities and pelvis.

- The patient places the arm of the side to be treated behind her neck as the practitioner, standing on the side opposite that to be treated, slides his cephalad hand under the patient's shoulders to grasp the treated-side axilla.

- The patient grasps the practitioner's cephalad arm at the elbow, with the treated-side hand, making the contact more secure.

- The patient's non-treated-side hand should be interlocked with the practitioner's cephalad hand.

- The patient's treated-side elbow should, at this stage, be pointing superiorly.

- The practitioner's caudad hand is placed firmly but carefully on the anterior superior iliac spine, on the side to be treated.

- The patient is instructed to very lightly side-bend towards the treated side.

- This should produce an isometric contraction in quadratus lumborum on the side to be treated.

- After 7 seconds the patient is asked to relax completely, and then to side-bend towards the non-treated side, as the practitioner simultaneously transfers his body weight from the cephalad leg to the caudad leg and leans backwards slightly, in order to side-bend the patient.

- This effectively stretches quadratus lumborum. The stretch is held for 30 seconds, allowing a lengthening of shortened musculature in the region.

- Repeat as necessary.

Method B. Quadratus lumborum side-lying MET (Fig. 5.25)

- The practitioner stands behind the side-lying patient, at waist level.

- The patient has the uppermost arm extended over the head to firmly grasp the top end of the table and, on an inhalation, abducts the uppermost leg until the practitioner palpates quadratus activity (elevation of around 30° usually).

- The patient holds the leg (and, if appropriate, the breath, see Box 5.2) isometrically in this manner, allowing gravity to provide resistance.

- After the 10-second (or so) contraction, the patient allows the leg to fall towards the floor, slightly behind him over the back of the table.

- The practitioner straddles this leg (to stabilise its position) and, cradling the pelvis with both hands (fingers interlocked over the crest of the pelvis), leans back to take out all slack of the soft tissues, including quadratus, easing the pelvis away from the lower ribs, during an exhalation.

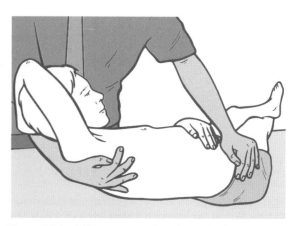

Figure 5.24   MET treatment of quadratus lumborum utilising 'banana' position.

- This stretch should be held for between 10 and 30 seconds.

- The method will be more successful if the patient is grasping the top edge of the table, so providing a fixed point from which the practitioner can induce stretch (see Fig. 5.25).

- Contraction followed by stretch is repeated once or twice more with the leg raised in front of the trunk, and once or twice with raised leg behind the trunk in order to activate, and subsequently stretch different quadratus fibres. This calls for the practitioner changing from the back to the front of the table for the best results.

- When the leg hangs to the back of the trunk the long fibres of the muscle are mainly affected; and when the leg hangs forward of the body the diagonal fibres are mainly involved.

- The direction of stretch should be varied so that it is always in the same direction as the long axis of the abducted leg.

Method C. Quadratus lumborum gravity-induced MET – self-treatment (see Fig. 3.2A–C)

- The patient stands, legs apart, bending sideways.

- The patient inhales and slightly raises the trunk (a few centimetres) at the same time as looking (moving the eyes only) away from the side to which side-flexion is taking place.

- On exhalation, the side-bend is allowed to slowly go further to its elastic limit, while the patient looks towards the floor, in the direction of the side-flexion. (Care is needed that very little, if any, forward or backward bending is taking place at this time.)

- This sequence is repeated a number of times.

Eye positions (visual synkinesis) influence the tendency to flex and side-bend (eyes look down) and extend (eyes look up) as discussed in Ch. 3 (Lewit 1999).

Gravity-induced stretches of this sort require holding the stretch position for at least as long as the contraction, and ideally longer. More repeti-

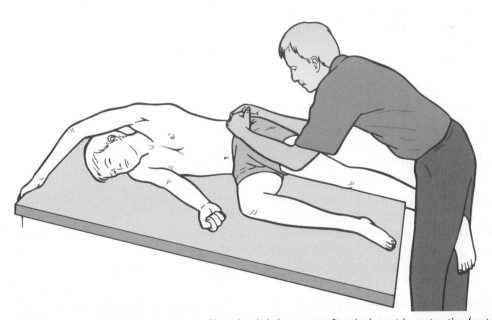

Figure 5.25 MET treatment of quadratus lumborum. Note that it is important after the isometric contraction (sustained raised/abducted leg) that the muscle be eased into stretch, avoiding any defensive or protective resistance which sudden movement might produce. For this reason, body weight rather than arm strength should be used to apply traction.

tions may be needed with a large muscle such as quadratus, and home stretches should be advised several times daily.

Method D. Quadratus lumborum MET

The side-lying treatment of latissimus dorsi described later in this chapter also provides an effective quadratus stretch when the stabilising hand rests on the pelvic crest (see Fig. 5.32).

8. Assessment and treatment of pectoralis major (11) and latissimus dorsi (12)

Latissimus and pectoral test A

Observation can be as accurate as palpation for evidence of pectoralis major shortening. The patient will have a rounded shoulder posture – especially if the clavicular aspect is involved. Or:

- The patient lies supine with upper arms on the table, hands resting palm down on the lower abdomen.

- The practitioner observes from the head and notes whether either shoulder is held in an anterior position in relation to the thoracic cage.

- If one or both shoulders are forward of the thorax, pectoralis muscles are short (see Fig. 5.26).

Latissimus and pectoral test B

- The patient lies supine with the head several feet from the top edge of the table, and is asked to rest the arms, extended above the head, on the treatment surface, palms upwards (see Fig. 5.27).

- If these muscles are normal, the arms should be able to easily reach the horizontal when directly above the shoulders, and also to be in contact with the surface for almost all of the length of the upper arms, with no arching of the back or twisting of the thorax.

- If either arm cannot reach the vertical above the shoulder, but is held laterally, elbow pulled outwards, then latissimus dorsi is probably short on that side. If an arm cannot

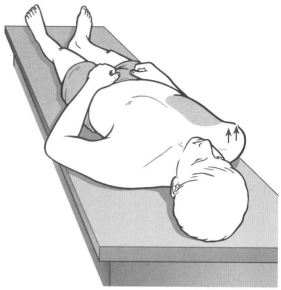

Figure 5.26   Observation assessment in which pectoral shortness on the right is suggested by the inability of the shoulder to rest on the table.

rest with the dorsum of the upper arm in contact with the table surface without effort, then pectoral fibres are almost certainly short.

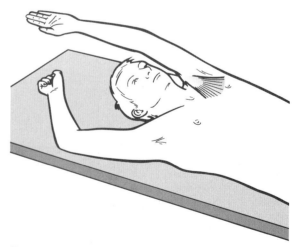

Figure 5.27   Assessment of shortness in pectoralis major and latissimus dorsi. Visual assessment is used: if the arm on the tested side is unable to rest along its full length, shortness of pectoralis major is probable; if there is obvious deviation of the elbow laterally, probable latissimus shortening is indicated.

Assessment of shortness in pectoralis major (Fig. 5.28)

- Assessment of the subclavicular portion of pectoralis major involves abduction of the arm to 90° (Lewit 1985b).

- In this position the tendon of pectoralis major at the sternum should not be found to be unduly tense, even with maximum abduction of the arm, unless the muscle is shortened.

- For assessment of sternal attachment the arm is brought into elevation and abduction, as the muscle, as well as the tendon on the greater tubercle of the humerus, is palpated.

- If the sternal fibres have shortened, tautness will be visible and tenderness of the tissues under palpation will be reported.

Assessment for strength of pectoralis major

- The patient is supine with arm in abduction at the shoulder joint, and medially rotated (palm is facing down) with the elbow extended.

- The practitioner stands at the head and secures the opposite shoulder with one hand to prevent any trunk torsion and contacts the dorsum of the distal humerus, on the tested side, with the other hand.

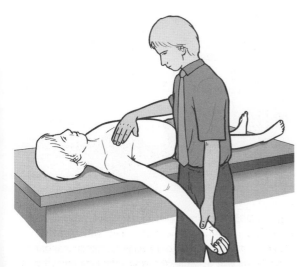

Figure 5.28 Palpation assessment for shortness of subclavicular portion of pectoralis major.

- The patient attempts to lift the arm and to adduct it across the chest, against resistance, as strength is assessed in the sternal fibres.

- Different arm positions can be used to assess clavicular and costal fibres. For example:
  - with an angle of abduction/elevation of 135° costal and abdominal fibres will be involved
  - with abduction/elevation of 45° the clavicular fibres will be assessed.

- The practitioner should palpate to ensure that the 'correct' fibres contract when assessments are being made.

- If this postural muscle tests as weak it may be useful to use Norris's (1999) approach (see description in Ch. 3) of strengthening it by application of a slow eccentric isotonic contraction, before proceeding to an MET stretching procedure.

Method A. MET treatment of short pectoralis major (Fig. 5.29A, B)

- The patient lies supine with the arm abducted in a direction which produces the most marked evidence of pectoral shortness (assessed by palpation and visual evidence of the particular fibres involved, as described in tests above).

- The more elevated the arm (i.e. the closer to the head), the more focus there will be on costal and abdominal fibres.

- With a lesser degree of abduction (to around 45°), the focus is more on the clavicular fibres.

- Between these two extremes lies the position which influences the sternal fibres most directly.

- The patient lies as close to the side of the table as possible, so that the abducted arm can be brought below the horizontal level in order to apply gravitational pull and passive stretch to the fibres, as appropriate.

- The practitioner stands on the side to be treated and grasps the humerus.

- A useful arm hold, which depends upon the relative size of the patient and the practitioner, involves the practitioner grasping the anterior aspect of the patient's flexed upper arm just above the elbow, while the patient cups the practitioner's elbow and holds this contact throughout the procedure (see Fig. 5.29B).

- *The patient's hand is placed on the contact (attachments of shortened fibres) area* on the thorax so that her hand acts as a 'cushion'. This is both more physically comfortable and also prevents physical contact with emotionally sensitive areas such as breast tissue.

- The practitioner's thenar or hyperthenar eminence is placed over the patient's 'cushion' hand in order to stabilise the area during the contraction and stretch, preventing movement of it.

- Commencing with the patient's arm in a position which takes the affected fibres to just short of their restriction barrier (for a chronic problem), the patient introduces a light contraction (20% of strength) involving adduction against resistance from the practitioner, for 7–10 seconds.

- As a rule the long axis of the patient's upper arm should be in a straight line with the fibres being treated.

- If a trigger point has previously been identified in pectoralis, the practitioner should ensure – by means of palpation if necessary, or by observation – that the fibres housing the triggers are involved in the contraction.

- As the patient exhales following complete relaxation of the area, a stretch through the new barrier is activated by the patient and maintained by the practitioner.

- Stretch is achieved via the positioning and leverage of the arm, while the contact hand on the thorax acts as a stabilising point only.

- There are two distinct phases to the stretch and these need to be carefully achieved to avoid irritation of the shoulder.

- The stretch needs to be one in which the arm is first pulled away (distracted) from the thorax, with the patient's assistance ('ease your arm away from your shoulder'), before the stretch is introduced. If the patient grasps the practitioner's elbow effectively this distraction is achieved by a simple lean backwards by the practitioner.

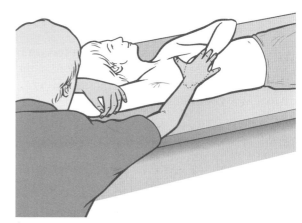

A

Figure 5.29A   MET treatment of pectoral muscle – abdominal attachment. Note that the fibres being treated are those which lie in line with the long axis of the humerus.

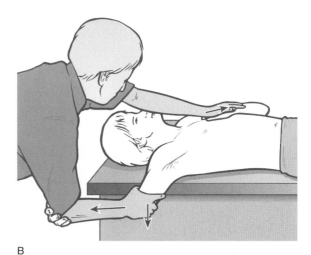

B

Figure 5.29B   An alternative hold for application of MET to pectoral muscle – sternal attachment. Note that the patient needs to be close to the edge of the table in order to allow the arm to be taken towards the floor once the slack has been removed, during the stretching phase after the isometric contraction.

- The stretch is then introduced and this involves the humerus being taken below the horizontal, achieved by means of the practitioner lowering his centre of gravity (bending the knees).

- During the stretching phase it is important for the entire thorax to be stabilised and the practitioner needs to be very sensitive to the point at which the muscle's end-of-range (length) barrier is engaged. No rolling or twisting of the thorax in the direction of the stretch should be permitted.

- To recapitulate: There are two phases of the stretching procedure, the first in which slack is removed by distracting the arm away from the contact/stabilising hand on the thorax, and the second involving movement of the arm towards the floor, initiated by the practitioner bending his knees.

- Stretching (after an isometric contraction) should be repeated two or three times in each position, so involving different pectoral fibres.

- All attachments should be treated, which calls for the use of different arm positions, as discussed above, each with different stabilising ('cushion') contacts as the various fibre directions and attachments are isolated.

(◎) Method B. Pectoralis major MET (Fig. 5.30)

- The patient lies supine close to the edge of the table on the side to be treated.

- The treated-side arm is taken into 90° of abduction at the shoulder and the elbow is flexed to 90°.

- The practitioner stands at waist level facing the head of the table.

- The practitioner's table-side hand is placed on the anterior shoulder area, holding this to the table throughout the procedure.

- The practitioner's non-table-side hand holds the ventral surface of the patient's wrist, with his forearm in contact along the length of the patient's forearm to provide a firm contact.

- The patient is asked to use no more than 20% of available strength to attempt to adduct the arm, pressing it against the resistance offered by the practitioners arm, for 7–10 seconds.

- On an exhalation the practitioner eases the arm into greater horizontal abduction, stretching pectoralis major.

- This is held or 30 seconds, before relaxing the stretch, repeating the contraction and stretching again.

(◎) Method C. Pectoralis major MET (Fig. 5.31)

- The patient is prone with her face in a face hole or cradle.

- Her right arm is abducted to 90° and the elbow flexed to 90°, palm towards the floor, with the upper arm supported by the table.

- The practitioner stands at waist level, facing cephalad, and places his non-table-side hand palm-to-palm with the patient's, so that the patient's forearm is in contact with the ventral surface of the practitioner's forearm.

- The practitioner's table-side hand rests on the patient's right scapula area, ensuring that no trunk rotation occurs.

- The practitioner eases the patient's arm into extension at the shoulder until he senses the first sign of resistance from pectoralis. It is important when extending the arm in this way to ensure that no trunk rotation occurs and that the anterior surface of the shoulder remains in contact with the table throughout.

- The patient is asked, using no more than 20% of strength, to attempt to bring her arm towards the floor and across her chest, with the elbow taking the lead.

- The attempt should be completely resisted by the practitioner, who also ensures that the patient's arm remains parallel to the floor throughout the 7–10 second isometric contraction.

- Following release of the contraction effort, and on an exhalation, the arm is taken into greater extension, with the patient's assistance, and held at stretch for not less than 20 seconds.

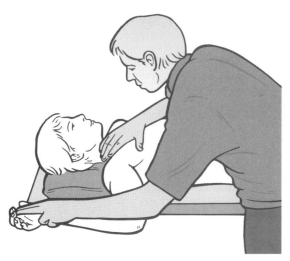

Figure 5.30   Pectoralis major MET stretch. (Redrawn from Kostopoulos D, Rizopoulos K 2001 *Manual of Trigger Point and Myofascial Therapy*, Slack, Thorofare, NJ, p 117.)

- This procedure should be repeated two or three times, slackening the muscle slightly from its end-range before each subsequent contraction, in order to reduce discomfort and for ease of application of the contraction (it is difficult to initiate a contraction from an end-range position, and is likely to cause the individual to inappropriately recruit other muscles than the one being targeted.)

- Variations in pectoralis fibre involvement can be achieved by altering the angle of abduction:
  - with a more superior angle (around 140°) the lower sternal and costal fibres are recruited
  - with a lesser angle (around 45°) the clavicular fibres will be committed.

Method D. Slow eccentric isometric contraction (SEIS) MET treatment of pectoralis major

- The patient lies supine with the arm abducted in a direction which produces the most marked evidence of pectoral shortness (assessed by palpation and visual evidence of the particular fibres involved, as described in the assessment tests above).

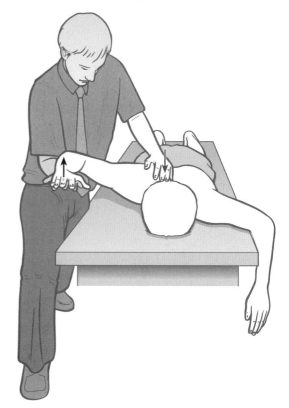

Figure 5.31   MET for pectoralis major in prone position.

- The patient is asked to maintain the arm in extension and adduction, at the resistance barrier, as the practitioner slowly eases (forces) it into flexion and abduction (taking the arm across the chest), so slowly isotonically stretching the antagonists to pectoralis major (such as – depending on the arm position – latissimus dorsi).

- After this the arm is replaced at the barrier and the stretching procedure described in method A is used to lengthen pectoralis major.

Latissimus dorsi (12) test for shortness

- To screen latissimus dorsi, the standing patient is asked to bend forward and allow the arms to hang freely from the shoulders as she holds a half-bend position, trunk parallel to the floor.

- If the arms are hanging other than perpendicular to the floor there is probably some muscular restriction involved, and if this involves latissimus the arms will be held closer to the legs than perpendicular (if they hang markedly forward of such a position then trapezius shortening is probable, see below).

- To further screen latissimus in this position, one side at a time, the practitioner stands in front of the patient (who remains in this half-bend position) and, stabilising the scapula area with one hand, grasps the arm at elbow level and gently draws the tested side (straight) arm forwards.

- It should, without undue effort or excessive bind in the tissues being held, allow itself to be taken to a position where the elbow is higher than the level of the back of the head.

- If this is not possible, then latissimus is short.

Method A. MET treatment of shortened latissimus dorsi

NOTE: The positioning for this method is virtually identical to that described for treatment of quadratus lumborum earlier, and illustrated in Fig. 5.24.

- The patient lies supine with the feet crossed (the side to be treated crossed under the non-treated-side leg at the ankle).

- The patient is arranged in a light side-bend away from the side to be treated so that the pelvis is towards that side, and the feet and head away from that side.

- The heels are placed just off the edge of the table, so anchoring the lower extremities.

- The patient places her arm on the side to be treated behind her neck, as the practitioner, standing on the side opposite that to be treated, slides his cephalad hand under the patient's shoulders to grasp the treated-side axilla.

- The patient grasps the practitioner's cephalad arm at the elbow, making this contact more secure. The patients treated-side elbow should point superiorly.

- The patient's non-treated-side hand should be interlocked with the practitioner's cephalad hand.

- The practitioner's caudad hand is placed on the anterior superior iliac spine on the side being treated, and the patient is instructed to very lightly take the pointed elbow towards the sacrum and also to lightly try to bend backwards and towards the treated side. This should produce a light isometric contraction in latissimus dorsi on the side to be treated.

- After 7–10 seconds the patient is asked to relax completely as the practitioner transfers his body weight from the cephalad leg to the caudad leg, to side-bend the patient further while simultaneously standing more erect and leaning in a caudad direction.

- This effectively lifts the patient's thorax from the table surface and introduces a stretch into latissimus (especially if the patient has maintained a grasp on the practitioner's elbow and the practitioner has a firm hold on the patient's axilla).

- This stretch is held for 15–30 seconds allowing a lengthening of shortened musculature in the region.

- Repeat at least once more.

Method B. MET of shortened latissimus dorsi (Fig. 5.32)

- The patient is side-lying, affected side up.

- The arm is taken into abduction to the point of resistance, so that it is possible to visualise, or palpate, the attachment of the shortened fibres on the lateral chest wall.

- The condition is treated in either the acute or chronic mode of MET, at or short of the barrier, as appropriate, as described earlier.

- As shown in Fig. 5.32, the practitioner stands near the head of the patient, and depending on the fibres to be stretched, slightly behind, at the head or slightly in front of the patient.

- The practitioner holds the patient's upper arm in the chosen position (as shown in Fig. 5.32 or in a more robust way, as demonstrated in the video-clip) while using the other hand to

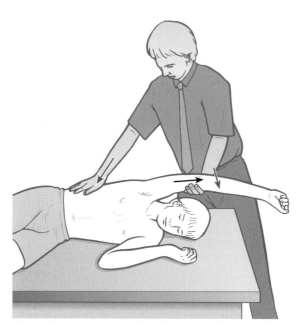

Figure 5.32   Treatment of latissimus dorsi. A variety of different positions are required for the stabilising hand (on the chest wall as well as on the crest of the pelvis) to allow for precise application of stretches of fibres with different attachments, following the sequence of isometric contractions.

stabilise the posterior thorax area, or the pelvic crest.[7]

- A build-up of tension should be palpated under the stabilising hand as the patient introduces an isometric contraction by attempting to bring the arm towards the ceiling, posteriorly and down (towards the lower spine), against firm resistance, using only a modest amount of effort (20%).

- After 7–10 seconds, the effort should be released as the patient relaxes completely, at which time the practitioner introduces stretch to, or through, the restriction barrier (acute/chronic), bringing the humerus into greater adduction, while applying a stretching/stabilising contact on the trunk,

---

[7] When the contact/stabilising hand is on the crest of the pelvis, the stretch using the arm as a lever will effectively also stretch quadratus lumborum.

anywhere between the lateral chest wall and the crest of the pelvis.

- A downward movement of the humerus, towards the floor, assists the stretch following a separation of the practitioner's two contact hands to remove all slack.

- As in the stretch of pectoralis major described above (method A), there should be two phases – a distraction, taking out the slack, and a movement towards the floor by the practitioner, flexing the knees, to induce a safe stretch.

- Repeat as necessary.

Latissimus should be retested following stretching to evaluate the degree of improvement.

9. Assessment and treatment of upper trapezius (13)

Lewit (1999) simplifies the need to assess for shortness of this muscle, by stating, 'The upper trapezius should be treated if tender and taut'. Since this is an almost universal state in modern life, it seems that everyone requires MET application to this muscle. Lewit also notes that a characteristic mounding of the muscle can often be observed when it is very short, producing the effect of 'Gothic shoulders', similar to the architectural supports of a Gothic church tower (see Fig. 2.16).

Upper trapezius shortness test A (Fig. 5.33)

See the description of the scapulohumeral rhythm test (Ch. 8) which helps identify excessive activity or inappropriate tone in levator scapula and upper trapezius, which, because they are postural muscles, indicates shortness (Fig. 8.13A, B).

Greenman (1996) describes a functional 'firing sequence' assessment which identifies general imbalance and dysfunction involving the upper and lower fixators of the shoulder (see Fig. 5.33).

- The patient is seated and the practitioner stands behind.

- The practitioner rests his right hand over the right shoulder area to assess the firing sequence of muscles during shoulder abduction.

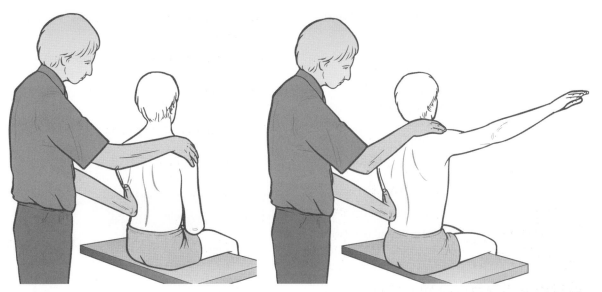

Figure 5.33 Palpation assessment for upper and lower fixators of the shoulder, including upper trapezius (Greenman 1996).

- The other hand can be placed either on the mid-thoracic region, mainly on the side being assessed, or spanning the lower back to palpate quadratus firing.

- The assessment should be performed several times so that various hand contacts are used to evaluate the behaviour of different muscles during abduction.

Greenman (1996) bases his findings on the work of Janda (1983), who described the 'correct' sequence for shoulder abduction, when seated, as involving:

- Supraspinatus
- Deltoid
- Infraspinatus
- Middle and lower trapezius
- Contralateral quadratus.

In dysfunctional states the most common substitutions are said to involve: shoulder elevation by *levator scapulae and upper trapezius*, as well as early firing by *quadratus lumborum, ipsilateral and contralateral*.

As explained by Janda, abduction of the arm, in this position, should not employ upper trapezius as a prime mover, although it does increase in tone during the procedure.

Inappropriate activity of any of the upper fixators results in shortness. When overactivity involves the lower fixators, weakness and possible lengthening results (Norris 1999).

See Ch. 2 for discussion of postural/phasic, etc. muscle characteristics.

Upper trapezius shortness test B

- The patient is seated and the practitioner stands behind with one hand resting on the shoulder of the side to be tested, stabilising it.

- The other hand is placed on the ipsilateral side of the head as the head/neck is taken into contralateral side-bending without force, while the shoulder is stabilised (see Fig. 5.34).

- The same procedure is performed on the other side with the opposite shoulder stabilised.

- A comparison is made as to which side-bending manoeuvre produced the greater range, and whether the neck can easily reach 45° of side-flexion in each direction, which it should.

- If neither side can achieve this degree of side-bending, then both trapezius muscles may be short.

- The relative shortness of one, compared with the other, is evaluated.[8]

Upper trapezius shortness test C

- The patient is supine with the neck fully (but not forcefully) side-bent contralaterally (away from the side being assessed).

- The practitioner is standing at the head of the table and uses a cupped hand contact on the ipsilateral shoulder (i.e. on the side being tested) to assess the ease with which it can be depressed (moved caudally) (Fig. 5.35).

- There should be an easy 'springing' sensation as the practitioner eases the shoulder towards the feet, with a *soft* end-feel to the movement.

- If depression of the shoulder is difficult or if there is a *harsh*, sudden end-point, upper trapezius shortness is confirmed.

- This same assessment (always with full lateral flexion) should be performed with the head fully rotated away from the side being tested, half turned away from the side being tested, and slightly turned *towards* the side being tested, in order to respectively assess the relative shortness and functional efficiency respectively of posterior, middle and anterior subdivisions of the upper portion of trapezius.

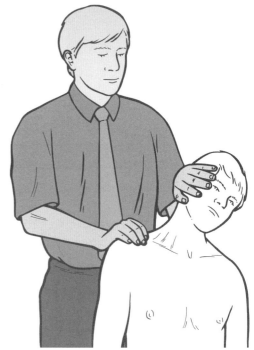

Figure 5.34   Assessment of the relative shortness of the right side upper trapezius. One side is compared with the other (for both the range of unforced motion and the nature of the end-feel of motion) to ascertain the side most in need of MET attention.

 Method A. MET treatment of chronically shortened upper trapezius (Fig. 5.35 A–C)

In order to treat all the fibres of upper trapezius, MET needs to be applied sequentially. In this clinical approach upper trapezius is subdivided into anterior, middle and posterior fibres. The flexed neck should be placed into three different positions of rotation (full rotation away from side being treated, half rotation away from side being treated, and slight rotation towards side being treated), always coupled with full side-bending away from the

side being assessed, for precise treatment of the posterior, middle and anterior fibres, respectively.

- The patient lies supine, arm on the side to be treated lying alongside the trunk, head/neck side-bent away from the side being treated to just short of the restriction barrier, while the practitioner stabilises the shoulder with one hand and cups the ipsilateral ear/mastoid area, with the other.

- With the flexed neck fully side-bent, and fully rotated contralaterally, the *posterior* fibres of upper trapezius are involved in the contraction (see below).

- This will facilitate subsequent stretching of this aspect of the muscle.

- With the flexed neck fully side-bent and half rotated, the *middle* fibres are involved in the contraction.

---

[8] If the shoulder towards which the head is being side-bent were stabilised, then assessment would be of the mobility of the cervical structures. By stabilising the side from which the bend is taking place, the muscular component is being evaluated.

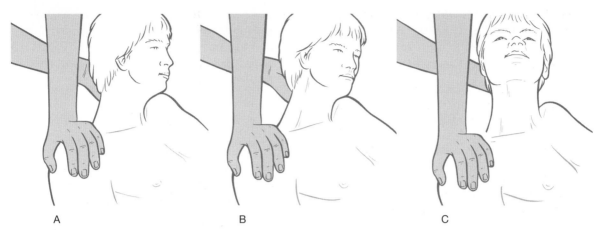

Figure 5.35 MET treatment of right-side upper trapezius muscle. **A** Posterior fibres, **B** middle fibres, **C** anterior fibres. Note that stretching in this (or any of the alternative positions which access the middle and posterior fibres) is achieved following the isometric contraction by means of an easing of the shoulder away from the stabilised head, with no force being applied to the neck and head itself.

- With the flexed neck fully side-bent and slightly rotated *towards* the side being treated, the *anterior* fibres of upper trapezius are engaged.

- The various contractions and subsequent stretches can be performed with practitioner's arms crossed, hands stabilising the mastoid area and shoulder (see Fig. 5.35).

- The patient introduces a light resisted effort (20% of available strength) to take the stabilised shoulder towards the ear (a shrug movement) and the ear towards the shoulder.

- The double movement (or effort towards movement) is important in order to introduce a contraction of the muscle from both ends simultaneously.

- The degree of effort should be mild and no pain should be felt.

- The contraction is sustained for 7–10 seconds and, upon complete relaxation of effort, the practitioner gently eases the head/neck into an increased degree of side-bending and rotation, where it is stabilised, as the shoulder is stretched caudally.

- As stretching is introduced, the patient can usefully assist in this phase of the treatment by initiating, on instruction, the stretch of the

muscle ('as you breathe out please slide your hand towards your feet').

- Patient participation in the stretch reduces the chances of a stretch reflex being initiated.

- Once the muscle is in a stretched position, the patient relaxes and the stretch is held for up to 30 seconds.

CAUTION: No stretch should be introduced from the cranial end of the muscle, as this could stress the neck. The head is stabilised at its side-flexion and rotation barrier.

Disagreement   There is some disagreement as to the head/neck rotation position as described in the treatment method above, which calls for side-bending and rotation away from the affected side to engage posterior and middle fibres:

- Liebenson (1996), suggests that the patient should 'lie supine with the head supported in anteflexion and laterally flexed away and rotated towards the side of involvement'.

- Lewit (1985b) suggests: 'The patient is supine ... the therapist fixes the shoulder from above with one hand, sidebending the head and neck with the other hand so as to take up the slack. He then asks the patient to look towards the side away from which the head is bent, resisting the patient's automatic tendency to move towards the side of the lesion.' (This method is described below.)

The author has used method A, described above, with good effect and urges readers to compare these approaches with those of Liebenson and Lewit, and to evaluate results for themselves.

Method B. MET treatment of acutely shortened upper trapezius, with visual synkinesis

Lewit (1985b) suggests the use of eye movements to facilitate initiation of a contraction before stretching, is an ideal method for *acute problems* in this region.

- The patient is supine, while the practitioner fixes the shoulder and the side-bent (away from the treated side) head and neck at the restriction barrier, and asks the patient to look, *moving the eyes only* (not the head), towards the side away from which the neck is bent.

- This eye movement is maintained, while the practitioner resists the slight isometric contraction this will have created.

- On an exhalation, and complete relaxation, the head/neck is taken to a new barrier and the process repeated.

- If the shoulder is brought into the process, this is firmly resisted as it attempts to lightly push into a shrug during the contraction phase.

- After this 10-second contraction, slack can again be removed as the head is repositioned, before a repetition of the procedure commences.

10. Assessment and treatment of scalenes (14) (see also Box 5.9)

Assessment of cervical side-bending (lateral flexion) strength (this sequence is not described in the text)

This involves the scalenes and levator scapulae (and to a secondary degree the rectus capitis lateralis and the transversospinalis group).

- The practitioner places a stabilising hand on the top of the shoulder to prevent movement and the other on the head above the ear, as the seated patient attempts to flex the head laterally against this resistance.

- Both sides are assessed.

Assessment A. Scalene functional observation

There is no easy test for shortness of the scalenes apart from observation, palpation and assessment of trigger point activity/tautness. However, a functional observation may prove useful.

- In most people who have marked scalene shortness there is commonly a tendency to overuse these (and other upper fixators of the shoulder and neck) as accessory breathing muscles (Peper & Tibbetts 1992, Middaugh et al 1994).

- There may also be a tendency to hyperventilation (with a possible history of anxiety, phobic behaviour, panic attacks and/or fatigue symptoms) (Goldstein 1996).

- These muscles seem to be excessively tense in many people with chronic fatigue and anxiety symptoms (George 1964).

Observation assessment consists of the practitioner placing his relaxed hands over the patient's shoulders so that the fingertips rest on the clavicles, at which time the seated patient is asked to inhale moderately. If the practitioner's hands noticeably rise towards the patient's ears during such inhalation then there exists inappropriate overuse of the scalenes, which indicates that they are stressed, which also means that, by definition, they will probably have shortened and would benefit from stretching treatment.

Assessment B. Scalene observation

Alternatively, during the history-taking interview, the patient can be asked to place one hand on the abdomen just above the umbilicus and the other flat against the upper chest (see Fig. 5.36). On inhalation, the hands are observed: if the upper hand initiates the breathing process and rises significantly towards the chin, rather than

Box 5.9 Notes on scalenes

- The scalenes are controversial muscles since they seem to be both postural and phasic (Lin et al 1994), their status being modified by the type(s) of stress to which they are exposed (see Ch. 3 for discussion of this topic).
- Janda (1988) reports that 'spasm and/or trigger points are commonly present in the scalenes as also are weakness and/or inhibition'.
- The attachment sites of the scalene muscles vary, as does their presence. The scalene posterior is sometimes absent, and sometimes blends with the fibres of medius.
- Scalene medius is noted to frequently attach to the atlas (Gray 1995) and sometimes extend to the 2nd rib (Simons et al 1999).
- The scalene minimus (pleuralis), which attaches to the pleural dome, is present in one-third (Platzer 1992) to three-quarters (Simons et al 1999) of people, on at least one side and, when absent, is replaced by a transverse cupular ligament (Platzer 1992).
- The brachial plexus exits the cervical column between the scalenus anterior and medius. These, together with the 1st rib, form the scalene hiatus (also called the 'scalene opening' or 'posterior scalene aperture') (Platzer 1992). It is through this opening that the brachial plexus and vascular structures for the upper extremity pass. When scalene fibres are taut, they may entrap the nerves (scalene anticus syndrome) or crowd the 1st rib against the clavicle and indirectly impinge on the vascular, or neurologic, structures (compromising of both neural and vascular structures is rare) (Stedman 1998). Any of these conditions may be diagnosed as 'thoracic outlet syndrome', 'a collective title for a number of conditions attributed to compromise of blood vessels or nerve fibres (brachial plexus) at any point between the base of the neck and the axilla' (Stedman 1998).

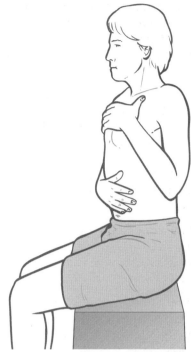

Figure 5.36 *Observation assessment of respiratory function. Any tendency for the upper hand to move cephalad, or earlier than the caudad hand, suggests scalene overactivity.*

moving slightly anteriorly, a pattern of upper chest breathing can be assumed, and therefore stress, and therefore shortness of the scalenes (and other accessory breathing muscles, notably sternomastoid).

MET treatment of short scalenes (Fig. 5.37A–C)

- The patient lies supine with a cushion or folded towel under the upper thoracic area so that, unless supported by the practitioner's

contralateral hand, the head would fall into extension.

- The head is rotated contralaterally (away from the side to be treated).
- There are three positions of rotation required:
  1. Full contralateral rotation, and side-flexion, of the head/neck produces involvement of the posterior scalene muscle.
  2. A contralateral 45° rotation, and side-flexion, of the head/neck involves the middle scalene.
  3. A position of only slight contralateral rotation and side-flexion involves the anterior scalene.
- The practitioner's free hand is placed on the side of the patient's face/forehead to restrain the isometric contraction, which will be used to initiate the release of the scalenes.
- The patient's head is in one of the degrees of rotation mentioned above, supported by the practitioner's contralateral hand.

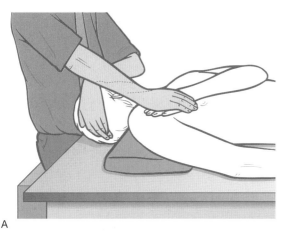

A

Figure 5.37A   MET for scalenus posticus. On stretching, following the isometric contraction, the neck is allowed to move into slight extension while a mild stretch is introduced by the contact hand which rests on the second rib, below the lateral aspect of the clavicle.

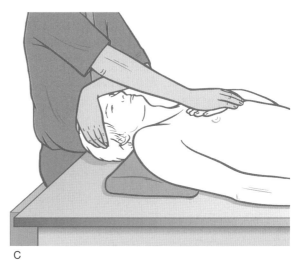

C

Figure 5.37C   MET treatment of the anterior fibres of the scalenes; hand placement is on the sternum.

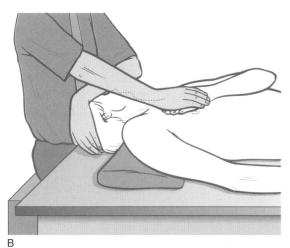

B

Figure 5.37B   MET treatment for the middle fibres of scalenes; hand placement (thenar or hypothenar eminence of relaxed hand) is on the 2nd rib below the centre of the clavicle.

- The patient is instructed to attempt to lift the forehead a fraction and to attempt to turn the head towards the affected side, resisted by the practitioner's hand to prevent both movements, together with appropriate breathing cooperation ('breathe in and hold your breath as you "lift and turn", and hold this for 7–10 seconds').

- Both the effort and the counterpressure should be modest and painless at all times.

- After a 7–10 second contraction, the head is placed into extension, and one hand remains on it to prevent movement during the scalene stretch. This hand should ideally be placed so that it restrains ('fixes') that part of the neck where scalenes attach.

- The patient's contralateral hand is placed (palm down) with the thenar eminence just inferior to the lateral end of the clavicle, on the affected side (for full rotation of the head, posterior scalenes).

- The practitioner's hand which was acting to produce resistance to the isometric contraction is now placed onto the dorsum of the patient's 'cushion' hand.

- As the patient slowly exhales, the practitioner's contact hand, resting on the patient's hand, which is itself resting on the upper thorax, pushes obliquely away and towards the foot on that same side, following the rib movement into its exhalation position, so stretching the attached musculature and fascia.

- This stretch is held for at least 20–30 seconds after each isometric contraction.

- The process is then repeated at least once more.

- The head is rotated 45° contralaterally and the 'cushion' hand (thenar eminence) contact, which will apply the stretch of the middle scalenes, is placed just inferior to the middle aspect of the clavicle.

- When the head is in the side flexed and in an almost upright facing position, for treatment of the anterior scalenes, the 'cushion' hand contact lies on the upper sternum itself.

- In all other ways the methodology is as described for the first position above.

NOTE: It is important not to allow heroic degrees of neck extension during any phase of this treatment. There should be some extension, but it should be appropriate to the age and condition of the individual.

A degree of eye movement can usefully assist scalene treatment and may be used as an alternative to the 'lift and turn' muscular effort described above, especially in conditions where pain and sensitivity demand a gentle approach.

If the patient makes the eyes look caudally (towards the feet), and towards the affected side, during the isometric contraction, she will increase the degree of contraction in the muscles. If during the resting phase, when stretch is being introduced, she looks away from the treated side, with eyes looking towards the top of the head, this will enhance the stretch of the muscle (Lewit 1999).

This whole procedure should be performed bilaterally several times in each of the three head positions.

Scalene stretches, with all their variable positions, clearly also influence many of the other anterior neck structures (such as platysma).

11. Assessment for shortness of sternocleidomastoid (15) (see also Box 5.10)

Assessment for sternocleidomastoid (SCM) is as for the scalenes – there is no absolute test for shortness but observation of posture (hyperlordotic neck, chin poked forward, upper crossed syndrome (Janda 1983, Lewit 1999)) and palpation of the degree of induration, fibrosis and trigger point

activity can all alert to probable shortness of SCM. This is an accessory breathing muscle and, as with the scalenes, will be shortened by inappropriate breathing patterns which have become habitual. Observation is an accurate assessment tool.

Since SCM is barely observable when normal, if the clavicular attachment is easily visible, or any part of the muscle is prominent, this can be taken as a clear sign of excessive tightness of the muscle. If the patient's posture involves the head being held forward of the body, often accompanied by cervical lordosis and dorsal kyphosis (see notes on upper crossed syndrome in Ch. 2), weakness of the deep neck flexors and tightness of SCM can be suspected.

Functional SCM test (Fig. 8.14A, B)

- The supine patient is asked to 'very slowly raise your head and touch your chin to your chest'.

- The practitioner stands to the side with his head at the same level as the patient.

- At the beginning of the movement of the head, as the patient lifts this from the table, the practitioner would (if SCM were short) note that the chin was lifted first, allowing it to jut forwards, rather than the forehead leading the arc-like progression of the movement.

- When shortness of SCM is very marked the chin pokes forward in a jerk as the head is lifted.

If the reading of this sign is unclear then Janda (1988) suggests that a slight resistance pressure be applied to the forehead, as the patient makes the 'chin to chest' attempt. If SCM is short this will ensure the jutting of the chin at the outset.

MET treatment of shortened SCM (Fig. 5.38)

- The patient is supine with the head supported in a neutral position by one of the practitioner's hands.

- The shoulders rest on a cushion or folded towel, so that when the head is placed on the table the neck will be in slight extension at

Box 5.10 Notes on sternocleidomastoid

- Sternocleidomastoid (SCM) is a prominent muscle of the anterior neck and is closely associated with the trapezius. SCM often acts as postural compensator for head tilt associated with postural distortions found elsewhere (spinal, pelvic or lower extremity functional or structural inadequacies, for instance) although they seldom cause restriction of neck movement.
- SCM is synergistic with anterior neck muscles for flexion of the head and flexion of the cervical column on the thoracic column, when the cervical column is already flattened by the prevertebral muscles. However, when the head is placed in extension and SCM contracts, it accentuates lordosis of the cervical column, flexes the cervical column on the thoracic column, and adds to extension of the head. In this way, SCM is both synergist and antagonist to the prevertebral muscles (Kapandji 1974).
- SCM trigger points are activated by forward head positioning, 'whiplash' injury, positioning of the head to look upwardly for extended periods of time and structural compensations. The two heads of SCM each have their own patterns of trigger point referral which include (among others) into the ear, top of head, into the temporomandibular joint, over the brow, into the throat, and those which cause proprioceptive disturbances, disequilibrium, nausea and dizziness. Tenderness in SCM may be associated with trigger points in the digastric muscle and digastric trigger points may be satellites of SCM trigger points (Simons et al 1999).
- Simons et al (1999) report:

    When objects of equal weight are held in the hands, the patient with unilateral trigger point [TrP]

involvement of the clavicular division [of SCM] may exhibit an abnormal Weight Test. When asked to judge which is heaviest of two objects of the same weight that look alike but may not be the same weight (two vapocoolant dispensers, one of which may have been used) the patient will [give] evidence [of] dysmetria by underestimating the weight of the object held in the hand on the same side as the affected sternocleidomastoid muscle. Inactivation of the responsible sternocleidomastoid TrPs promptly restores weight appreciation by this test. Apparently, the afferent discharges from these TrPs disturb central processing of proprioceptive information from the upper limb muscles as well as vestibular function related to neck muscles.

- Lymph nodes lie superficially along the medial aspect of the SCM and may be palpated, especially when enlarged. These nodes may be indicative of chronic cranial infections stemming from a throat infection, dental abscess, sinusitis or tumour. Likewise, trigger points in SCM may be perpetuated by some of these conditions (Simons et al 1999).
- Lewit (1999) points out that tenderness noted at the medial end of the clavicle and/or at the transverse process of the atlas is often an indication of SCM hypertonicity. This will commonly accompany a forward head position and/or tendency to upper chest breathing, and will almost inevitably be associated with hypertonicity, shortening and trigger point evolution in associated musculature, including scalenes, upper trapezius and levator scapula (see crossed syndrome notes in Ch. 2).

---

which time the degree of extension of the neck should be slight, 10–15° at most.

- The patient's contralateral hand rests on the upper aspect of the sternum to act as a cushion when pressure is applied during the stretch phase of the operation (as in scalene and pectoral treatment described above).

- The patient's head is fully but comfortably rotated, contralaterally.

- The patient is asked to lift the fully rotated head a small degree towards the ceiling, and to hold the breath.

- When the head is raised there is no need for the practitioner to apply resistance as gravity effectively provides this.

- After 7–10 seconds of isometric contraction, the patient is asked to slowly release the effort (and the breath) and to place the head (still in rotation) on the table, so that a small degree of extension occurs.

- The practitioner's hand should be placed over the patient's 'cushion' hand (which rests on the sternum) in order to apply oblique pressure/stretch to the sternum, to ease it away from the head and towards the feet.

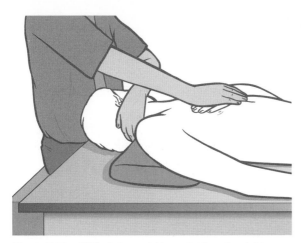

Figure 5.38   MET of sternocleidomastoid on the right.

- The hand not involved in applying pressure to the sternum caudally should be in contact with the mastoid process in order to gently restrain the tendency the head will have to follow this stretch, but *should not under any circumstances apply pressure to stretch the head/neck while it is in this vulnerable position of rotation and slight extension.*

- This stretch of SCM, which is applied as the patient exhales, is maintained for not less than 30 seconds to begin the release/stretch of hypertonic and fibrotic structures.

- Repeat at least once.

- The other side should then be treated in the same manner.

⚠ **CAUTION:** Care is required, especially with middle-aged and elderly patients, in applying this useful stretching procedure. Appropriate tests should be carried out to evaluate cerebral circulation problems. The presence of such problems indicates that this particular MET method should be avoided as described.

12. Assessment and treatment of levator scapulae (16)

Test A (spring test) for levator scapula shortness

- The patient lies supine with the arm of the side to be tested stretched out with the supinated hand and lower arm tucked under the buttocks, to help restrain movement of the shoulder/scapula.

- The practitioner's contralateral arm is passed across and under the neck to cup the shoulder of the side to be tested, with the forearm supporting the neck.[9]

- The practitioner's other hand supports and guides the head.

- The forearm is used to lift the neck into *full pain-free flexion* (aided by the hand on the head).

- Once fully flexed, the neck/head is placed fully towards side-flexion and rotation, *away* from the side being treated.

- With the shoulder held caudally and the neck/head in the position described (at the resistance barrier), stretch is being placed on levator from both ends.

- If dysfunction exists and/or levator scapula is short, there will be discomfort reported at the attachment on the upper medial border of the scapula, and/or pain reported near the levator attachment on the spinous process of C2.

- The hand on the shoulder should then gently 'spring' it caudally.

- If levator is short there will be a *harsh*, wooden, 'blocked' feel to this action.

- If it is normal there will be a soft springing response.

Test B for levator scapula shortness (observation)

- A functional assessment involves applying the evidence we have seen (Ch. 2) of the imbalances that commonly occur between the upper and lower stabilisers of the scapula.

---

[9] Lewit (1992) achieves the same control by having the supine patient place their flexed elbow above their head, in contact with the practitioner's thigh or abdomen. This allows pressure through the long axis of the humerus to fix the scapula, while both hands are free to take the head/neck into its desired position.

- In this process, shortness is often noted in pectoralis minor, levator scapulae and upper trapezius (as well as SCM), while weakness develops in serratus anterior, rhomboids, middle and lower trapezius – as well as the deep neck flexors.

- Observation of the patient from behind will often show a 'hollow' area between the shoulder blades, where interscapular weakness has occurred, as well as an increased (above normal) distance between the medial borders of the scapulae and the thoracic spine, if the scapulae have 'winged' away from it.

Test C for levator dysfunction

- To see the imbalance described in test B in action, Janda (1996) has the patient in the press-up position (see Fig. 8.15).

- On very slow lowering of the chest towards the floor from a maximum push-up position, the scapula(e) on the side(s) where stabilisation has been compromised will move laterally and superiorly – often into a winged position – rather than medially towards the spine.

- This is diagnostic of weak lower stabilisers, which implicates tight upper stabilisers, including levator scapulae, as probably inhibiting them.

- If there is such evidence then levator scapula will have shortened.

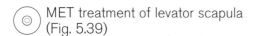 ### MET treatment of levator scapula (Fig. 5.39)

Treatment of levator scapula using MET enhances the lengthening of the extensor muscles attaching to the occiput and upper cervical spine. The position described below is used for treatment, either at the limit of easily reached range of motion, or a little short of this, depending upon the degree of acuteness or chronicity of the dysfunction.

- The patient lies supine with the arm of the side to be tested stretched out alongside the trunk with the hand supinated.

- The practitioner, standing at the head of the table, passes his contralateral arm under the

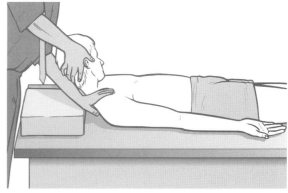

Figure 5.39 MET test A and treatment position for levator scapula (right side).

neck to rest on the patient's shoulder on the side to be treated, so that the practitioner's forearm supports the patient's neck.

- The practitioner's other hand supports and directs the head into subsequent positioning (see below).

- The practitioner's forearm lifts the neck into full flexion (aided by the other hand).

- The head is turned fully into side-flexion and rotation *away* from the side being treated.

- With the shoulder (or the scapula – see next bullet point) held caudally by the practitioner's hand, and the head/neck in full flexion, side-flexion and rotation (each at its resistance barrier), all available slack will have been removed from levator, from both ends.

- An alternative (and preferred) hand contact would be for the practitioner to place his hand palm upward, with the scapula lying on the hand and its superior border being engaged by the thenar and hyperthenar eminences.

- The patient is asked to take the head backwards towards the table, and slightly to the side from which it was turned, against the practitioner's unmoving resistance, while at the same time a slight (20% of available strength) shoulder shrug (or superior movement of the scapula) is asked for, and resisted.

- Following the 7–10 second isometric contraction and complete relaxation of all elements of this combined contraction, the neck is taken to further flexion, side-bending and rotation, where it is maintained, as the shoulder (or scapula) is depressed caudally with the patient's assistance, following the instruction, 'As you breathe out, take your shoulder blade towards your pelvis'.

- The stretch is held for 30 seconds.

- The process is repeated at least once.

CAUTION: Avoid overstretching this sensitive area.

Facilitation of tone in lower shoulder fixators using pulsed MET (Ruddy 1962)

Method A

In order to commence rehabilitation and proprioceptive re-education of a weak serratus anterior:

- The practitioner places a single digit contact very lightly against the lower medial scapula border, on the side of the treated upper trapezius, of the seated or standing patient.

- The patient is asked to attempt to ease the scapula, at the point of digital contact, towards the spine.

- An instruction is given such as: 'Press against my finger with your shoulder blade, towards your spine, just as hard [i.e. very lightly] as I am pressing against your shoulder blade, for less than a second'.

- Once the patient has learned to establish control over the particular muscular action required to achieve this subtle movement (which can take a significant number of attempts), and can do so for 1 second at a time, repetitively, she is ready to begin the sequence based on Ruddy's methodology (see Ch. 3).

- The patient is told something such as: 'Now that you know how to activate the muscles which push your shoulder blade lightly against my finger, I want you to try to do this 20 times in 10 seconds, starting and stopping, so that no actual movement takes

place, just a contraction and a stopping, repetitively'.

- This repetitive contraction will activate the rhomboids, middle and lower trapezii and serratus anterior – all of which are likely to be inhibited if upper trapezius is hypertonic.

- The repetitive contractions also produce an automatic reciprocal inhibition of upper trapezius, and levator scapula.

- The patient can be taught to make a light finger or thumb contact against the medial scapula (by placing the opposite arm behind the back) so that home application of this method can be performed several times daily.

Method B

- A similar process of facilitation of the lower fixators of the scapula combined with inhibition of overactivity of the upper fixators (levator scapula, upper trapezius, etc.) can be achieved by introducing the same sequence with a finger contact on the lower angle of the scapula.

- An instruction can be offered, such as: ' Pulse your shoulder blade towards the floor in a rhythmic way, one pulse per second, for 20 repetitions, then rest and repeat the process'.

- It is important that the patient be taught to achieve these pulsations without undue movement occurring. Ruddy (1962) used the term, 'No wobble, no bounce' to help to achieve this.

Pulsed MET treatment for eye muscles (Ruddy 1962)

Ruddy's treatment method for the muscles of the eye is outlined in Box 5.11.

13. Assessment and treatment of shortness in infraspinatus (17)

Infraspinatus shortness test A

- The patient is asked to reach backwards, upwards and across to touch the upper border of the opposite scapula, so producing external rotation of the humeral head.

- If this effort is painful infraspinatus shortness should be suspected.

Infraspinatus shortness test B (Fig. 5.40)

- Visual evidence of shortness is obtained by having the patient supine, the upper arm of the side to be tested at right angles to the trunk, elbow flexed so that lower arm is parallel to the trunk, pointing caudally with the palm downwards.

- This brings the arm into internal rotation and places infraspinatus at stretch.

- The practitioner ensures that the shoulder remains in contact with the table during this assessment by means of light compression.

- If infraspinatus is short, the lower arm will not be capable of resting parallel to the floor, obliging it to point somewhat towards the ceiling.

Assessment for infraspinatus weakness

- The patient is seated.

- The practitioner stands behind.

- The patient's arms are flexed at the elbows and held to the side, and the practitioner provides isometric resistance to external rotation of the lower arms (externally rotating them and also the humerus at the shoulder).

- If this effort is painful, an indication of probable infraspinatus shortening exists.

- The relative strength is also judged.

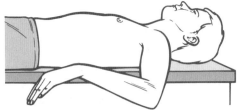

Figure 5.40   Assessment and self-treatment position for infraspinatus. If the upper arm cannot rest parallel to the floor, possible shortness of infraspinatus is indicated.

Box 5.11 Ruddy's treatment for the muscles of the eye (Ruddy 1962)

Osteopathic eye specialist Dr T. Ruddy described a practical treatment method for application of MET principles to the muscles of the eye:

- The pads of the practitioner's index, middle and ring finger and the thumb are placed together to form four contacts into which the eyeball (eye closed) can rest (middle finger is above the cornea and the thumb pad below it).

- These contacts resist the attempts the patient is asked to make to move the eyes downwards, laterally, medially and upwards – as well as obliquely between these compass points – up and half medial, down and half medial, up and half lateral, down and half lateral, etc.

- The fingers resist and obstruct the intended path of eye motion.

- Each movement should last for a count 'one' and then rest between efforts for a similar count, and in each position there should be 10–20 repetitions before moving on around the circuit.

Ruddy maintained the method released muscle tension, permitted better circulation, and enhanced drainage. He applied the method as part of treatment of many eye problems.

Ruddy's self-treatment method

- The patient is asked to close the eyes and to move the gaze (eyes closed) around the clock face – 12 o'clock, 1 o'clock, etc., until a full circle has been covered. When a particular direction of gaze produces a sense of discomfort, even if mild, it is assumed that the muscles antagonist to those active in moving towards that direction, are short, hypertonic.

- The patient creates a 'circle' by placing the thumb, index, middle and ring fingers of either hand together and placing these to surround the closed eyeball. These digits provide a barrier against which the eye can be pulsed, towards the direction of mild discomfort previously noted; 10–20 very small, pulsed movements are made in that direction, after which the eyes are relaxed and the direction again tested for discomfort. It should be far easier and more relaxed.

- This procedure is carried out on each eye, wherever a direction of discomfort is noted.

- If weak, the method discussed by Norris (1999) (see Ch. 3) should be used to increase strength (isotonic eccentric contraction performed slowly).

NOTE: In this, as in other tests for weakness, there may be a better degree of cooperation if the practitioner applies the force, and the patient is asked to resist as much as possible. Force should always be built slowly and not suddenly.

MET treatment of infraspinatus (Fig. 5.41)

- The patient is supine, upper arm at right angles to the trunk, elbow flexed so that lower arm is parallel to the trunk, pointing caudally, with the palm downwards.

- This brings the arm into internal rotation and places infraspinatus at stretch.

- The practitioner ensures that the posterior shoulder remains in contact with the table by means of light compression.

- The patient slowly and gently lifts the dorsum of the wrist towards the ceiling, against resistance from the practitioner, for 7–10 seconds.

- After this isometric contraction, on relaxation, the forearm is taken towards the floor

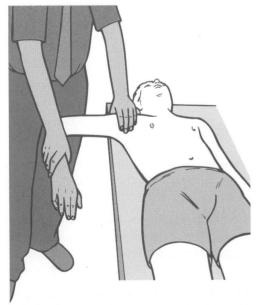

Figure 5.41 MET treatment of infraspinatus. Note that the practitioner's left hand maintains a downward pressure to stabilise the shoulder to the table during this procedure.

(combined patient and practitioner action), so increasing internal rotation at the shoulder and stretching infraspinatus (mainly at its shoulder attachment).

- Care needs to be taken to prevent the shoulder from rising from the table as rotation is introduced, so giving a false appearance of stretch in the muscle.

- The stretch is held for 30 seconds.

And/or:

- In order to initiate stretch of infraspinatus at the scapular attachment, the patient is seated with the arm (flexed at the elbow) fully internally rotated and taken into full adduction across the chest.

- The practitioner holds the upper arm and applies sustained traction from the shoulder in order to prevent subacromial impingement.

- The patient is asked to use a light (20% of strength) effort to attempt to externally rotate and abduct the arm, against resistance offered by the practitioner, for 7–10 seconds.

- After this isometric contraction, and with the traction from the shoulder maintained, the arm is taken into increased internal rotation and adduction (patient and practitioner acting together) with the stretch held for at least 20 seconds.

14. Assessment and treatment of subscapularis (18)

Subscapularis shortness test A

Direct palpation of subscapularis is often required to define problems in it, since pain patterns in the shoulder, arm, scapula and chest may all derive from subscapularis or from other sources.

- The patient is supine and the practitioner grasps the affected-side hand and applies traction while the fingers of the other hand palpate over the edge of latissimus dorsi in order to make contact with the ventral surface of the scapula, where subscapularis can be palpated.

- There may be a marked reaction from the patient when this is touched, indicating acute sensitivity.

Subscapularis shortness test B (Fig. 5.39)

- The patient is supine with the arm abducted to 90°, the elbow flexed to 90°, and the forearm in external rotation, palm upwards.

- The whole arm is resting at the restriction barrier, with gravity as its counterweight.

- If subscapularis is short the forearm will be unable to easily rest parallel to the floor, but will be somewhat elevated.

- Care is needed to prevent the anterior shoulder becoming elevated in this position (moving towards the ceiling) and so giving a false normal picture.

Assessment of weakness in subscapularis

- The patient is prone with humerus abducted to 90° and elbow flexed to 90°, hand directed caudally.

- The humerus should be in internal rotation so that the forearm is parallel to the trunk, palm towards the ceiling.

- The practitioner stabilises the scapula with one hand and with the other applies pressure to the patient's wrist and forearm as though taking the humerus towards external rotation, while the patient resists.

The relative strength is judged and the method discussed by Norris (1999) (see Ch. 3) should be used to increase strength (isotonic eccentric contraction performed slowly).[10]

◎ MET treatment of subscapularis

- The patient is supine with the arm abducted to 90°, the elbow flexed to 90°, and the forearm in external rotation, palm upwards.

---

[10] There could be other reasons for a restricted degree of external rotation, and accurate assessment calls for direct palpation as in (A) above.

- The whole arm is resting at the restriction barrier, with gravity as its counterweight (care is needed to prevent the anterior shoulder becoming elevated in this position, i.e. moving towards the ceiling, and so giving a false normal picture).

- The patient raises the forearm slightly, against minimal resistance from the practitioner, for 7–10 seconds and, following relaxation, gravity or slight assistance from the operator takes the arm into greater external rotation, through the barrier, where it is held for 30 seconds.

15. Assessment for shortness of supraspinatus (19)

Supraspinatus shortness test

- The practitioner stands behind the seated patient, with one hand stabilising the shoulder on the side to be assessed while the other hand reaches in front of the patient to support the flexed elbow and forearm.

- The patient's upper arm is adducted to its easy barrier and the patient then attempts to abduct the arm.

- If pain is noted in the posterior shoulder region during this attempt, this is diagnostic of supraspinatus dysfunction and, by implication because it is a postural muscle, of probable shortness.

Assessment for supraspinatus weakness

- The patient sits or stands with arm abducted 15°, elbow extended.

- The practitioner stabilises the shoulder with one hand while the other hand offers a resistance contact which, if forceful, would adduct the arm.

- The patient attempts to resist this, and the degree of effort required to overcome the patient's resistance is graded as weak or strong.

The relative strength is judged and the method discussed by Norris (1999) (see Ch. 3) should be used to increase strength (isotonic eccentric contraction performed slowly).

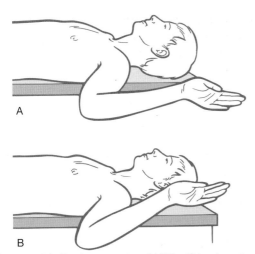

A

B

Figure 5.42A, B Assessment and MET self-treatment position for subscapularis. If the upper arm cannot rest parallel to the floor, possible shortness of subscapularis is indicated.

MET treatment of supraspinatus (Fig. 5.43)

- The practitioner stands behind the seated patient, with one hand stabilising the shoulder on the side to be treated while the other hand reaches in front of the patient to support the flexed elbow and forearm.

- The patient's upper arm is adducted to its easy barrier and the patient then attempts to abduct the arm using 20% of strength against practitioner resistance.

- After a 7–10-second isometric contraction, the arm is taken gently towards its new resistance barrier into greater adduction, with the patient's assistance.

- Repeat several times, holding each painless stretch for not less than 30 seconds.

16. Assessment and treatment of flexors of the arm (20)

Biceps tendon shortness test A

The long biceps tendon can be considered to be stressed if pain arises when the semi-flexed arm is raised against resistance.

Biceps tendon shortness test B

- The patient fully flexes the elbow and the practitioner holds it in one hand while holding the patient's hand in the other.

- The patient is asked to resist as the practitioner attempts to externally rotate the elbow and to straighten the arm.

- If unstable, the tendon may momentarily leave its groove and pain will result.

Biceps tendon shortness test C

- The patient sits with extended arm (taking it backwards from the shoulder) and half flexes the elbow so that the dorsum of the hand approximates the contralateral buttock.

- The patient attempts to flex the elbow further against resistance.

- If pain is noted, there is stress on the tendon and the flexor muscles are probably shortened.

MET treatment for shortness in biceps tendon

Lewit (1992) describes the following method:

- The patient sits in front of the practitioner, with the affected arm behind the back, the

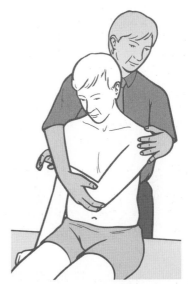

Figure 5.43 Position for test A and MET treatment of supraspinatus.

dorsal aspect of that hand passing beyond the buttock on the opposite side.

- The practitioner grasps this hand, bringing it into pronation, to take up the slack (see Fig. 5.44).

- The patient is instructed to attempt to take the hand back into supination.

- This is resisted for about 10 seconds by the practitioner, and the relaxation phase is used to take it further into pronation, with simultaneous extension of the elbow.

- Repeat several times more.

Self-treatment is possible, with the patient applying counterpressure with the other hand.

Flexors of the forearm – MET treatment
NOTE: see CD-ROM for SEIS method

A painful medial humeral epicondyle usually accompanies tension in the flexors of the forearm.

- The patient is seated facing the practitioner, with flexed elbow supported by the practitioner's fingers.

- The patient's hand is dorsiflexed at the wrist, so that the palm is upwards and fingers face the shoulder (see Fig. 5.45).

- The practitioner guides the wrist into greater flexion to an easy barrier, with pronation exaggerated by pressure on the ulnar side of the palm.

- This is achieved by means of the practitioner's thumb being placed on the dorsum of the patient's hand, while the fingers stabilise the palmar aspect, fingertips pressing this towards the floor on the patient's ulnar side of the palm.

- The patient attempts to gently supinate the hand against resistance for 7–10 seconds following which, after relaxation (depending on whether it is an acute or chronic problem), dorsiflexion is increased to, or through, the new barrier.

- Repeat as needed.

This method is easily capable of adaptation to self-treatment by means of the patient applying the counterpressure.

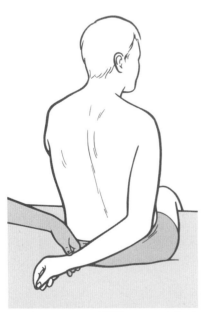

Figure 5.44 Assessment and MET treatment for dysfunction affecting biceps tendon.

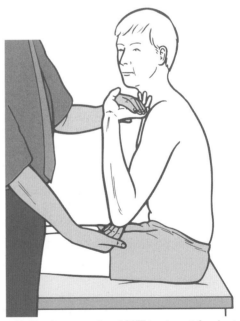

Figure 5.45 Assessment and MET treatment for shortness of the flexors of the forearm.

Biceps brachii – assessment and MET treatment

If extension of the arm is limited, the flexors are probably short.

- Treatment of biceps brachii involves the affected arm being held in extension at the easy barrier.

- The practitioner holds the patient's wrist in order to restrain a light effort to flex the elbow for 7–10 seconds after which, following appropriate relaxation of the effort, the arm is extended to or through (depending on whether it is an acute or chronic problem), the new resistance barrier.

- Repeat several times.

17. Assessment and treatment of paravertebral muscles (21)

Paravertebral muscle shortness test A

- The patient is seated on a treatment table, legs extended, pelvis vertical.

- Flexion is introduced in order to approximate forehead to knees.

- An even 'C'-shaped curve should be observed and a distance of about 4 inches (10 cm) from the knees achieved by the forehead.

- No knee flexion should occur and the movement should be a spinal one, not involving pelvic tilting (see Fig. 5.46).

Interpretation of what is observed is described below.

Paravertebral muscle shortness test B

- The assessment position is then modified to remove hamstring shortness from the picture by having the patient sit at the end of the table, knees flexed over it.

- Once again the patient is asked to perform full flexion, without strain, so that forward bending is introduced to bring the forehead towards the knees.

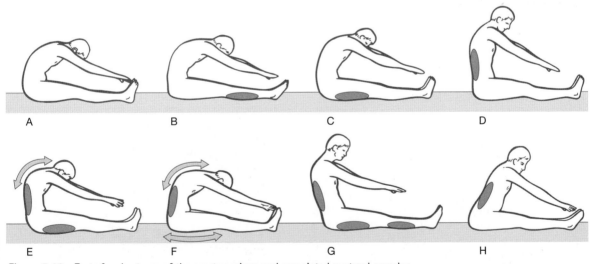

A   B   C   D

E   F   G   H

Figure 5.46 Tests for shortness of the erector spinae and associated postural muscles.
A Normal length of erector spinae muscles and posterior thigh muscles.
B Tight gastrocnemius and soleus; the inability to dorsiflex the feet indicates tightness of the plantar–flexor group.
C Tight hamstring muscles, which cause the pelvis to tilt posteriorly.
D Tight low-back erector spinae muscles.
E Tight hamstrings; slightly tight low-back muscles and overstretched upper back muscles.
F Slightly shortened lower back muscles, stretched upper back muscles and slightly stretched hamstrings.
G Tight low-back muscles, hamstrings and gastrocnemius/soleus.
H Very tight low-back muscles, with lordosis maintained even in flexion.

- The pelvis should be fixed by the placement of the patient's hands on the pelvic crest.

- If bending of the trunk is greater in this position than in test A above, then there is probably shortened hamstring involvement.

Interpretation

- During these assessments, areas of shortening in the spinal muscles may be observed as 'flatness', or even, in the lumbar area, as a reversed curve.

- For example, on forward bending a lordosis may be maintained in the lumbar spine, or flexion may be very limited even without such lordosis.

- There may be evidence of obvious overstretching of the upper back and relative tightness of the lower back.

- All areas of 'flatness' are charted since these represent an inability of those segments to flex, which involves the erector spinae muscles as a primary or a secondary feature.

- Even if the flexion restriction relates to articular factors, the erector group may benefit from MET.

- If the soft tissues are primary features of the flexion restriction then MET attention is even more indicated.

NOTE: Lewit (1999) points out that patients with a long trunk and short thighs may perform the flexion movement without apparent difficulty, even if the erectors are short, whereas if the trunk is short and the thighs long, even if the erectors are supple, flexion will not allow the head to approximate the knees.

In the modified position, with patient's hands on the crest of the pelvis, and the patient 'hunching' her spine, Lewit suggests observation of the presence or otherwise of lumbar kyphosis for evidence of shortness in that region. If it fails to appear, erector spinae shortness in the lumbar region is likely. This, together with the presence of flat areas, provides significant evidence of shortness.

Paravertebral muscle shortness test C (Fig. 5.47)

- Once all flat areas are noted and charted, the patient is placed in prone position.

- The practitioner squats at the side and observes the spinal 'wave' as deep breathing is performed.

- There should be a wave of movement starting at the sacrum and finishing at the base of the neck on inhalation.

- Areas of restriction ('flat areas'), lack of movement, or where motion is not in sequence should be noted and compared with findings from tests A and B above.

- Periodic review of the relative normality of this wave is a useful guide to progress (or lack of it) in normalisation of the functional status of the respiratory and spinal structures.

MET treatment of erector spinae muscle

- The patient sits on the treatment table, back towards the practitioner, legs hanging over the side, and hands clasped behind the neck.

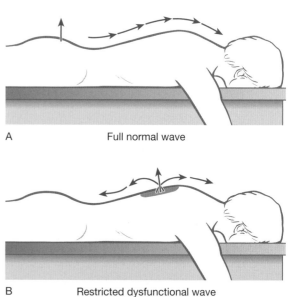

A   Full normal wave

B   Restricted dysfunctional wave

Figure 5.47   Observation of the prone breathing wave indicates areas of paravertebral stiffness or vertebral fixation. Rigid areas tend to move as a block, rather than as a wave.

- The practitioner stands on the side towards which the patient will be positioned, or behind the patient, and passes a hand across the front of the patient's chest, to rest on the contralateral shoulder, or to grasp the patient's upper arm (for variations see Figs 6.1A–F and 6.2A, B).

- The patient is drawn into flexion, side-bending and rotation to take out slack in the area being treated.

- The practitioner's free hand monitors the area of tightness (as evidenced by 'flatness' in the flexion test) and ensures that the various forces localise at the point of maximum contraction/tension.

- When the patient has been taken to the comfortable limit of flexion and/or side-flexion, and or rotation, he is asked either to look (moving the eyes only) towards the direction from which movement has been made, or to do so while also introducing a very slight degree of effort towards returning to the upright position, against firm resistance from the practitioner.

- During the contraction it may be useful to have the patient 'breathe into' the tight spinal area which is being palpated and monitored by the practitioner. This will cause an additional increase in isometric contraction of the shortened muscles.

- The patient is then asked to release the breath, and completely relax.

- The practitioner waits for the patient's second full exhalation and then takes the patient further in all the directions of restriction, towards the new barrier, but not through it.

- This whole process is repeated several times, at each level of restriction/flatness.

- The patient may also be asked to gently attempt to move towards the restriction barrier. This involves contraction of the antagonists.

- After relaxation of the effort, the new barrier is again approached.

Thoracolumbar dysfunction

This important region was discussed briefly in the section dealing with quadratus lumborum (heading 7 above), and deserves special attention due to its particularly vulnerable 'transition' status involving the powerful effect that spasm and tightness of the major stabilising muscles of the region can have on it: notably psoas, the thoracolumbar erector spinae and quadratus lumborum, as well as the influence of rectus abdominis in which weakness is all too common (see lower crossed syndrome notes in Ch. 2).

Screening for lumbodorsal dysfunction involves having the patient straddle the table (so locking the pelvis) in a slightly flexed posture (slight kyphosis). Rotation in either direction then enables segmental impairment to be observed at the same time that the spinous processes are monitored.

Restriction of rotation is the most common characteristic of this dysfunction.

MET treatment of thoracolumbar dysfunction

Psoas and/or quadratus lumborum should be assessed and if found to be dysfunctional (most probably shortened), treated as described earlier in this chapter.[11]

NOTE: Thoracic spinal restriction treatment is covered in Ch. 6, which evaluates MET and joints.

Assessment for shortness in erector spinae muscles of the neck (22)

- The patient is supine and the practitioner stands at the head of the table, or to the side, supporting the neck in one hand, and the occiput in the other, to afford complete support for both.

- When the head/neck is eased into flexion the chin should easily be able to be brought into contact with the suprasternal area, *without force*.

---

[11] Not all the muscles involved in thoracolumbar dysfunction pattern described above may need treatment, since when one or other is treated appropriately the others commonly normalise. Underlying causes must also always receive attention.

- If there remains a noticeable gap between the tip of the chin (ignore double chin tissues!) and the upper chest wall, then the neck extensors are considered to be short.

Assessment of weakness of deep neck flexors

NOTE: In applying this test it is helpful for the supine patient if the practitioner maintains a hand contact on the lower thorax to stabilise the trunk, especially if weak abdominal muscles are a feature.

- The patient is asked to flex the neck to approximately 45°, and to maintain this position for 10 seconds.

- If this is not possible, or if visible tremor is noted as the patient attempts to maintain the position, weakness of the deep neck flexors can be assumed.

- It is also possible to test relative strength by offering resistence against the forehead as the patient attempts to flex the neck.

If weakness is shown, in conjunction with shortness of the extensor muscles of the neck, then weakness should be treated initially (see discussion in Ch. 2 regarding weakness and MET, and recommendations by Norris in particular.

Toning the deep neck flexors using slow eccentric isotonic stretching (SEIS) (see Ch. 3)

- The neck of the supine patient is taken into flexion, as described for the weakness test above.

- The practitioner stands at the head of the table and supports the neck with one hand. This hand should be placed just below the occiput so that it supports the suboccipital and upper neck region.

- The other hand is on the patient's forehead.

- The patient is asked to 'tuck your chin in' (to activate the deep neck flexors) and this additional flexion is 'locked in' by the practitioner's hand on the forehead.

- The patient is asked to resist the effort the practitioner will make to extend the neck over his hand, slowly.

- This action is performed and then repeated.

The effect is to tone the deep neck flexors and to inhibit the shortened extensors, which can then be taken into stretch, as described in the MET method below.

MET treatment of short neck extensor muscles

- The neck of the supine patient is flexed to its easy barrier of resistance (if acute), or short of this (if chronic), and the patient is asked to extend the neck ('take the back of your head back to the table, gently') using minimal effort on an inhalation, against resistance.

- If the hand positions as described in the test above are not comfortable, then try placing the hands, arms crossed, so that a hand rests on the anterior surface of each shoulder, while the head rests on the crossed forearms.

- After the contraction, the neck is flexed further to the new barrier of resistance, ensuring that the suboccipital muscles receive focused stretching attention.

- A further aid during the contraction phase may be achieved by having the practitioner contact the top of the patient's head with his abdomen, and to use this contact to prevent the patient tilting the head upwards.

- This allows for an additional isometric contraction which involves the short extensor muscles at the base of the skull ('Try to tip your chin upwards').

- The subsequent stretch, as above, will involve these muscles as well.

- Repetitions of the stretch to the new barrier should be performed until no further gain is possible, or until the chin easily touches the chest on flexion.

NOTE: No force should be used, or pain produced during this procedure.

MET treatment methods for joint problems

A variety of MET treatment methods for pelvic and spinal joint restrictions, as well as the shoulder, clavicular and cervical area, will be found in Ch. 6, and these can be used alongside the more general, muscle-orientated, approaches detailed in this chapter.

References

Bandy W, Irion J, Briggler M 1997 The effect of time and frequency of static stretching on flexibility of the hamstring muscles. Physical Therapy 77: 1090–1096

Basmajian J 1974 Muscles alive. Williams and Wilkins, Baltimore

Bergmark A 1989 Stability of the lumbar spine: a study in mechanical engineering. Acta Orthopaedica Scandinavica 230(suppl): 20–24

Block S 1993 Fibromyalgia and the rheumatisms. Controversies in Rheumatology 119(1): 61–78

Bogduk N 1997 Clinical anatomy of the lumbar spine and sacrum, 3rd edn. Churchill Livingstone, Edinburgh

Bogduk N, Pearcy M, Hadfield G 1992 Anatomy and biomechanics of psoas major. Clinical Biomechanics 7: 109–119

Bourdillon J 1982 Spinal manipulation, 3rd edn. Heinemann, London

Cailliet R 1962 Low back pain syndrome. Blackwell, Oxford

Chaitow L 1991 Soft tissue manipulation. Healing Arts Press, Rochester

Chaitow L 2003 Modern neuromuscular techniques, 2nd edn. Churchill Livingstone, Edinburgh

Dommerholt J 2000 Posture. In: Tubiana R, Amadio P (eds) Medical problems of the instrumentalist musician. Martin Dunitz, London, pp 405–406

Duna G, Wilke W 1993 Diagnosis, etiology and therapy of fibromyalgia. Comprehensive Therapy 19(2): 60–63

Dvorak J, Dvorak V 1984 Manual medicine – diagnostics. George Thieme Verlag, New York

Evjenth O 1984 Muscle stretching in manual therapy. Alfta Rehab, Alfta, Sweden

Feland J, Myrer J, Schulthies S et al 2001 The effect of duration of stretching of the hamstring muscle group for increasing range of motion in people aged 65 years or older. Physical Therapy 81: 1100–1117

Fryette H 1954 Principles of osteopathic technic. In: Yearbook of the Academy of Applied Osteopathy, 1954, Indianapolis

George S 1964 Changes in serum calcium, serum phosphate and red cell phosphate during hyperventilation. New England Journal of Medicine 270: 726–728

Gerwin R, Dommerholt J 2002 Treatment of myofascial pain syndromes. In: Weiner R (ed) Pain management; a practical guide for clinicians. CRC Press, Boca Raton, pp 235–249

Gluck N, Liebenson C 1997 Paradoxical muscle function. Journal of Bodywork and Movement Therapies 1(4): 219–222

Goldenberg D 1993 Fibromyalgia, chronic fatigue syndrome and myofascial pain syndrome. Current Opinion in Rheumatology 5: 199–208

Goldstein J 1996 Betrayal by the brain. Haworth Press, New York

Gray 1995 Gray's anatomy, 38th edn. Churchill Livingstone, Edinburgh

Greenman P 1989 Principles of manual medicine, 1st edn. Williams and Wilkins, Baltimore

Greenman P 1996 Principles of manual medicine, 2nd edn. Williams and Wilkins, Baltimore

Janda V 1983 Muscle function testing. Butterworths, London

Janda V 1988 In: Grant R (ed) Physical therapy of the cervical and thoracic spine. Churchill Livingstone, New York

Janda V 1996 Evaluation of muscular imbalance. In: Liebenson C (ed) Rehabilitation of the spine. Williams and Wilkins, Baltimore

Jull G 1994 Active stabilisation of the trunk. Course notes. Edinburgh

Kapandji I 1974 The physiology of the joints, vol 3, 2nd edn. Churchill Livingstone, Edinburgh

Kendall F P, McCreary E K, Provance P G 1993 Muscles, testing and function, 4th edn. Williams and Wilkins, Baltimore

Kuchera W A, Kuchera M L 1992 Osteopathic principles in practice. Kirksville College of Osteopathic Medicine Press, Missouri

Lehmkuhl L, Smith L 1983 Brunnstrom's clinical kinesiology, 4th edn. F A Davis, Philadelphia

Lewit K 1985a Muscular and articular factors in movement restriction. Manual Medicine 1: 83–85

Lewit K 1985b Manipulative therapy in rehabilitation of the motor system. Butterworths, London

Lewit K 1992 Manipulative therapy in rehabilitation of the locomotor system, 2nd edn. Butterworths, London

Lewit K 1999 Manipulative therapy in rehabilitation of the locomotor system, 3rd edn. Butterworths, London

Lewit K, Simons D 1984 Myofascial pain: relief by post-isometric relaxation. Archives of Physical Medicine and Rehabilitation 65: 452–456

Liebenson C 1996 Rehabilitation of the spine. Williams and Wilkins, Baltimore

Lin J-P et al 1994 Physiological maturation of muscles in childhood. Lancet (June 4): 1386–1389

McGill S M, Juker D, Kropf P 1996 Quantitative intramuscular myoelectric activity of quadratus lumborum during a wide variety of tasks. Clinical Biomechanics 11: 170–172

Maffetone P 1999 Complementary sports medicine. Human Kinetics, Champaign IL

Mennell J 1964 Back pain. T and A Churchill, Boston

Middaugh S et al 1994 Muscle overuse and posture as factors in the development and maintenance of chronic musculoskeletal pain. In: Grzesiak R, Ciccone D (eds), Psychological vulnerability to chronic pain. Springer, New York, pp 55–89

Mitchell F, Moran P, Pruzzo N 1979 Manual of osteopathic muscle energy technique. Valley Park, Missouri

Moore M et al 1980 Electromyographic investigation manual of muscle stretching techniques. Medicine and Science in Sports and Exercise 12: 322–329

Norris C 1999 Functional load abdominal training (part 1). Journal of Bodywork and Movement Therapies 3(3): 150–158

Norris C 2000 The muscle designation debate. Journal of Bodywork and Movement Therapies 4(4): 225–241

Peper E, Tibbetts V 1992 Fifteen-month follow up with asthmatics utilizing EMG/Incentive inspirometer feedback. Biofeedback and Self-Regulation 17(2): 143–151

Platzer W 1992 Color atlas/text of human anatomy, vol 1, Locomotor system, 4th edn. Thieme, Stuttgart

Richard R 1978 Lésions ostéopathiques du sacrum. Maloine, Paris

Richardson C, Jull G, Hodges P, Hides J 1999 Therapeutic exercise for spinal segmental stabilisation in low back pain. Churchill Livingstone, Edinburgh

Rolf I 1977 Rolfing – integration of human structures. Harper and Row, New York

Rosenthal E 1987 Alexander technique and how it works. Medical Problems in the Performing Arts 2: 53–57

Rubin B et al 1990 Treatment options in fibromyalgia syndrome. Journal of the American Osteopathic Association 90(9): 844–845

Ruddy T 1962 Osteopathic rapid rhythmic resistive technic. Academy of Applied Osteopathy Yearbook, 1962, pp 23–31

Schamberger W 2002 The malalignment syndrome. Churchill Livingstone, Edinburgh, p 90

Scudds R A, Landry M, Birmingham T et al 1995 The frequency of referred signs from muscle pressure in normal healthy subjects (abstract). J Musculoskeletal Pain 3 (Suppl 1): 99

Shrier I, Gossal K 2000 Myths and truths of stretching. Individualised recommendations for healthy muscles. The Physician Sports Medicine 28(8): 1–7

Simons D, Travell J, Simons L 1999 Myofascial pain and dysfunction: the trigger point manual, vol 1, 2nd edn. Williams and Wilkins, Baltimore

Stedman 1998 Stedman's electronic medical dictionary. Version 4.0. Williams and Wilkins, Baltimore

Stotz A, Kappler R 1992 Effects of osteopathic manipulative treatment on tender points associated with fibromyalgia. Journal of the American Osteopathic Association 92(9): 1183–1184

Taylor D, Dalton J, Seaber A, Garrett W 1990 Viscoelastic properties of muscle-tendon units: the biomechanical effects of stretching. American Journal of Sports Medicine 18: 300–309

Taylor D, Brooks D E, Ryan J B 1997 Visco-elastic characteristics of muscle: passive stretching versus muscular contractions. Medicine and Science in Sports and Exercise 29(12): 1619–1624

TePoorten B 1960 The piriformis muscle. Journal of the American Osteopathic Association 69: 150–160

Travell J, Simons D 1992 Myofascial pain and dysfunction: the trigger point manual, vol 2. Williams and Wilkins, Baltimore

Tyler T, Zook L, Brittis D, Gleim G 1996 A new pelvic tilt detection device: roentgenographic validation and application to assessment of hip motion in professional ice hockey players. Journal of Orthopaedic and Sports Physical Therapy 24(5): 303–308

van Wingerden J-P 1997 The role of the hamstrings in pelvic and spinal function. In: Vleeming A (ed) Movement, stability and low back pain. Churchill Livingstone, New York

Vleeming A, Mooney A, Dorman T, Snijders C, Stoekart R 1989 Load application to the sacrotuberous ligament: influences on sacroiliac joint mechanics. Clinical Biomechanics 4: 204–209

Williams P 1965 Lumbosacral spine. McGraw Hill, New York

MET and the treatment of joints

6

CHAPTER CONTENTS

Joints and MET	**199**
End-feel	200
Mechanisms	200
Evidence	200
Muscles or joints?	203
Preparing joints for manipulation using MET	**203**
Joint mobilisation using MET	**204**
Basic criteria for treating joint restriction with MET	**205**
Precise focus of forces – example of lumbar dysfunction	207
Focus rather than force	207
Harakal's cooperative isometric technique	208
No stretching as a feature of joint MET application	208
More on MET and the low back	**209**
Questions and answers	**212**
Cervical application of MET	**212**
General procedure using MET for cervical restriction	212
Upper cervical dysfunction assessment and MET treatment	212
Stiles' comments regarding whiplash injury and MET	213
Greenman's exercise in cervical palpation and MET application	214
Exercise in cervical palpation	215
MET treatment of the cervical area to treat translation restriction	216
MET in joint treatment	**216**
Spencer shoulder sequence incorporating MET	217
Modified PNF 'spiral stretch' techniques	221
MET treatment of acromioclavicular and sternoclavicular dysfunction	223
MET for rib dysfunction	226
Assessment and MET treatment of sacroiliac (SI) and iliosacral (IS) restrictions	232
MET treatment for temporomandibular joint (TMJ) dysfunction	243
References	**245**

Joints and MET

In the previous chapter, MET application to a multitude of muscles, relating to most of the joints in the body, were described. Release of hypertonicity in these major muscles clearly has an effect on range of motion of joints with which they are involved. In most of these MET uses, stretching was involved (unless the condition was acute).

In this chapter, specific application of MET to spinal, pelvic, cervical, shoulder, acromioclavicular and sternoclavicular joints, and TMJ, are described. In these examples no stretching is used, merely a movement after the isometric contraction (or use of pulsed MET), to a new barrier, without force.

In order to apply the principles embodied in MET methodology to any joint dysfunction that is not specifically covered in the text, all that is required is an appreciation of restriction barriers of the joint. In essence this means having an awareness of what the normal range of movement and end-feel is for that joint. This requires an appreciation of the physiological and anatomical barriers that a particular joint enjoys.

With that information, and a keen sense of end-feel (what the end of a movement *should* feel like, compared with what is actually presented) should come an appreciation of what is needed in order to position a joint for receipt of MET input, irrespective of which joint is involved. If end-feel is sharp or sudden, it probably represents protective spasm of joint pathology, such as arthritis. The benefits of MET to such joints will be limited to what the pathology will allow; however, even in arthritic settings, a release of soft tissues commonly produces benefits.

End-feel

Kaltenborn (1985) summarises normal end-feel variations as follows:

- Normal soft end-feel results from soft tissue approximation (as in flexing the knee) or soft tissue stretching (as in ankle dorsiflexion).

- Normal firm end-feel is the result of capsular or ligamentous stretching (internal rotation of the femur for example).

- Normal hard end-feel occurs when bone meets bone as in elbow extension.

Kaltenborn defines abnormal end-feel variations as follows:

- A firm, elastic feel is noted when scar tissue restricts movement or when shortened connective tissue is present.

- An elastic, less soft end-feel occurs when increased muscle tonus prevents free movement.

- An empty end-feel is noted when the patient stops the movement, or requests that it be stopped, before a true end-feel is reached, usually as a result of extreme pain such as might occur in active inflammation, or a fracture, or because of psychogenic factors.

- As noted above, a sudden, hard end-feel is commonly due to interosseous changes such as arthritis.

- By engaging the barrier (*always* the barrier, never short of the barrier for joint conditions) and using appropriate degrees of isometric effort, the barriers can commonly be pushed back.

Mechanisms

As mentioned earlier, the mechanisms that have until recently been assumed to be operating in MET were postisometric relaxation (PIR) and reciprocal inhibition (RI). See Ch. 4 for more recent interpretations of the research into 'how MET works'.

Remember also Ruddy's pulsed MET variations, which are useful in treating joint problems (see Ch. 3). There does not appear to be any research evidence for the use of pulsed MET; however, there are clinical usage and anecdotal reports accumulated over approximately 60 years.

Apart from those joints and areas discussed in this chapter, no additional specific joint guidelines are described (apart from in a physical therapy setting in Ch. 9) because it is assumed that the reader will be able to employ the principles as explained, and the examples as given (using visual images on the CD-ROM as aids if necessary), to adapt and extrapolate the use of MET methods to any/most other joint conditions, and to personally evaluate the potentials of this classic osteopathic approach.

Evidence

Research evidence in relation to MET in general, including joint mobilisation, is presented in Ch. 4, where it is shown that features such as changes in viscoelasticity, and increased tolerance to stretch, appear to be the main mechanisms involved in enhancing range of motion (ROM) of soft tissues. Joint restrictions can also be modified by use of MET-type soft tissue stretching and mobilisation of the osteoligamentous system, as demonstrated by increased ROM (Lardner 2001).

With soft tissues, factors such as duration of stretch, and number of repetitions, appear to be the main variables that determine such outcomes.

A 30-second duration of stretch seems to be a key element in whether or not MET procedures are successful in changing muscle ROM, with some evidence that a single, long-held, 30-second stretch offers the same benefits as two 15-second, or five 6-second, stretches (Bandy et al 1997).

There are particular suggestions regarding length of stretch where age is a factor. For example Feland et al (2001) demonstrated that in elderly subjects a 60-second stretch, repeated four times, was more effective in increasing knee extension ROM than a 15- or 30-second stretch (also repeated four times).

It is clear from the evidence in relation to stretching in general that, while the ROM of joints increases following appropriate stretching of particular muscles, the individual responses of different joints to stretching varies. Examples of joint ROM increases following MET include:

- The *hip joint* was more responsive to flexion ROM improvement (±9°) on average, than was the ankle joint, where only a modest increase (±3°) in dorsiflexion was achieved (Shrier & Gossal 2000).

- Lenehan et al (2003) were able to show a greater than 10° increase in rotation ROM of the *thoracic spine,* after just one MET isometric contraction.

- Schenk et al (1994) investigated the effect of MET over a 4-week period, on *cervical* ROM of 18 asymptomatic subjects with limitations (10° or more) of active motion, in one or more planes. Those treated underwent seven treatment sessions in which the joint was positioned against the restrictive barrier, using three repetitions of light 5-second isometric contractions. Pre- and post-ROM was measured using a cervical ROM device, and the post-test range was measured 1 day after the last session. Those in the MET group achieved significant gains in rotation (approximately 8°), and smaller non-significant gains in all other planes. The control group demonstrated little change.

- As shown in their research into *cervical rotation,* Fryer and Ruskowski (2004) demonstrated a 6.65° increase in ROM using MET. However, the results differed depending

on the length of the sustained isometric contraction (see below).

Length of contraction for increasing joint ROM

Fryer & Ruskowski (2004) evaluated different lengths of contraction in a study involving 52 asymptomatic individuals.

- Results showed that a 5-second isometric contraction, using mild degrees of effort, was more effective in increasing cervical ROM than a 20-second contraction.

- ROM increased in those using 5-second contractions by 6.65° (after three repetitions of the isometric contraction).

- ROM only increased in those using 20-second contractions by 4.34° (after three repetitions of the isometric contraction).

- A sham group (bogus 'functional' technique) increased by 1.41°.

MET versus HVLT

High-velocity, low-amplitude thrust treatment has been compared with MET in treatment of cervical joint problems (Scott-Dawkins 1997).

- 30 patients with chronic cervical pain were randomised to receive either HVLT or MET manipulation.

- Each group was treated twice weekly for 3 weeks.

- 'Patients treated with HVLT experienced a greater immediate relief of pain but at the end of the treatment period there was no difference in pain levels, with pain decreasing in both groups to the same extent.'

MET treatment of low-back pain

Research at the Karolinska Hospital in Stockholm investigated the effects of MET application in a group of long-term, low-back pain (lumbar area only) sufferers, specifically excluding patients with signs of disc compression, spondylitis or sacroiliac lesions, but not those with radiographic evidence of common degenerative signs – such as spondylosis deformans (Brodin 1987).

The group comprised 41 patients (24 female, 17 male) who had suffered pain in one or two lumbar segments, with reduced mobility that had lasted for at least 2 months. The patients were randomly assigned to two groups, one receiving no treatment and the other receiving MET treatment three times weekly for 3 weeks. The MET approach used is described by Brodin as 'a modification of the technique described by Lewit ... a variation of Mitchell's MET'.

Both groups of patients recorded their pain level at rest and during activity according to a 9-graded scale each week.

Results   After 3 weeks, the group receiving treatment showed significant pain reduction, statistically greater than in the non-treated group, as well as an increase in mobility of the lumbar spine:

- Of the 21 in the treated group, four remained the same or were worse, while 17 were improved, of whom seven became totally pain free.

- Only one in the non-treated group ($n = 20$) became totally pain free, while 16 remained the same or were worse. A total of four of this group, including the one who was totally improved, showed some improvement.

MET approaches used in this study

- The patient was side-lying, with the lumbar spine rotated by moving the upper shoulder backwards, with the table-side shoulder drawn forwards until the restricted segment of the spine was engaged.

- The practitioner stabilised the patient's pelvis and the patient then pushed the shoulder forwards, using a very small amount of effort, against resistance from the practitioner, for 7 seconds.

- During relaxation, the practitioner increased the degree of lumbar rotation to the new barrier, and repeated the isometric resistance phase again, until no further gain was made, usually involving four or five repetitions.

- Additionally active, rhythmic, small rotatory movements against the resistance barrier were carried out. See the description in Ch. 3

of 'pulsed MET' (Ruddy 1962) which calls for this type of active engagement of the barrier.

- Aspects of respiratory and visual synkinesis were also employed (see Ch. 3).

- Patients were advised to use pain-free movements and positions during everyday life.

The author states: 'From this study we can conclude that in pre-selected cases, muscle energy technique is an effective treatment for lower back pain [particularly when] mobility is decreased, or its end-feel abnormally distinct' (Brodin 1982).

Acute low-back pain and MET

A detailed description of MET use in treatment of acute low-back pain is given by Wilson & Peyton (2003). They conclude: 'Results from this pilot study suggest that MET, combined with supervised neuromuscular re-education and resistance training exercises, may be superior to supervised neuromuscular re-education and resistance training exercises alone, in improving function in patients with acute low back pain.'

The procedures used in this study are outlined in Ch. 8.

MET treatment of joints damaged by haemophilia

Just how useful MET can be in treating joint problems in severely ill patients is illustrated by a Polish study of the effects of the use of MET in a group of haemophiliac patients, in whom bleeding had occurred into the joints. There had also been bleeding into muscles such as iliopsoas, quadriceps and gastrocnemius (Kwolek 1989).

The study notes that: 'As a result of haemorrhage into the joints and muscles the typical signs and symptoms of inflammation develop; if they are untreated, or treated incorrectly, or rehabilitation is neglected, motion restriction, deformation, athrodesis, muscle atrophy, scarring and muscular contractures may occur.'

Standard medical treatment used included electromagnetic field applications, heat, paraffin baths and massage, as well as (where appropriate) the use of casts for limbs and other medical and surgical procedures.

All patients received instruction as to self-application of breathing, relaxation and general fitness exercise, as well as rehabilitation methods for the affected joints using postisometric relaxation methods (MET). These were performed twice daily, for a total of 60 minutes.

Range of movement was assessed, and it was found that those patients using PIR (MET) methods achieved an improvement in range of movement of between 5° and 50° in 87% of the 49 joints treated – mainly involving ankles, knees and elbows (there was a reduction in motion range of 5–10° in just six joints). These impressive results for MET, in a group of severely ill and vulnerable patients, highlights the safety of the method, since anything approaching aggressive intervention in treating such patients would be contraindicated.

The researchers, having pointed to frequent complications arising in the course of more traditional approaches, concluded: 'The 87% improvement in movement range of 5° to 50°, and the lack of complications when rehabilitating articulations with haemophiliac arthropathy, speaks in favour of routine application of the post isometric relaxation methods for patients with haemophilia.'

Muscles or joints?

While Janda (1988) acknowledges that it is not known whether dysfunction of muscles causes joint dysfunction or vice versa, he points to the undoubted fact that each massively influences the other, and that it is possible that a major element in the benefits noted following joint manipulation derives from the effects such methods (high-velocity thrust, mobilisation, etc.) have on associated soft tissues.

Steiner (1994) has discussed the influence of muscles in disc and facet syndromes. He describes a possible sequence as follows:

- A strain involving body torsion, rapid stretch, loss of balance, etc., produces a myotatic stretch reflex response in, for example, a part of the erector spinae.

- The muscles contract to protect excessive joint movement, and spasm may result if (for any of a range of reasons, see notes on facilitation in Ch. 2) there is an exaggerated response and they fail to resume normal tone following the strain.

- This limits free movement of the attached vertebrae, approximates them and causes compression and bulging of the intervertebral discs, and/or a forcing together of the articular facets.

- Bulging discs might encroach on a nerve root, producing disc syndrome symptoms.

- Articular facets, when forced together, produce pressure on the intra-articular fluid, pushing it against the confining facet capsule which becomes stretched and irritated.

- The sinuvertebral capsular nerves may therefore become irritated, provoking muscular guarding, initiating a self-perpetuating process of pain–spasm–pain.

Steiner continues: 'From a physiological standpoint, correction or cure of the disc or facet syndromes should be the reversal of the process that produced them, eliminating muscle spasm and restoring normal motion.' He argues that before discectomy, or facet rhizotomy, is attempted, with the all too frequent 'failed disc syndrome surgery' outcome, attention to the soft tissues and articular separation to reduce the spasm should be tried, in order to allow the bulging disc to recede, and/or the facets to resume normal motion.

Clearly, osseous manipulation (high-velocity thrust) often has a place in achieving this objective (Gibbons & Tehan 1998), but clinical experience suggests that a soft tissue approach that either relies largely on MET, or at least incorporates MET as a major part of its methodology, is likely to produce excellent results in at least some such cases, and fortunately in this era of evidence-based medicine, research validation of this is available (see Chs 4 and 8).

Preparing joints for manipulation using MET

What if high-velocity thrust or mobilisation methods of joint manipulation are the appropriate method of choice in treatment of a restricted joint? How can MET fit into the picture?

Muscle energy methods are versatile, and while they certainly have applications which are aimed at normalising soft tissue structures, such as shortened or tense muscles, with no direct implications as to the joints associated with these, they can also be used to help to improve joint mobility via their influence on dysfunctional soft tissues, which may be the major obstacle to the restoration of free movement.

MET may be employed to relax tight, tense musculature, or even spasm, and can also help in reduction of fibrotic changes in chronic soft tissue problems, as well as toning weakened structures which may be present in the antagonists of shortened soft tissues.

MET may therefore be employed in a *premanipulative* mode. In this instance, the conventional manipulative procedure is prepared for, as it would normally be, whether this involves leverage or a thrust technique. The practitioner – having adopted an appropriate position, made suitable manual contacts, prepared the tissues for the high-velocity or mobilisation adjustment, and engaged the restriction barrier by taking out available slack – could then ask the patient to 'push back' from this position against solid resistance. The practitioner will have engaged the barrier in this preparation for manipulation, and will have taken out the slack that was available in the soft tissues of the joint(s), in order to achieve this position.

When the patient is asked to firmly but painlessly resist or 'push back', against the practitioner's contact hands, this produces a patient-indirect (practitioner pushing towards the resistance barrier while the patient pushes away from it) isometric contraction, which would have the effect of contracting the presumably shortened muscles associated with the restricted joint. After holding this effort for several seconds, both practitioner and patient would simultaneously release their efforts, in a slow, deliberate manner.

This could be repeated several times, with the additional slack being taken out after appropriate relaxation by the patient.

Having engaged and re-engaged the barrier a number of times, the practitioner would decide when adequate release of restraining tissues had taken place and would then make the high-velocity adjustment or mobilisation movement, as normal.

Hartman (1985) states that: 'If the patient is in the absolute optimum position for a particular thrust technique during one of these repetitions [of MET], the joint in question will be felt to release. Even if this has not occurred, when retesting the movement range there is often a considerable increase in range and quality of play.' He suggests that the practitioner use the temporary rebound reflex relaxation in the muscles, which will have followed the isometric contraction, to perform the manipulative technique. This will allow successful completion of the adjustment with minimal force. This refractory period of relaxation lasts for quite a few seconds and is valuable in all cases, but especially where the patient is tense or resistant to a manipulative effort.

Joint mobilisation using MET

The emphasis of MET on soft tissues should not be taken to indicate that intra-articular causes of dysfunction are not acknowledged. Indeed, Lewit (1985) addressed this controversy in an elegant study which demonstrated that some typical restriction patterns remain intact even when the patient is observed under narcosis with myorelaxants. He tries to direct attention to a balanced view when he states: 'The naive conception that movement restriction in passive mobility is necessarily due to articular lesion has to be abandoned. We know that taut muscles alone can limit passive movement, and that articular lesions are regularly associated with increased muscular tension.'

He then goes on to point to the other alternatives, including the fact that many joint restrictions are not the result of soft tissue changes, using as examples those joints not under the direct control of muscular influences, such as tibiofibular, sacroiliac and acromioclavicular. He also points to the many instances where joint play is more restricted than normal joint movement. Since joint play is a feature of joint mobility that is not subject to muscular or voluntary control, the conclusion has to be made that there are indeed joint problems in which the soft tissues represent a secondary rather than primary factor in any general dysfunctional pattern of pain and/or restricted range of motion (blockage).

He continues: 'This is not to belittle the role of the musculature in movement restriction, but it is important to re-establish the role of articulation, and even more to distinguish clinically between movement restriction caused by taut muscles, and that due to blocked joints, or very often, to both.' Fortunately MET seems capable of offering assistance in normalisation of both forms of dysfunction.

Basic criteria for treating joint restriction with MET (Fig. 6.1A–F)

In treating joint restriction with MET, Sandra Yates (1991) suggests the following simple criteria be maintained:

1. The joint should be positioned at its physiological barrier (specific in three planes if spinal segments are being considered: flexion or extension, side-bending and rotation).

2. The patient should be asked to statically contract muscles towards their freedom of motion (i.e. away from the barrier(s) of restriction) as the practitioner resists totally any movement of the part. The contraction, Yates suggests, should be held for about 3 seconds (many MET experts suggest longer – up to 10 seconds).

3. The patient is asked to relax for 2 seconds or so, between the contraction efforts, at which time the practitioner re-engages the joint at its new motion barrier(s).

This process is repeated until free movement is achieved, or until no further gain is apparent following a contraction.

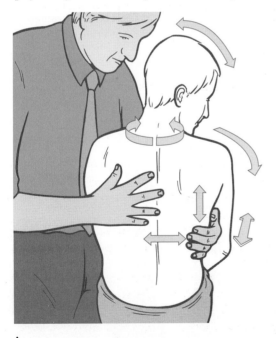

A

Figure 6.1A   General assessment for restriction in thoracic spine, showing the possible directions of movement – flexion, extension, side-bending and rotation right and left, translation forwards, backwards, laterally in both directions, compression and distraction. MET treatment can be applied from any of the restriction barriers (or any combination of barriers) elicited in this way, with the area stabilised at the point of restriction.

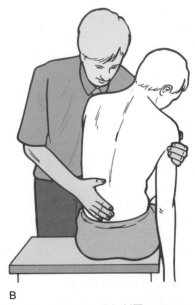

B

Figure 6.1B   Assessment and possible MET treatment position for restriction in side-bending and rotation to the right, involving the lumbar spine.

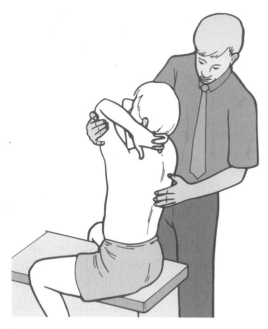

C

Figure 6.1C Assessment and possible MET treatment position for flexion restriction (inability to adequately extend) in the mid-thoracic area. MET treatment should commence from the perceived restriction barrier.

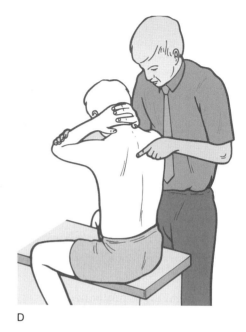

D

Figure 6.1D Assessment and possible MET treatment position for extension restriction (inability to adequately flex) in the upper thoracic area. MET treatment should commence from the perceived restriction barrier.

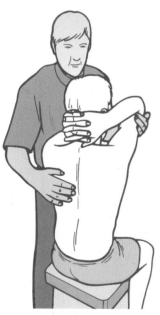

Figure 6.1E Assessment and possible MET treatment position for side-bending restriction (inability to adequately side-bend left) in the mid-thoracic area. MET treatment should commence from the perceived restriction barrier.

E

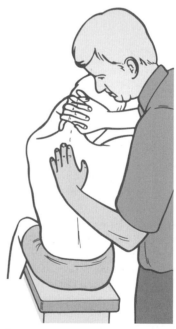

Figure 6.1F Assessment and possible MET treatment position for rotation restriction (inability to adequately rotate right) in the upper thoracic area. MET treatment should commence from the perceived restriction barrier.

F

Precise focus of forces – example of lumbar dysfunction

Stiles (1984a), like most other practitioners using muscle energy methods, places emphasis on the importance of accurate and precise structural diagnosis, if MET is to be used effectively in treatment of joint dysfunction. By careful motion palpation, determination is made as to restricted joints or areas, and which of their motions is limited.

Precise, detailed localisation is required if there is to be accuracy in determining the direction in which the patient is to apply their forces, so that the specific restricted barrier can be engaged. If MET applications are poorly focused, it may be possible to actually create hypermobility in neighbouring segments, instead of normalising the restricted segment, by inappropriately introducing stretch into already adequately mobile tissues, above or below the restricted area.

For example, if a particular restriction is present between lumbar vertebrae – say limitation in gapping of the L4–L5 left-side facets on flexion – should a general MET mobilisation attempt be used that is not localised to this segment, and which involved the joints above and/or below the restricted segment, hypermobility of these joints could result, leading, on retesting for general mobility, to an incorrect assumption that the restriction had been reduced.

In order to localise the effort at the appropriate segment, the patient would require to be positioned so as to precisely engage the barrier in that joint. For example:

- One of the practitioner's hands would palpate the facets of L4–L5, while the seated patient is guided into a flexed and side-bent position which brings the affected segment to its barrier of motion (see Fig. 6.1B).

- At that point an instruction would be given for the patient to attempt to return to an upright position so involving the muscles (agonists) restraining the joint from movement to its normal barrier.

- At the same time the practitioner's force would restrain any movement.

- This isometric contraction should ideally be maintained for 3–5 seconds (Stiles's timing) with no more than perhaps 20% of the patient's strength being employed in the effort (ideally synchronised to breathing, see Box 5.2).

- After this, when all efforts have ceased, the barrier should have retreated, so that greater flexion and side-bending can be achieved, without effort, before re-engaging the barrier.

Repetition would continue several times, until the maximum degree of motion had been obtained.

Alternatively:

- Precisely the opposite method could also be employed, in which, having engaged the barrier, the patient would be asked to attempt to move through it, while being restrained. This would bring into play reciprocal inhibition of any overly contracted muscles that might be restraining normal range of motion. In treating an acute condition, using reciprocal inhibition reduces to the likelihood of pain being produced during the procedure.

Focus rather than force

Goodridge (1981) cautions that: 'Monitoring of force is more important than intensity of force. Localisation depends on the practitioner's palpatory proprioceptive perception of movement (or resistance to movement) at or about the specific articulation.' He continues: 'Monitoring and confining forces to the muscle group, or level of somatic dysfunction involved, are important in achieving desirable changes. Poor results are most often due to improperly localised forces, usually too strong.'

Precise localisation of restrictions, and identification of muscular contractions and fibrotic changes, depend on careful palpation, a set of skills requiring constant refinement and maintenance by virtue of use. Identification of the particulars of each restriction can only be achieved via the development of the skills required to assess joint mechanics, combined with a sound anatomical knowledge.

Assessment, via motion palpation, is also called for. If forces are misdirected, then results will not only be poor but may also exacerbate the problem. In joint problems, localisation of the point of restriction seems to be the major determining factor of the success (or otherwise) of MET (as in all manipulation).

Harakal's cooperative isometric technique (Harakal 1975) (see Fig. 6.2A–D)

When there is a specific or general restriction in a spinal articulation (for example):

- The area should be placed in neutral (usually with the patient seated).

- The permitted range of motion should be determined by noting the patient's resistance to further motion.

- The patient should be rested for some seconds at a point just short of the resistance barrier, termed the 'point of balanced tension', in order to 'permit anatomic and physiologic response' to occur.

- The patient is asked to reverse the movement towards the barrier by 'turning back towards where we started', thus contracting any agonist muscles that may be influencing the restriction.

- The degree of patient participation at this stage can be at various levels, ranging from 'just think about turning' to 'turn as hard as you would like', or by giving specific more instructions.

- Following a holding of this effort for a few seconds, and then relaxing completely, the patient is taken further in the direction of the previous barrier, to a new point of restriction determined by resistance to further motion, as well as tissue response (feel for 'bind').

- The procedure is repeated until no further gain is being achieved.

It would also, of course, be appropriate to use the opposite direction of rotation, for example asking the patient to 'turn further towards the direction you are moving', so utilising the antagonists to the muscles which may be restricting free movement.

No stretching as a feature of joint MET application

NOTE: An important issue in this description is that it does not involve any attempt whatsoever to

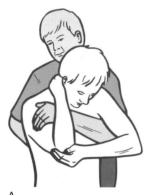

A

Figure 6.2A Harakal's approach requires the dysfunctional area (mid-thoracic in this example, in which segments cannot easily side-bend right and rotate left) to be taken to a position just short of the assessed restriction barrier. This is termed a point of 'balanced tension' where, after resting for a matter of seconds, an isometric contraction is introduced as the patient attempts to return towards neutral (sitting upright) against the practitioner's resistance.

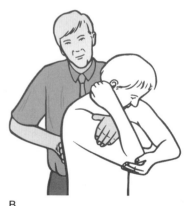

B

Figure 6.2B Following this effort, the restriction barrier should have eased and the patient can be guided through it towards a new point of balanced tension, just short of the new barrier, and the procedure is repeated.

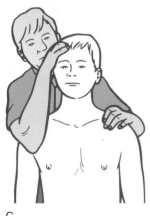

Figure 6.2C In this example the patient, who cannot easily side-bend and rotate the neck towards the left, is held just short of the present barrier in order to introduce an isometric contraction by turning the head to the right against resistance.

C

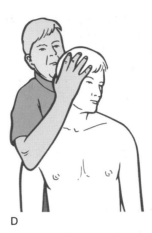

Figure 6.2D Following the contraction described in Fig. 6.2C, it is possible for the practitioner to ease the neck into a greater degree of side-bending and rotation towards the left.

D

move the tissues forcefully. Following the isometric contraction, and complete relaxation, the joint is carefully positioned at its new barrier, without force. This is in complete contrast to MET applied to a muscle, in which lengthening is the objective, and where stretching beyond the barrier would be both appropriate and essential to a positive outcome.

More on MET and the low back

Grieve (1984) describes a low-back approach, using MET, that provides insights that can be adapted for use in other spinal regions. He discusses a spine, capable of full flexion, but in which palpable left side-bending and left rotation fixation exists (i.e. it is locked in left side-bending rotation, and therefore cannot freely side-bend and rotate to the right) in the lumbar spine.

Grieve's low-back approach (Fig. 6.3)

In Grieve's example:

- The patient sits on a stool, feet apart and flat on the floor.

- The patient's left arm hangs between his knees, taking him into slight flexion and right rotation/side-bending.

- The practitioner stands at the patient's left side, with his left leg straddling the patient's left leg.

- The practitioner reaches across and holds the patient's right shoulder, while the right hand palpates the vertebral interspace between the spinous processes immediately below the restricted vertebra for its ability to rotate to the right.

- The patient is asked to slump forwards in this twisted posture until the segment under inspection is most prominent, posteriorly.

- At this point the practitioner presses his left pectoral area against the patient's left shoulder and, with the patient still flexed, the spine is side-bent by the practitioner, without resistance, so that the patient's right hand approximates the floor.

- The practitioner then rotates the patient to the right until maximum tension (bind) is felt to build at the segment being palpated. This is the restriction barrier.

At this time the first MET procedure is brought into play:

- The patient is asked to attempt to reach the floor with his right hand, and this effort is resisted by the practitioner – in order to produce reciprocal inhibition.

- The isometric contraction may last for 5–10 seconds, after which the patient relaxes.

- As the patient exhales, the practitioner increases the side-bending and rotation to the right, before increasing the degree of flexion

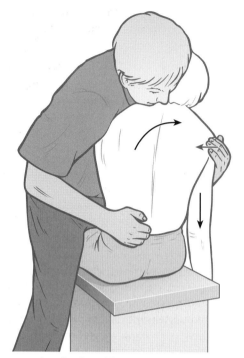

Figure 6.3 Localisation of forces before using MET to release low-back restriction.

to the barrier of resistance. No force is used, simply removal of whatever additional degree of slack has been produced by the isometric effort.

- The procedure of attempting to increase these directions of spinal movement (side-bending and rotation to the right and flexion) is then repeated, against resistance, until no additional gain is achieved.

- After the repetitions, the patient (who is still flexed and rotated, and side-bent to the right) attempts to push against the practitioner's chest with the left shoulder (i.e. attempts to rotate left and side-bend left, as well as to extend).

- This effort is maintained for 5–10 seconds before relaxation, re-engagement of the barrier, and repetition.

- This contraction involves those structures which have shortened, and so the isometric

contraction produces postisometric relaxation in them.

- After each such contraction the slack is again taken out by taking the patient further into right side-bending, rotation and flexion.

- The practitioner's position alters after the isometric efforts to the left and right, so that he now stands behind the patient with a hand on each shoulder.

- Grieve then suggests that the patient be asked to perform a series of stretching movements to the floor, first with the left hand and then with the right hand, against resistance, before being brought into an upright position by the practitioner, against slight resistance of the patient.

- The condition is then reassessed.

Discussion of Grieve's method

Notice that Grieve uses both reciprocal inhibition and postisometric relaxation in this manoeuvre. He states: 'Whether autogenic (PIR) or reciprocal inhibition is used is totally dependent on which technique effects the best neurophysiological change in the joint environment.'

In practice, however, it may not be clear which to choose; the author's experience is that PIR incorporating use of the agonists – those structures thought to be most restricted and negatively influencing joint movement – produces the most beneficial results. Reciprocal inhibition methods are, nevertheless, valuable – for example, in situations in which PIR is painful, or where agonist and antagonist both require therapeutic attention (e.g. following trauma such as whiplash in which all soft tissues will have been stressed).

In short, PIR works best in chronic settings and RI in acute settings, but both can be used effectively in either type of condition if the guideline is adhered to that no pain should be produced, and if no attempt is made to force or 'stretch' joint structures.

Unlike the approach adopted in treating muscles, joint applications of MET require that the barrier is engaged, with no attempt to push through it.

Additional choices

Goodridge (1981) describes two additional MET procedures (the same pattern of dysfunction, described above, is assumed):

- *If the left transverse process of L5 is more posterior, when the patient is flexed, one postulates that the left caudad facet did not move anteriorly and superiorly along the left cephalad facet of S1, as did the right caudad facet.*
- *There would therefore seem to be restrictions in movements in the directions of flexion, lateral flexion (side-bending) to the right, and rotation to the right.*
- *It is conceptualised that the restricted motion involves hypertonicity (or shortening) of some muscle fibres.*
- *Therefore, the practitioner devises a muscle energy procedure to decrease the tone of (or to lengthen) the affected shortened or hypertonic fibres.*

Method (Fig. 6.3)

- The position described by Grieve (see above) is adopted.

- The patient is seated, left hand hanging between thighs, with the practitioner at his left, the patient's right hand lateral to his right hip and pointing to the floor.

- The practitioner's right hand monitors either L5 spinous or transverse process.

- The patient's left shoulder is contacted against the practitioner's left axillary fold, and upper chest.

- The practitioner's left hand is holding the patient's right shoulder.

- The patient slouches in order to flex the lumbar spine, so that the apex of the posterior convexity is located at the L5–S1 articulation.

- The practitioner induces first a right side-bend, and then right rotation (patient's right hand approaches the floor) and localises movement at L5, when a sense of bind and restriction is noted there by the palpating hand.

- The patient is then asked to attempt to move in one or more directions, singly or in combination.

- These movements might involve left side-bending, rotation left and/or extension, all against practitioner's counterforces.

- The patient is, in all of these efforts, contracting muscles on the left side of the spine, but is not changing the distance between the origin and insertion in muscles on either side of the spine.

- This achieves postisometric relaxation, and subsequent contractions would be initiated after appropriate taking up of slack and engagement of the new barrier.

- *Additionally,* as in the Grieve example above, having attained the position of flexion, right side-bending and right rotation, localised at the joint in question, the patient is asked to move both shoulders in a translation to the left, against resistance from the practitioner's chest and left anterior axillary fold.

- Neither of the shoulders should rise or fall as this is done, during the translation effort.

- While the patient is attempting to move in this manner, the practitioner palpates the degree of increased right side-bending which it induces, at L5–S1.

- As the patient eases off from this contraction, as described, the practitioner should be able to increase right rotation and side-bending until once again resistance is noted.

- The objective of Goodridge's alternative method is the same as in Grieve's example, but the movement involves a concentric-isotonic procedure, because it allows right lateral flexion of the thoracolumbar spine during the effort.

As this method demonstrates, some MET methods are very simple, while others involve conceptualisation of multiple movements and the localisation of forces to achieve their ends. The principles remain the same, however, and can be applied to any muscle or joint dysfunction, since the degree of effort, duration of effort and muscles utilised provide so many variables which can be tailored to meet most needs.

Questions and answers

What if pain is produced when using MET in joint mobilisation?

- Evjenth & Hamberg (1984) have a practical solution to the problem of pain being produced when an isometric contraction is employed. They suggest that the degree of effort be markedly reduced and the duration of the contraction increased from 10 seconds to 30 seconds. If this fails to allow a painless contraction, then use of the antagonist muscle(s) for the isometric contraction is another alternative.

Following the contraction, when the joint is being moved to a new resistance barrier, what variations are possible if this produces pain?

- If, following an isometric contraction, and movement towards the direction of restriction, there is pain, or if the patient fears pain, Evjenth suggests, 'then the therapist may be more passive and let the patient actively move the joint'.

- Pain experienced may often be lessened considerably if the therapist applies gentle traction while the patient actively moves the joint.

- Sometimes pain may be further reduced if, in addition to applying gentle traction, the therapist simultaneously either aids the patient's movement at the joint, or provides gentle resistance while the patient moves the joint.

Cervical application of MET

Edward Stiles (1984b) has described some of the most interesting applications of MET in treatment of joint restrictions. Some of his thoughts on cervical assessment and treatment are explained below.

General procedure using MET for cervical restriction

Prior to any testing, Stiles suggests a general manoeuvre in which the patient is sitting upright. The practitioner stands behind and holds the head in the midline, with both hands stabilising it, and possibly employing his chest to prevent neck extension.

The patient is told to try (gently) to flex, extend, rotate and side-bend the neck, in all directions, alternately. (No particular sequence is necessary as long as all directions are engaged a number of times.) Each muscle group should undergo slight contraction against unyielding force. This relaxes the tissues in a general manner. Traumatised muscles will commonly relax without much pain via this method.

Upper cervical dysfunction assessment and MET treatment

NOTE: If assessment is being made of cervical rotational efficiency/restriction a simple screening device is available. When the head/neck is in full flexion, and rotation is introduced, all rotation below C2 is blocked. Therefore, if rotation is tested in full flexion and there is a limitation to one side, this probably represents a problem in the atlanto-occipital or atlanto-axial joints. When the head is fully extended on the neck, then the atlanto-occipital and C1/2 joints are locked and any rotation restriction relates to problems below that level.

- To test for dysfunction in the upper cervical region, the patient lies supine.

- The practitioner flexes the head on the neck to its end of range with one hand while the other cradles the neck. (As noted above, flexion stabilises the cervical area below C2 so that evaluation of atlanto-axial rotation may be carried out. The region C1 and C2 is usually responsible for half the gross rotation of the neck.)

- With the neck flexed (effectively 'locking' everything below C2), it is then passively rotated to both left and right.

- If the range is greater on one side, then this is indicative of a probable restrictive barrier, which may be amenable to MET. If rotation towards the left is normally about 85°, but in this instance it is restricted, then palpation of muscle tissues at the level of the facets of C2 (just below the level of joint dysfunction) should indicate contraction or tension locally on the right.

- This may or may not be tender, but the likelihood is that it will be so if there is dysfunction. (Pain is often more noticeable at the level of any more mobile joint rather than where the actual restriction is noted. This may be ascertained by palpation and motion palpation, feeling the tissues as the joint is moved.)

- If dysfunction is suspected at the atlanto-axial joint, then C2 is stabilised, in order to isolate C1 for treatment.

- A fingertip is placed on the left transverse process of C2 so that it cannot turn left when the patient's head is turned left.

- The second finger of the practitioner's left hand (which is cradling the neck in flexion) creates a barrier to prevent left rotation of C2, and the head is then taken gently into left rotation. C1 and the head move, and C2 remains fixed.

- The barrier will be engaged when C2 starts to move (i.e. 'bind' is noted by the palpating finger).

- The slack is removed, and at that point the patient is asked to try to turn the head gently to the right, *away from* the barrier.

- The practitioner's right hand, supporting the right side of the patient's head, prevents this right rotation.

- The patient's light rotation force is exerted against the practitioner's hand and this is maintained for about 5–7 seconds.

- Both patient and practitioner release their efforts simultaneously, and the practitioner then attempts to take the head and C1 further to the left, without force, to engage the new barrier.

- This process is repeated two or three times.

- The monitoring and stabilising pressure on C2 should be minimal but unyielding, since the patient's effort is not a strong one (this must be stressed to the patient).

- The patient will be using the muscles that are either in spasm or contracted (preventing rotation left) and, according to Stiles, 'the exertion builds up tension in the contracted muscles; the Golgi receptor system starts reporting the increased tension in relation to surrounding muscles, and spasm is reflexively inhibited.'

- This is a practitioner-direct approach, involving postisometric relaxation.

Stiles' comments regarding whiplash injury and MET

Post-whiplash X-ray pictures are often normal, as are neurological examinations. Pain, often of major proportions, is nevertheless present. Careful examination should show some segments that are not capable of achieving a full range of movement. These would normally correlate with palpable tissue change and sensitivity. More often than not there is a restriction in which a vertebra is caught in flexion (forward bending). Less commonly, extension fixations may be noted. Each vertebra should be tested to note its ability to flex, extend, side-bend and rotate. MET is applied to whatever specific restrictions are found, as in the example described above.

Wherever a restriction is noted in any particular direction, MET should be used. For example:

- If C3–C4 facets close properly as the neck is side-bent to the left, a characteristic physiological 'springing' will be noted as the barrier is reached.

- If on the right, however, there is dysfunction as the neck is side-bent to that side, the facets will not be felt to close, and a pathological barrier will be noted, characterised by a lack of 'give', or increased resistance. This restriction may be expressed in two ways:

1. The positional diagnosis would be that the segment is flexed and side-bent to the left (and therefore, because of the nature of spinal coupling mechanics, rotated left) (Fryette 1954, Mimura et al 1989).
2. The functional diagnosis would be that the joint will not extend, side-bend, or rotate to the right.

- The patient should be in the same position used in diagnosis (supine, neck slightly flexed).

- The practitioner's right middle fingers would be placed over the right pillars of C3–C4 and the neck taken to the maximum position of side-bending rotation to the right, engaging the barrier.

- The left hand is placed over the patient's left parietal and temporal areas.

- With this hand offering counterforce, the patient is invited to side-bend and rotate to the left, for a few seconds. This employs the muscles which are presumably shortened, preventing the joint from easily side-bending and rotating to the right.

- Postisometric relaxation of these muscles should follow the 5–7-second mild contraction, after which the neck can be taken to its new barrier, and the same procedure repeated two or three times.

- An alternative would be for the patient to engage the barrier, while the practitioner resists, so incorporating reciprocal inhibition.

- A further alternative would be to have the patient use Ruddy's pulsating contractions (described in Ch. 3).

Greenman's exercise in cervical palpation and MET application

The following exercise sequence is based on the work of Philip Greenman (1996), and is suggested as an excellent way of becoming familiar with both the mechanics of the neck joints, and safe and effective MET applications to whatever is found to be restricted.

In performing this exercise it is important to be aware that normal physiology dictates that side-bending and rotation in the cervical area (C3–C7) is usually 'type 2' (see Box 6.1), which means that segments that are side-bending will automatically rotate towards the same side (i.e. a side-bend to the right means that rotation will take place to the right). Most cervical restrictions are compensations and will involve several segments, all of which will adopt this type 2 pattern.

Exceptions occur if a segment is traumatically induced into a different format of dysfunction, in

---

Box 6.1 Spinal coupling concepts

Fryette (1954) described spinal biomechanics and defined basic 'laws' as follows:
- Law 1 – side-bending with the spine in neutral results in rotation to the contralateral side (i.e. rotation into the convexity). This is known as 'type 1' coupling.
- Law 2 – side-bending with the spine in hyperextension or hyperflexion results in rotation to the ipsilateral side (i.e. into the concavity). This is known as 'type 2' coupling.
- Law 3 – when motion is introduced to a joint in one plane its mobility in other planes is reduced.

In the past MET has been taught with this model utilised to predict probable directions of motion. Gibbons & Tehan (1998) have extensively examined current research and maintain that:
1. Coupled motion occurs in all regions of the spine
2. Coupled motion occurs independently of muscular activity but muscular activity might influence the direction and the magnitude of coupled movement
3. Coupling of side-bending and rotation in the lumbar spine is variable in degree and direction
4. There are many variables that can influence the degree and direction of coupled movement and include pain, vertebral level, posture and facet tropism
5. There does not appear to be any simple and consistent relationship between conjunct rotation and intervertebral motion segment level in the lumbar spine.

However, they state that the evidence of research and the literature is that 'in the cervical spine, below C2, Fryette's laws do seem to be applicable'. The use of these biomechanical laws therefore allows application of Greenman's cervical spine method, as described in this chapter, to be used with confidence.

which case there could be side-bending to one side and rotation to the other – termed 'type 1', which it is claimed is the physiological pattern for the rest of the spine, unless the region is in flexion or extension, when type 2 coupling could occur (Greenman 1996, Ward 1997). The concept of general spinal coupling taking place in a predictable manner (apart from in the cervical region) has been challenged (Gibbons & Tehan 1998). This is discussed in Box 6.1.

Exercise in cervical palpation (Fig. 6.4A, B)

To easily palpate for side-bending and rotation, a side-to-side *translation* ('shunt') movement is used, with the neck in moderate flexion or extension. When the neck is in absolute neutral (no flexion or extension – an unusual state in the neck), true translation side-to-side is possible.

As a segment is translated to one side it automatically creates a side-bending effect and, because of the anatomical and physiological rules governing it, rotation to the same side occurs (Fryette 1954, Mimura et al 1989, Gibbons & Tehan 1998).

In order to evaluate cervical function using this knowledge, Greenman suggests that the practitioner places the fingers as follows, on each side of the spine (see Fig. 6.4A):

- The index finger pads rest on the articular pillars of C6, just above the transverse processes of C7, which can be palpated just anterior to the upper trapezius.

- The middle finger pads will be on C6, and the ring fingers on C5, with the little finger pads on C3.

Then:

1. With these contacts (practitioner seated at the head of the supine patient) it is possible to examine for sensitivity, fibrosis, hypertonicity, as well as being able to apply lateral translation to cervical segments with the head in neutral, flexion or extension. In order to do this effectively, it is necessary to stabilise the superior segment to the one being examined. The heel of the hand helps to control movement of the head.

2. With the head/neck in relative neutral (no flexion and no extension), translation to the right and then left is introduced (any segment) to assess freedom of movement (and by implication, side-bending and rotation) in each direction. Say C5 is being stabilised with the finger pads, as translation to the left is introduced, the ability of C5 to freely side-bend and rotate on C6 is being evaluated when the neck is in neutral. If the joint (and/or associated soft tissues) is normal, this translation will cause a gapping of the left facet and a 'closing' of the right facet as left translation is performed, and vice versa. There will be a soft end-feel to the movement, without harsh or sudden braking. If, however, translation of the segment towards the right from the left produces a sense of resistance/bind, then the segment is restricted in its ability to side-bend left and (by implication) to rotate left.

3. If such a restriction is noted, the translation should be repeated, but this time with the head in extension instead of neutral. This is achieved by lifting the contact fingers on C5 (in this example) slightly towards the ceiling before reassessing the side-to-side translation.

4. The head and neck are then taken into flexion, and left-to-right translation is again assessed.

The objective is to ascertain which position (neutral, flexion, extension) creates the greatest degree of bind as the translation barrier is engaged. Is movement more restricted in neutral, extension or flexion?

If this restriction is greater with the head extended, the diagnosis is of a joint restricted or locked in flexion, side-bent right and rotated right (meaning that there is difficulty in the joint extending and of side-bending and rotating to the left).

If this (C5 on C6 translation left to right) restriction is greater with the head flexed, then the joint is said to be restricted or locked in extension, and side-bent right and rotated right (meaning there is difficulty in the joint flexing, side-bending and rotating to the left).

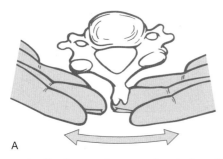

Figure 6.4A   The finger pads rest as close to the articular pillars as possible, in order to be able to palpate and guide vertebral motion in a translatory manner.

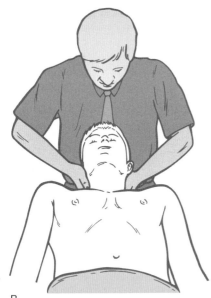

Figure 6.4B   With the neck/head in a neutral position, the practitioner sequentially guides individual segments into translation in both directions in order to sense indications of restriction and tissue modification. If a restriction is sensed, its increase or decrease is evaluated by retesting with the segment held in greater flexion and then extension. MET would be applied from the position of greatest unforced bind/restriction, using muscles which would either take the area through (antagonists to shortened muscles) or away from (shortened muscles themselves – the agonists) the barrier.

MET treatment of the cervical area to treat translation restriction

Using MET, and using the same example (C5 on C6 as above, translation right is restricted with the greatest degree of restriction noted in extension) the procedure would be as follows:

- One hand palpates both of the articular pillars of the inferior segment of the pair that testing (above) has shown to be dysfunctional.

- In this instance, this hand will stabilise the C6 articular pillars, holding the inferior vertebra so that the superior segment can be moved on it.

- The other hand will introduce movement to, and control the head and neck above, the restricted vertebra.

- The articular pillars of C6 are held and are lifted towards the ceiling, introducing extension, while the other hand introduces side-bending and rotation to the left of the head and cervical spine down to C5, until the restriction barrier is reached.

- A slight isometric contraction is asked for, with the patient incorporating side-bending, rotation to the right, and/or flexion.

- The patient is asked to try to lightly turn his head to the right, and to side-bend it right, while straightening the neck (or any one of these movements individually, if the combination is painful).

- The effort should be firmly restrained.

- After 5–7 seconds the patient relaxes, and extension, side-bending and rotation to the left are increased to the new resistance barrier, with no force at all.

- Repeat several times.

NOTE: Eye movement can be used instead of muscular effort in cases where effort results in pain. Looking upwards will encourage isometric contraction of the extensors and vice versa, and looking towards a direction encourages contraction of the muscles on that side (see Ch. 3).

MET in joint treatment

As we have seen, joints are treatable via MET, and some additional examples are given below. It is, however, not possible to provide a comprehensive body-wide, joint-by-joint description of MET application in joint restriction, especially in a text focusing its attention on soft tissue dysfunction. Nevertheless, sufficient information is provided in this chapter to allow the interested therapist/practitioner to pursue this approach further, providing insights into possible technique applications involving spinal joints quite specifically, as well as generally, and also, more surprisingly perhaps, for dealing with joints that have no obvious muscular control, the iliosacral and acromio-clavicular joints, both of which commonly respond well to MET use.

As a learning exercise in practical clinical application of MET to a dysfunctional joint, the well-known osteopathic Spencer shoulder sequence has been modified (see below). This sequence is based on a clinically useful and practical approach, first described nearly a century ago and still taught in most osteopathic schools in its updated form utilising MET or positional release methods.

Spencer shoulder sequence incorporating MET (Fig. 6.5A–F)

The Spencer shoulder treatment is a traditional osteopathic procedure (Spencer 1976, Patriquin 1992) that has in recent years been modified by the addition to its mobilisation procedures (described below) of MET. Clinical research has validated application of the Spencer sequence in a study involving elderly patients.

- In a study 29 elderly patients with pre-existing shoulder problems were randomly assigned to a treatment (Spencer sequence osteopathic treatment) or a control group (Knebl 2002).

- The histories of those in the two groups were virtually identical: approximately 76% had a history of arthritis, 21% bursitis, 21% neurological disorders, 10% healed fractures.

- 63% had reduced shoulder ROM as their chief complaint, and 33% pain (4% had both reduced ROM and pain).

- Treatment of the control (placebo) group involved the patients being placed in the same seven positions (see descriptions and Figs 6.5A–F) as those receiving the active treatment; however, the one element that was not used in the control group was MET (described as the 'corrective force') as part of the protocol. Home exercises were also prescribed.

- Over the course of 14 weeks there were a total of eight 30-minute treatment sessions. Functional, pain and ROM assessments were conducted during alternate weeks, as well as 5 weeks after the end of treatment.

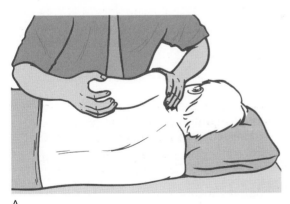

A

Figure 6.5A Shoulder extension.

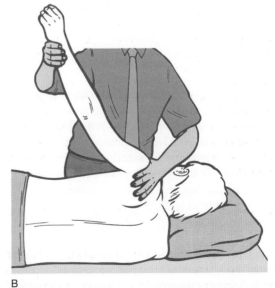

B

Figure 6.5B Circumduction and traction

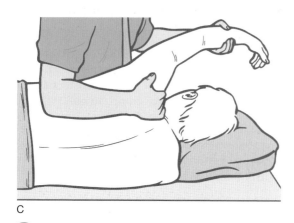

C

Figure 6.5C   Shoulder flexion

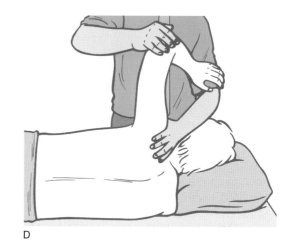

D

Figure 6.5D   Start position for both abduction and adduction of shoulder.

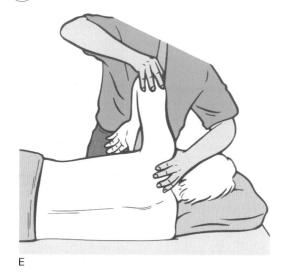

E

Figure 6.5E   Circumduction with compression.

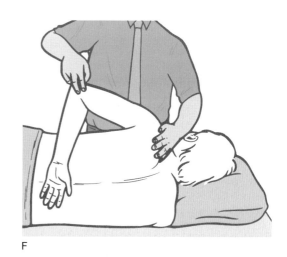

F

Figure 6.5F   Internal rotation of the shoulder.

- Over the course of the study both groups demonstrated significantly increased ROM and a decrease in perceived pain. However after treatment: 'Those subjects who had received osteopathic manipulative treatment [i.e. muscle-energy-enhanced Spencer sequence] demonstrated continued improvement in ROM, while the ROM of the placebo group decreased.'

The researchers concluded: 'Clinicians may wish to consider OMT [i.e. muscle energy technique combined with Spencer sequence] as a modality for elderly patients with restricted ROM in the shoulder.'

A. Assessment and MET treatment of shoulder extension restriction (Fig. 6.5A)

- The practitioner's cephalad hand cups the shoulder of the side-lying patient, firmly compressing the scapula and clavicle to the thorax, while the patient's flexed elbow is held in the practitioner's caudad hand, as the arm is taken into extension towards the optimal 90° of extension.

- The first indication of resistance to movement should be sensed, indicating the beginning of the end of range of that movement.

- At that 'first sign of resistance' barrier the patient is instructed to push the elbow towards the feet, or anteriorly, or to push further towards the direction of extension – utilising no more than 20% of available strength, building up force slowly.

- This effort is firmly resisted by the practitioner, and after 7–10 seconds the patient is instructed to slowly cease the effort.

- After complete relaxation, and on an exhalation, the practitioner moves the shoulder further into extension, to the next restriction barrier, and the MET procedure is repeated, possibly using a different direction of effort.

B. Assessment and MET treatment of shoulder flexion restriction (Fig. 6.5B)

- The patient has the same starting position as in A, above.

- The practitioner stands at chest level, half-facing cephalad. The practitioner's non-table-side hand grasps the patient's forearm while the table-side hand holds the clavicle and scapula firmly to the chest wall.

- The practitioner slowly introduces shoulder flexion in the horizontal plane, as range of motion to 180° is assessed, by which time the elbow will be in extension.

- At the position of very first indication of restriction in movement (palpated by the hand stabilising the shoulder, and by the hand/arm moving the patient's arm towards the direction being assessed), the patient is instructed to pull the elbow towards the feet, or to direct it posteriorly, or to push further towards the direction of flexion – utilising no more than 20% of available strength, building up force slowly.

- This effort is firmly resisted, and after 7–10 seconds the patient is instructed to slowly cease the effort.

- After complete relaxation, and on an exhalation, the practitioner moves the shoulder further into flexion, to the next restriction barrier, where the MET procedure is repeated.

- A degree of active patient participation in the movement towards the new barrier may be helpful.

C. Articulation and assessment of circumduction with compression (Fig. 6.5C)

- The patient is side-lying with flexed elbow.

- The practitioner's cephalad hand cups the patient's shoulder, firmly compressing scapula and clavicle to the thorax.

- The practitioner's caudad hand grasps the patient's elbow and takes the shoulder through a slow clockwise circumduction, while adding compression through the long axis of the humerus.

- This is repeated several times in order to assess range, freedom and comfort of the circumduction motion, as the humeral head moves on the surface of the glenoid fossa.

- The same procedure is then performed anticlockwise.

- If any restriction is noted, Ruddy's pulsed MET may be usefully introduced, in which the patient attempts to execute a series of minute contractions, towards the restriction barrier, 20 times in a period of 10 seconds, before articulation is continued.

- Or a simple effort towards or away from the direction of restriction may be introduced against resistance, as described in previous Spencer positions.

- This would be followed by resumption of the circumduction movement until another barrier was identified.

D. Articulation and assessment of circumduction with traction (Fig. 6.5D)

- The patient is side-lying with arm straight.

- The practitioner's cephalad hand cups the patient's shoulder, compressing scapula and clavicle to the thorax, while the caudad hand grasps the patient's wrist and introduces slight traction, before taking the arm through slow clockwise circumduction.

- This articulates the joint while assessing range of motion in circumduction, as well as the status of the joint capsule.

- The same process is repeated anticlockwise.

- If any restriction is noted, Ruddy's pulsed MET (as described above), or a regular MET contraction against resistance, can usefully be introduced before articulation is continued.

E. Assessment and MET treatment of shoulder abduction restriction (Fig. 6.5E)

- The patient is side-lying.

- The practitioner cups the patient's shoulder and compresses the scapula and clavicle to the thorax with the cephalad hand, while cupping flexed elbow with the caudad hand.

- The patient's hand is supported on the practitioner's cephalad forearm/wrist to stabilise the arm.

- The elbow is moved towards the patient's head, to abduct the shoulder, and range of motion is assessed.

- A degree of internal rotation is involved in this abduction.

- Pain-free easy abduction should be close to 180°.

- Any restriction in range of motion is noted.

- At the position of the very first indication of resistance to movement, the patient is instructed to pull the elbow towards the waist, or to push further towards the direction of abduction, utilising no more than 20% of available strength, building up force slowly.

- This effort is firmly resisted, and after 7–10 seconds the patient is instructed to slowly cease the effort simultaneously with the practitioner.

- After complete relaxation, and on an exhalation, the practitioner, using his contact on the elbow, moves the shoulder further into abduction, to the next restriction barrier, where the MET procedure is repeated if necessary (i.e. if there is still restriction).

- A degree of active patient participation in the movement towards the new barrier may be helpful.

F. Assessment and MET treatment of shoulder adduction restriction (not illustrated)

- The patient is side-lying.

- The practitioner cups the patient's shoulder and compresses the scapula and clavicle to the thorax with the cephalad hand, while cupping the elbow with the caudad hand.

- The patient's hand is supported on the practitioner's cephalad forearm/wrist to stabilise the arm.

- The elbow is taken in an arc forward of the chest so that it moves both cephalad and medially, as the shoulder adducts and externally rotates.

- The action is performed slowly, and any signs of resistance are noted.

- At the position of the very first indication of resistance to movement, the patient is instructed to pull the elbow towards the ceiling, or to push further towards the direction of adduction – utilising no more than 20% of available strength, building up force slowly.

- This effort is firmly resisted, and after 7–10 seconds the patient is instructed to slowly cease the effort.

- After complete relaxation, and on an exhalation, the elbow is moved to take the shoulder further into adduction, to the next restriction barrier, where the MET procedure is repeated if restriction remains.

- A degree of active patient participation in the movement towards the new barrier may be helpful.

G. Assessment and MET treatment of internal rotation restriction (Fig. 6.5F)

- The patient is side-lying.

- The patient's flexed arm is placed behind his back to evaluate whether the dorsum of the hand can be painlessly placed against the dorsal surface of the ipsilateral lumbar area (see Fig. 6.5F).

- This arm position is maintained throughout the procedure.

- The practitioner stands facing the side-lying patient and cups the patient's shoulder and compresses the scapula and clavicle to the thorax with his cephalad hand while cupping the flexed elbow with the caudad hand.

- The practitioner slowly brings the patient's elbow (ventrally) towards his body, and notes any sign of restriction as this movement, which increases internal rotation, is performed.

- At the position of first indication of resistance to this movement, the patient is instructed to pull his elbow away from the practitioner, either posteriorly, or medially, or both simultaneously – utilising no more than 20% of available strength, building up force slowly.

- This effort is firmly resisted, and after 7–10 seconds the patient is instructed to slowly cease the effort simultaneously with the practitioner.

- After complete relaxation, and on an exhalation, the elbow is moved to take the shoulder further into abduction and internal rotation, to the next restriction barrier, where the MET procedure is repeated.

Variable directions of effort

In any of the Spencer assessments, treatment of identified restrictions may involve isometric contractions towards, or away from, the barrier, or in any other directions that result in an increased range of movement. Alternatively, pulsed MET may be employed.

Modified PNF 'spiral stretch' techniques (see Fig. 6.6A, B)

Proprioceptive neuromuscular facilitation (PNF) methods have been incorporated into useful assessment and treatment sequences (McAtee &

Charland 1999). These methods have been modified to take account of MET principles (Chaitow 2001).

Spiral MET method 1. Shoulder 'spiral' stretch into extension to increase the range of motion in flexion, adduction and external rotation (Fig. 6.6A)

- The patient lies supine and ensures that her shoulders remain in contact with the table throughout the procedure.

- The head is turned left.

- The patient flexes, adducts and externally rotates the (right) arm fully, maintaining the elbow in extension (palm facing the ceiling).

- The practitioner stands at the head of the table and supports the patient's arm at proximal forearm and elbow.

- The patient is asked to begin the process of returning the arm to her side, in stages, against resistance.

- The amount of force used by the patient should not exceed 25% of available strength.

- The first instruction is to pronate and internally rotate the arm ('turn your arm so that your palm faces the other way'), followed by abduction and then extension ('bring your arm back outwards and to your side').

- All these efforts are combined by the patient into a sustained effort which is resisted by the practitioner so that a 'compound' isometric contraction occurs, involving infraspinatus, middle trapezius, rhomboids, teres minor, posterior deltoid and pronator teres.

- On complete relaxation the practitioner, with the patient's assistance, takes the arm further into flexion, adduction and external rotation, stretching these muscles to a new barrier.

- The same procedure is repeated two or three times.

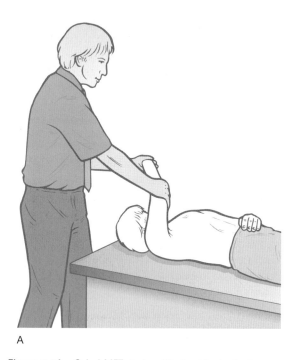

A

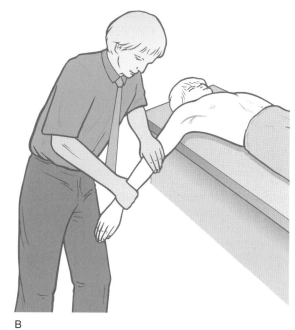

B

Figure 6.6A   Spiral MET starts with shoulder in flexion, adduction and external rotation. Following compound isometric contraction all these directions are taken to new barriers.

Figure 6.6B   Spiral MET2 starts with shoulder in extension, abduction and internal rotation. Following compound isometric contraction all these directions are taken to new barriers.

Spiral MET method 2. Shoulder 'spiral' stretch into flexion to increase the range of motion in extension, abduction and internal rotation (Fig. 6.6B)

- The patient lies supine and ensures that her shoulders remain in contact with the table throughout the procedure.

- She extends, abducts and internally rotates the (right) arm fully, maintaining the elbow in extension (wrist pronated).

- The practitioner stands at the head of the table and supports the patient's arm at proximal forearm and elbow.

- The patient is asked to begin the process of returning the arm to her side, in stages, against resistance. The amount of force used by the patient should not exceed 25% of available strength.

- The first instruction is to supinate and externally rotate the arm ('turn your arm outwards so that your palm faces the other way'), followed by adduction and then flexion ('bring your arm back towards the table, and then up to your side').

- All these efforts are combined by the patient into a sustained effort that is resisted by the practitioner, so that a 'compound' isometric contraction occurs, involving the clavicular head of pectoralis major, anterior deltoid, coracobrachialis, biceps brachii, infraspinatus and supinator.

- On complete relaxation the practitioner, with the patient's assistance, takes the arm further into extension, abduction and internal rotation, stretching these muscles to a new barrier.

- The same procedure should be repeated two or three times.

MET treatment of acromioclavicular and sternoclavicular dysfunction

Whereas spinal and most other joints are seen to be moved by, and to be under, the postural influence of muscles, and therefore to an extent to be capable of having their function modified by muscle energy techniques, articulations such as those of the sternoclavicular, acromioclavicular and iliosacral joints seem far less amenable to such influences. Hopefully, some of the methods detailed below will modify this impression, since MET is widely used in the osteopathic profession to help normalise the functional integrity of these joints.

In regard to the sacroiliac (SI) joint the work of Vleeming et al (1995) and Lee (2000), in particular, has shown that force closure of the joint provides stability. Simple logic suggests that if laxity of soft tissues removes stability, excessive tone and/or tightness, shortness of the soft tissues in question (which includes latissimus dorsi and the hamstrings) could produce restrictions to normal SI joint motion. It can be hypothesised that similar influences doubtless apply to other joints that lie outside voluntary control, such as the acromioclavicular (AC) joint (possibly involving structures such as upper trapezius, pectoralis minor, subclavius and/or the scalenes?).

Acromioclavicular dysfunction (Fig. 6.7A, B)

Stiles (1984b) suggests beginning evaluation of AC dysfunction at the scapulae, the mechanics of which closely relate to AC function.

- The patient sits erect and the spines of both scapulae are palpated by the practitioner, standing behind. The hands are moved medially, until the medial borders of the scapulae are identified, at the level of the spine of the scapula.

- Using the palpating fingers as landmarks, the levels are checked to see whether they are the same. Inequality suggests AC dysfunction.

- The side of dysfunction remains to be assessed, and each side is then tested separately (see Fig. 6.7A).

- To test the right-side AC joint, the practitioner is behind the patient, with the left hand palpating over the joint. The right hand holds the patient's right elbow. The arm is lifted in a direction, 45° from the sagittal and frontal planes.

- As the arm approaches 90° elevation, the AC joint should be carefully palpated for hinge movement, between the acromion and the clavicle.

- In normal movement, with no restriction, the palpating hand should move slightly caudad, as the arm is abducted beyond 90°. If the AC is restricted, the palpating hand/digit will move cephalad and little or no action will be noted at the joint itself as the arm goes beyond 90° elevation.

- Muscle energy technique is employed with the arm held at the restriction barrier, as for testing above.

- If the scapula on the side of dysfunction had been shown to be more proximal than that on the normal side, then the humerus is placed in external rotation, which takes the scapula caudad against the barrier, before the isometric contraction commences.

- If, however, the scapula on the side of the AC dysfunction was more distal than the scapula on the normal side, then the arm is internally rotated, taking the scapula cephalad against the barrier before the isometric contraction commences.

- The left hand (we assume this to be a right-sided problem in this example) stabilises the distal end of the clavicle, with caudad pressure being applied by the left thumb which rests on the proximal surface of the scapula. The first finger of the left hand lies on the distal aspect of the clavicle.

- The combination of the rotation of the arm as appropriate (externally if the scapula on that side was high and internally if it was low) as well as the caudad pressure exerted by the left hand on the clavicle and the scapula, provides an unyielding counterforce.

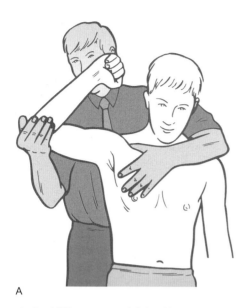

A

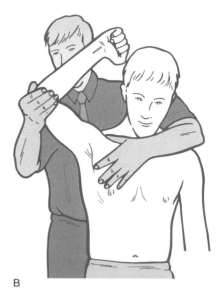

B

Figure 6.7A   MET treatment of right-side acromioclavicular restriction. Patient attempts to return the elbow to the side against resistance.

Figure 6.7B   Following the isometric contraction, the arm is elevated further while firm downward pressure is maintained on the lateral aspect of the clavicle.

- The arm will have been raised until the first sign of inappropriate movement at the AC joint was noted (as a sense of 'bind'). This is the barrier, and at this point the various stabilising holds (internal or external arm rotation, etc.) are introduced.

- An unyielding counterpressure is applied at the point of the patient's elbow by the right hand, and the patient is asked to try to take that elbow towards the floor with less than full strength.

- After 7–10 seconds the patient and practitioner relax, and the arm is once more taken towards the barrier.

- Again, greater internal or external rotation is introduced to take the scapula higher or lower, as appropriate, as firm but not forceful pressure is sustained on the clavicle and scapula in a caudad direction.

- The mild isometric contraction is again called for, and the procedure repeated several times. (It is worth recalling that respiratory accompaniment to the efforts described is helpful, with inhalation accompanying effort, and exhalation accompanying relaxation and the engagement of the new barrier.)

- The procedure is repeated until no further improvement is noted in terms of range of motion or until it is sensed that the clavicle has resumed normal function.

◎   Assessment and MET treatment of restricted abduction in the sternoclavicular joint ('Shrug' test)

- As the clavicle abducts, it rotates posteriorly.

- To test for this motion, the patient lies supine, or is seated, with arms at side (Fig. 6.8A).

- The practitioner places his index fingers on the superior surface of the medial end of the clavicle.

- The patient is asked to shrug the shoulders as the practitioner palpates for the expected caudal movement of the medial clavicle. If it fails to do so, there is a restriction preventing normal abduction.

MET treatment of restricted abduction in the sternoclavicular joint (Fig. 6.8B)

- The practitioner stands behind the seated patient with his thenar eminence on the superior margin of the medial end of the clavicle to be treated.

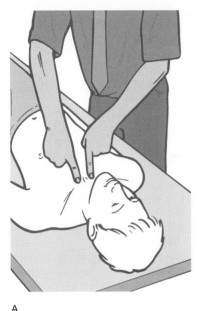

Figure 6.8A Assessment ('shrug test') for restriction in clavicular mobility.

A

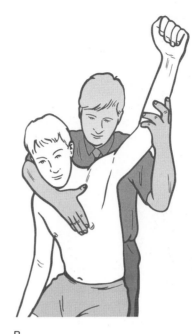

Figure 6.8B MET treatment of restricted sternoclavicular joint. Following an isometric contraction, the arm is elevated and extended while firm downward pressure is maintained on the medial aspect of the clavicle with the thenar eminence.

B

- The other hand grasps the patient's flexed elbow and holds this at 90°, with the upper arm externally rotated and abducted.

- The patient is asked to adduct the upper arm for 5–7 seconds against resistance, using about 20% of available strength.

- Following the effort and complete relaxation, the arm is abducted further, and externally rotated further, until a new barrier is sensed, with the practitioner all the while maintaining firm caudad pressure on the medial end of the clavicle.

- The process is repeated until free movement of the medial clavicle is achieved.

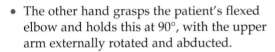 Assessment ('prayer' test) and MET treatment of restricted horizontal flexion of the upper arm (sternoclavicular restriction)

- The patient lies supine and the practitioner stands to one side with the index fingers resting on the anteromedial aspect of each clavicle.

- The patient is asked to extend his arms forwards in front of his face in a 'prayer' position, palms together, pointing to the ceiling (Fig. 6.9A).

- On the patient pushing the hands forwards towards the ceiling, the clavicular heads should drop towards the floor and not rise up to follow the hands. If one or both fail to drop, there is a restriction.

◎ MET treatment of restricted horizontal flexion of the upper arm (sternoclavicular restriction)

- The patient is supine and the practitioner stands on the contralateral side facing the patient at shoulder level. The practitioner places the thenar eminence of his cephalad hand over the medial end of the dysfunctional clavicle, holding it towards the floor. His caudad hand lies under the shoulder on that side to embrace the dorsal aspect of the lateral scapula (Fig. 6.9B).

- The patient is asked to stretch out the arm on the side to be treated so that the hand can rest behind the practitioner's neck or shoulder.

- The practitioner leans back to take out all the slack from the extended arm and shoulder while at the same time lifting the scapula on that side slightly from the table. At this time the patient is asked to pull the practitioner towards himself, against firm resistance, for 7–10 seconds.

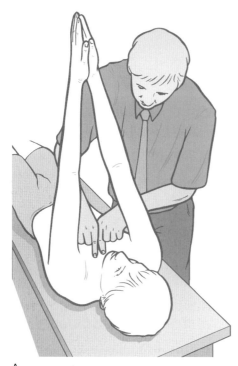

A

Figure 6.9A   Assessment ('prayer test') for restricted horizontal flexion of the sternoclavicular joint.

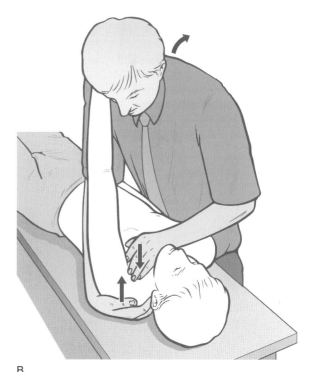

B

Figure 6.9B   MET treatment of horizontal flexion restriction. After isometric contraction (patient attempts to pull practitioner towards himself) the practitioner simultaneously lifts the shoulder while maintaining firm downwards pressure (to the floor) with the hypothenar eminence on the medial aspect of the clavicle.

- Following complete release of all the patient's efforts, the downwards (to the floor) thenar eminence pressure is maintained (painlessly) and more slack is taken out (practitioner keeps in place all elements of the procedure throughout, only the patient releases effort between contractions).

- The process is repeated once or twice more or until the 'prayer' test proves negative.

NOTE: No pain should be noted during this procedure.

MET for rib dysfunction (Greenman 1996, Goodridge & Kuchera 1997)

In order to use MET successfully to normalise rib dysfunction the nature of the problem requires identification. In this section of the chapter only a limited number of rib problems are considered, in order to illustrate MET usefulness.

Terminology

There are various somewhat confusing ways of describing the manner in which a rib, or group of ribs, is restricted. For example:

- A rib that fails to move fully into its inhalation position can be variously described as being 'locked in exhalation', 'an exhalation restriction', 'limited in inhalation', or 'depressed'.

- A rib that fails to move fully into its exhalation position can variously be described as being 'locked in inhalation', 'an inhalation restriction', 'limited in exhalation', or 'elevated'.

In this text the shorthand terms 'elevated' and 'depressed' will be used.

Study is recommended of Greenman (1996) and Ward (1997) for a wider range of MET choices for treating such restrictions.

As a rule, clinical experience suggests that unless there has been direct trauma, rib restrictions are compensatory, and involve groups of ribs. Osteopathic clinical experience also suggests that, when treating a group of depressed ribs, the 'key' rib to receive primary attention should be the most superior of these. If this is successfully released it will tend to 'unlock' the remaining ribs in that group. Similarly, if a group of elevated ribs is being treated, the key rib is likely to be the most inferior of these, which if successfully released will unlock the remaining ribs in that group.

If palpation commences at the most cephalad aspect of the thorax, the 2nd rib is the most easily palpated. The ribs should be sequentially assessed, and if a depressed rib is noted this is clearly the most cephalad, and is the one to be treated (see below). Similarly, if an elevated rib is identified, the ribs continue to be evaluated until a normal pair is located, and the dysfunctional rib cephalad to these is treated.

MET methods described below are one way of releasing such restrictions. However, there are also extremely useful positional release methods for treating such problems, based on Jones's strain/counterstrain methods (Jones 1981, Chaitow 2002).

As in all forms of somatic dysfunction, causes should be sought and addressed, in addition to mobilisation of restrictions, using MET or other methods, as described in this text.

Rib palpation test: rib 1 (Fig. 6.10)

- The patient is seated and the practitioner stands behind.

- The practitioner places his hands so that the fingers can draw posteriorly the upper trapezius fibres lying superior to the 1st rib.

- The tips of the practitioner's middle and index (or middle and ring) fingers can then most easily be placed on the superior surface of the posterior shaft of the 1st rib.

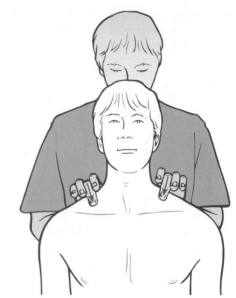

Figure 6.10   Palpation of 1st rib anterior to upper trapezius fibres.

- Symmetry is evaluated as the patient breathes lightly.

- The commonest dysfunction is for one of the pair of 1st ribs to be 'locked' in an elevated position ('inhalation restriction').

- The superior aspect of this rib will palpate as tender and attached scalene structures are likely to be short and tight (Greenman 1996).

Or:

- The patient is seated and the practitioner stands behind.

- The practitioner places his hands so that the fingers can draw posteriorly the upper trapezius fibres lying superior to the 1st rib.

- The tips of the practitioner's middle and index (or middle and ring) fingers can then most easily be placed on the superior surface of the posterior shaft of the 1st rib.

- The patient exhales and shrugs his shoulders and the palpated 1st ribs behave asymmetrically (one moves superiorly more than the other), or the patient inhales fully and the palpated 1st ribs behave asymmetrically (one moves more than the other).

- The commonest restriction of the 1st rib is into elevation and the likeliest soft tissue involvement is of anterior and medial scalenes (Goodridge & Kuchera 1997).

◎ Rib palpation test: ribs 2–10 (Fig. 6.11)

- The patient is supine or seated.

- The practitioner stands at waist level facing the patient's head, with a single finger contact on the superior aspect of one pair of ribs.

- The practitioner's dominant eye determines the side of the table from which he is approaching the observation of rib function (right-eye dominant calls for standing on the patient's right side).

- The fingers are observed as the patient inhales and exhales fully (eye focus is on an area between the palpating fingers so that peripheral vision assesses symmetry of movement).

- If, on inhalation, one of a pair of ribs fails to move as far as its pair, it is described as a depressed rib, unable to move fully to its end of range on inhalation (an 'exhalation restriction').

- If, on exhalation, one of a pair of ribs fails to fall as far as its pair, it is described as an *elevated rib*, unable to move fully to its end of range on exhalation (an 'inhalation restriction').

Rib palpation test: ribs 11 and 12 (Fig. 6.12)

- Assessment of 11th and 12th ribs is usually performed with the patient prone and palpation performed with a hand contact on the posterior shafts to evaluate full inhalation and exhalation motions.

- The 11th and 12th ribs usually operate as a pair so that if any sense of reduction in posterior motion is noted on one side or the other, on inhalation, the pair is regarded as depressed, unable to fully inhale ('exhalation restriction').

- If any sense of reduction in anterior motion is noted on one side or the other, on exhalation, the pair (or individual rib) is regarded as elevated, unable to fully exhale ('inhalation restriction').

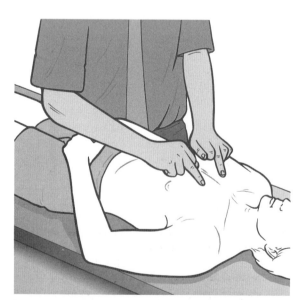

Figure 6.11   Palpation of ribs 2–10.

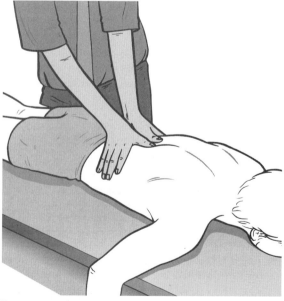

Figure 6.12   Palpation of ribs 11 and 12.

General principles of MET for rib dysfunction

Before using MET on rib restrictions identified in tests such as those outlined above, appropriate attention should be given to the attaching musculature, for example the scalenes for the upper ribs, and pectorals, latissimus, quadratus lumborum and others for the lower ribs (see Ch. 5).

Additionally, before specific attention is given to rib restrictions, evaluation and appropriate treatment should be given to any thoracic spine dysfunction that may be influencing the function of associated ribs. Attention should also be given to postural and breathing habits that may be contributing to thoracic spine and/or rib dysfunction, and appropriate re-education and exercise protocols prescribed (Chaitow et al 2002).

MET treatment for restricted 1st rib (Fig. 6.13)

- The patient is seated.

- To treat a right elevated 1st rib, the practitioner's left foot is placed on the table and the patient's left arm is 'draped' over the practitioner's flexed knee.

- The practitioner's left arm is flexed, with the elbow placed anterior to the patient's shoulder and with the left hand supporting the patient's (side of) head.

- The practitioner makes contact with the tubercle of the 1st rib with the fingers or thumb of his right hand, taking out available soft tissue slack as steady force is applied in an inferior direction.

- The practitioner eases his flexed leg to the left and simultaneously uses his left hand to encourage the patient's neck into a side-flexion and rotation to the right, so unloading scalene tension on that side and encouraging the 1st rib shaft to move anteriorly and inferiorly.

- The contact thumb or fingers on the rib tubercle/shaft take out available slack, and the patient is asked to 'inhale and hold your breath for a few seconds and at the same time gently press your head towards the left against

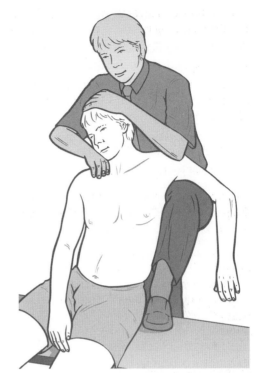

Figure 6.13 Position for MET treatment of restricted (elevated) 1st rib on the right.

my hand'. This 5–7-second effort will activate and isometrically contract the scalenes.

- On releasing the breath, slack is taken out of the soft tissues as all the movements which preceded the contraction are repeated.

- Two or three repetitions usually results in greater rib symmetry and functional balance.

MET treatment for restricted 2nd to 10th ribs

◎ **MET method for elevated ribs (Fig. 6.14)**

- The most inferior of a group of elevated ribs should be identified.

- The patient is supine and the practitioner stands at the head of the table, slightly to the left of the patient's head, with the right hand (for left-side rib dysfunction) supporting the patient's upper thoracic region, forearm supporting the neck and head.

- The left hand is placed so that the thenar eminence rests on the superior aspect of the costochondral junction of the designated rib, close to the mid-clavicular line (for upper ribs; for ribs 7–10 the contact would be more lateral, closer to the mid-axillary line), directing the rib caudally.

- The upper thoracic and cervical spine is then eased into flexion, as well as side-flexion towards the treated side, until motion is sensed at the site of the rib stabilisation.

- If introduction of side-flexion is difficult, the patient should be asked to ease the left hand (in this example) towards the feet until motion is noted at the palpated rib.

- The patient should then be asked to 'inhale fully and hold your breath' (producing an isometric contraction of the intercostals as well as the scalenes) and to attempt to return the trunk and head to the table, against the practitioner's firm resistance.

- On release and full exhalation, slack is removed from the local tissues (with the thenar eminence holding the rib towards its caudad position) as increased flexion and side-flexion is introduced.

- This sequence is repeated once or twice only, and usually results in release of the group of 'elevated' ribs.

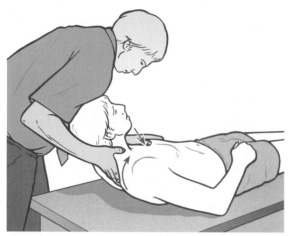

Figure 6.14   MET treatment of elevated rib.

◎ **MET method for depressed ribs (Fig. 6.15)**

In this protocol various muscles are used for different depressed rib restrictions (see method below), based on their attachments. Goodridge & Kuchera (1997) list (and recommend patient positioning to treat) the appropriate muscles as:

1. *Rib 1: anterior and middle scalenes.* The patient's ipsilateral arm is flexed, forearm resting on forehead, head rotated away from the side to be treated (towards the left in this example). The patient is instructed to attempt to flex the neck and head further, against resistance for 5–7 seconds.

2. *Rib 2: posterior scalene.* The patient's ipsilateral arm is flexed, forearm resting on the forehead, head rotated away from the side to be treated (towards the left in this example). The patient is instructed to attempt to move the elbow and head anteriorly against resistance for 5–7 seconds (see Fig. 6.15).

3. *Ribs 3–5: pectoralis minor.* The patient's head is in neutral, the arm flexed and placed alongside of the head. The patient is asked to bring the elbow towards the sternum against resistance for 5–7 seconds.

4. *Ribs 6–9: serratus anterior.* The patient's head is in neutral, the elbow flexed, the dorsum of the hand resting on the forehead. The patient is asked to bring the hand anteriorly against resistance for 5–7 seconds.

5. *Ribs 10–12: latissimus dorsi.* The patient is prone; the arm, elbow flexed, lies in abduction between 90° and 130°, depending on localisation of forces to rib being treated. The patient is asked to abduct the arm against resistance (see Fig. 6.16).

Method:

- The most superior of an identified group of depressed ribs is treated.

- The patient is supine and the practitioner stands on the contralateral side, and places his table-side arm across the patient's trunk, inserting the hand beneath the patient's torso so that he can engage, with fingertips, the superior aspect of the costal angle of the designated rib (the most superior of the group).

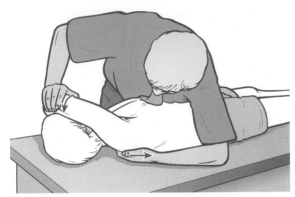

Figure 6.15   MET treatment of depressed 2nd rib.

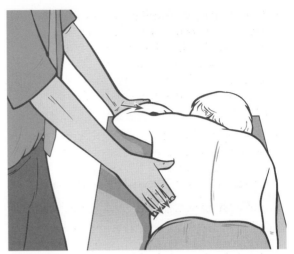

Figure 6.16   MET treatment of depressed 11th and/or 12th ribs.

- The patient's head or arm is placed in the most suitable position so that an isometric contraction will engage the muscle(s) most likely to influence the key rib (see the list and suggestions above).

- The patient is asked to move the head or arm as appropriate (see list above), against practitioner resistance, while holding the breath (this produces an isometric contraction of the intercostals), for 5–7 seconds.

- On complete relaxation the fingers draw the rib inferiorly, to take out available slack, and the process is repeated at least once more before reassessment of rib movement is carried out.

MET treatment for depressed 11–12th ribs (Fig. 6.16)

- The patient is prone, and the practitioner stands on the ipsilateral side, facing the patient.

- For left-side depressed 11th rib, the patient places his left arm above his head and the practitioner holds that elbow with his cephalad hand.

- The practitioner locates the depressed 11th rib and draws it superiorly to its barrier, with his finger pads.

- The patient is asked to breathe in and hold the breath, while simultaneously attempting to bring the elevated and abducted left elbow sideways, back towards the side, against resistance.

- After 5–7 seconds, and complete relaxation by the patient, the rib is drawn superiorly towards its new barrier via the finger contact.

- A repetition of the procedure should then be carried out and the rib reassessed for motion.

MET treatment for elevated 11–12th ribs (Fig. 6.17)

- The patient is prone, arms at his side, and the practitioner stands on the contralateral side to the dysfunctional ribs.

- For right-side 11th and 12th elevated ribs, the practitioner places the thenar and hypothenar eminences of his cephalad hand on the medial aspects of the shafts of both the 11th and 12th ribs (these two ribs usually act in concert in the way they become dysfunctional).

- The practitioner's caudad hand grasps the patient's right ASIS.

- The patient is asked to exhale fully, and hold this out, and to reach towards the right foot with the right hand, so introducing side-bending to the right, taking the elevated ribs towards their normal position.

- At the end of the exhalation the patient is asked to bring the ASIS firmly into the practitioner's hand ('push your pelvis towards the table').

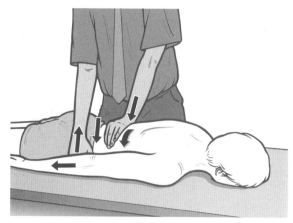

Figure 6.17   MET treatment of elevated 11th and/or 12th ribs.

- After 5–7 seconds and complete relaxation, the practitioner takes out all slack with his contact hand and the process is repeated, before retesting.

⊚ General thoracic cage release using MET (Fig. 6.18)

- The patient is supine and the practitioner stands at waist level facing cephalad, and places his hands over the middle and lower thoracic structures, fingers along the rib shafts.

- Treating the structure being palpated as a cylinder, the hands test the preference this cylinder has to rotate around its central axis, one way and then the other:
  - 'Does the lower thorax rotate with more difficulty to the right or to the left?'

- Once the direction of greatest rotational restriction has been established, the side-bending one way or the other is evaluated:
  - 'Does the lower thorax side-flex with more difficulty to the right or to the left?'

- Once these two pieces of information have been established, the combined positions of restriction, so indicated, are introduced.

- By side-bending and rotating *towards the tighter* directions, the combined directions of restriction are engaged, at which time the patient is asked to inhale and hold the breath,

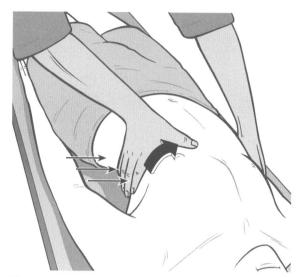

Figure 6.18   General MET for release of lower thorax and diaphragm.

and to 'bear down' slightly (Valsalva manoeuvre). These efforts introduce isometric contractions of the diaphragm and intercostal muscles.

- On release and complete exhalation and relaxation the diaphragm should be found to function more normally, accompanied by a relaxation of associated soft tissues and a more symmetrical rotation and side-flexion potential of the previously restricted tissues.

Assessment and MET treatment of sacroiliac (SI) and iliosacral (IS) restrictions

In order to usefully apply MET to SI and/or IS (or other pelvic) dysfunction, it is necessary to assess the implicated joint accurately. This seems to be easier said than done.

A survey of Australian osteopaths (Peace & Fryer 2004) evaluated what tests were most commonly used, and whether correlation existed between the tests and clinical experience. The results revealed that, amongst the 168 responders (representing approximately 30% of those surveyed), the commonest assessment tools for the SIJ involved:

- Asymmetry of bony landmarks (most commonly PSIS, ASIS and iliac crests)

- Motion tests (most commonly prone sacral springing, standing flexion and ASIS compression)

- Pain provocation tests (prone sacral spring, ASIS compression and SIJ spring/'thigh thrust'). Additionally, piriformis assessment was reported as being commonly tested for tenderness and tissue texture change.

Few, if any, of the tests mentioned have been shown to consistently offer accurate clinical information, and some have been shown to produce positive results in asymptomatic individuals (Dreyfuss et al 1994, Meijne & van Neerbos 1999, Kokmeyer & van der Wurff 2002).

Additionally, factors such as differences in leg length, body type and dimension, and assymetrical bone structure, as well as the limited experience and skill of the examiner, create questions as to the clinical usefulness of static assessment findings (Cibulka & Koldehoff 1999, Levangie 1999, Lewit & Rosina 1999).

It is further suggested that the distinction, initially made by Mitchell et al (1979) regarding the need to differentiate between IS and SI dysfunction, remains clinically useful.

CAUTION: Evidence derived from, for example, the standing flexion test (as described below) might be compromised by concurrent shortness in the hamstrings, since this will effectively give either:

- A false positive sign at the contralateral SIJ when there is unilateral hamstring shortness. For example, left hamstring shortness could prevent left iliac movement during flexion, helping to encourage a compensating right iliac movement during flexion, or

- False negative signs if there is bilateral hamstring shortness. That is, there may be IS motion which is being masked by the restriction placed on the ilia via bilateral hamstring shortness.

The hamstring shortness tests, as described in Ch. 5, should therefore be carried out before a standing flexion test, and if shortness is found these structures should be normalised, as far as is possible, prior to the IS flexion tests, described below, being used.

The lead author suggests that form and force closure assessments (as described below) be carried out before moving on to use of other test procedures, in order to establish that the SIJ is indeed responsible for the individual's symptoms. In order to understand the concept of form and force closure the functional stability of the SIJ, particularly during the gait cycle, is briefly summarised in Box 6.2.

Form and force assessment

Supine functional SI assessments (form/ force closure) (Vleeming et al 1995, 1996, 1997, Barker et al 2004, Lee 1997, 2000) (Fig. 6.20A, B)

- The patient is supine and is instructed to raise one leg.

- If there is evidence of compensatory rotation of the pelvis towards the side of the raised leg, during performance of the movement, or if pain is reported in the SIJ during the effort, dysfunction is suggested.

Form closure assessment:

- The same leg should then be raised after the practitioner has applied compressive, medially directed, force across the pelvis, with a hand on the lateral aspect of each innominate at the level of the ASIS (this augments form closure of the SIJ) (Fig. 6.20A).

- If this *form* closure strategy, applied by the practitioner, enhances the ability to easily raise the leg, this suggests that structural factors within the joint may require externally enhanced support, such as a trochanter belt.

Force closure assessment:

- To test for the influence of *force* closure, the same leg is raised with the patient simultaneously attempting to slightly flex and rotate the trunk towards the side being tested, against the practitioner's resistance, which is applied to the contralateral shoulder (Fig. 6.20B).

- This increases oblique muscular activity and force-closes the ipsilateral SIJ (which is being assessed).

Box 6.2 The sacroiliac joint during gait

As the right leg swings forward the right ilium rotates backward in relation to the sacrum (Greenman 1996). Simultaneously, sacrotuberous and interosseous ligamentous tension increases to brace the sacroiliac joint (SIJ) in preparation for heel strike.

Just before heel strike, the ipsilateral hamstrings are activated, thereby tightening the sacro-tuberous ligament (into which they merge) to further stabilise the SIJ.

Vleeming et al (1997) have demonstrated that, as the foot approaches heel strike there is a downward movement of the fibula, increasing (via biceps femoris) the tension on the sacrotuberous ligament, while simultaneously tibialis anticus fires, in order to dorsiflex the foot in preparation for heel strike.

Tibialis anticus links via fascia to peroneus longus under the foot, thus completing this elegant sling mechanism (the 'anatomical stirrup') which both braces the SIJ and engages the entire lower limb in that process.

Biceps femoris, peroneus longus and tibialis anticus together form this longitudinal muscle–tendon–fascial sling, which is loaded to create an energy store to be used during the next part of the gait cycle.

As Lee (1997) points out, 'Together, gluteus maximus and latissimus dorsi tense the thoracolumbar fascia and facilitate the force closure mechanism through the SIJ' (see functional form and force assessment, in this chapter).

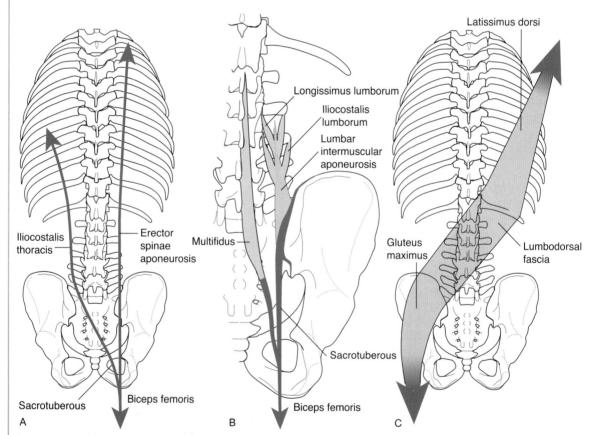

Figure 6.19   A The biceps femoris (BF) is directly connected to the upper trunk via the sacrotuberous ligament, the erector spinae aponeurosis (ESA) and iliocostalis thoracis (IT). **B** Enlarged view of the lumbar spine area showing the link between biceps femoris (BF), the lumbar intermuscular aponeurosis (LIA), longissimus lumborum (LL), iliocostalis lumborum (IL) and multifidus (Mult). **C** Relations between gluteus maximus (GM), lumbodorsal fascia (LF) and latisimus dorsi (LD). (Reproduced with permission from Vleeming et al 1999.)

Box 6.2 Continued

During the latter stage of the single support period of the gait cycle, biceps femoris activity eases, as compression of the SIJ reduces and the ipsilateral iliac bone rotates anteriorly.

As the right heel strikes, the left arm swings forward – and the right gluteus maximus activates to compress and stabilise the SIJ.

There is a simultaneous coupling of this gluteal force with the contralateral latissimus dorsi by means of thoracolumbar fascia in order to assist in counter-rotation of the trunk on the pelvis.

In this way, an oblique muscle–tendon–fascial sling is created across the torso, providing a mechanism for further energy storage to be utilised in the next phase of the gait cycle.

As the single support phase ends and the double support phase initiates, there is a lessened loading of the SIJs and gluteus maximus reduces its activity, and as the next step starts, the leg swings forward and nutation at the SIJ starts again.

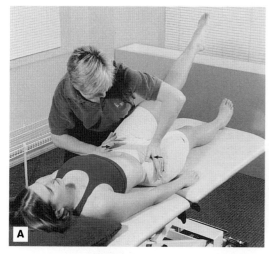

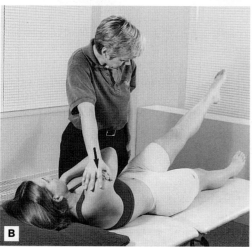

Figure 6.20 Functional test of supine-active straight leg raise: **A** with form closure augmented; **B** with force closure augmented. (Reproduced from Lee 2000, p 89.)

- If the initial leg raising suggests SI dysfunction, and this is markedly reduced or absent with force-closure, the prognosis is good if appropriate balancing of soft tissue status can be achieved, and the patient engages in appropriate rehabilitation exercise.

Prone functional SIJ assessment (form/force closure) (Vleeming et al 1995, 1996, 1997, Barker et al 2004, Lee 1997, 2000) (Fig. 6.21A, B)

- The prone patient is asked to extend the leg at the hip by approximately 10°.

- Hinging should occur at the hip joint, and the pelvis should remain in contact with the table throughout.

- If there is an excessive degree of pelvic rotation in the transverse plane (anterior pelvic rotation), or if pain is reported in the SIJ during the effort, possible SIJ dysfunction is suggested.

Form closure assessment:

- If *form* features (i.e. structural) of the SIJ are at fault, the prone straight leg raise will be more normal (and painless) when medial compression of the joint is introduced by the practitioner applying firm bilateral medial pressure towards the SIJs, with hands on the innominates (Fig. 6.21A).

Force closure assessment:

- *Force* closure may be enhanced during the assessment if latissimus dorsi can be recruited to increase tension on the thoracolumbar fascia.

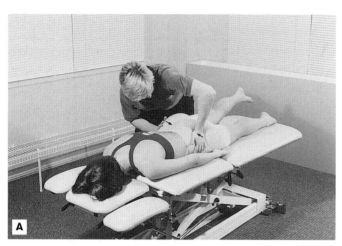

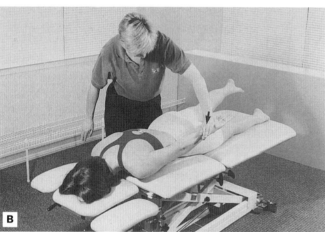

Figure 6.21   Functional test of prone-active straight leg raise: **A** with form closure augmented; **B** with force closure augmented. (Reproduced from Lee 2000, p 90.)

- Lee (1997) states, 'This is done by [the practitioner] resisting extension of the medially rotated [contralateral] arm prior to lifting the leg' (Fig. 6.21B).

- As in the supine straight leg raising (SLR) test, if force closure enhances more normal (and less painful) SIJ function, the prognosis for improvement is good; to be achieved by means of appropriate balancing of soft tissue status, rehabilitation exercises and reformed use patterns.

It is suggested that normalisation of the status of dysfunctional postural muscles, attaching to the pelvis (from above and below), by means of stretching, toning and trigger point deactivation, as well as via postural re-education, will contribute greatly to removal of many instances of SIJ pain.

In addition, methods such as iliosacral joint and general pelvic normalisation, as described below, can prove extremely useful clinically, but only after soft tissue balance has been initiated.

Tests and MET treatment for pelvic and sacroiliac joint dysfunction

Test A: pelvic balance   The practitioner stands or squats behind the standing patient and places the medial side of his hands on the lateral pelvis below the crests, pushing inwards and upwards until the index fingers lie superior to the crest:

- If these are judged to be level then no anatomical leg length discrepancy exists.

- If an inequality of height of pelvic crests is observed, the heights of the greater trochanters should also be assessed, by direct palpation.

- If both the pelvic crest height and the height of the greater trochanter on the same side appear to be greater than the opposite side, an anatomical leg length difference is likely (Greenman 1996).

- If pelvic crest height *or* trochanter height are greater on one side than the other, pelvic imbalance is a possible explanation, commonly involving postural muscle shortening and imbalance, or actual osseous asymmetry.

Test B: iliosacral assessment   The PSIS positions are assessed just below the pelvic dimples:

- Are they symmetrical?
- Is one superior or anterior to the other?

Anteriority may involve shortness of the external rotators on that side (iliopsoas, quadratus femoris, piriformis) or internal rotators on the other side (gluteus medius, hamstrings).
  Inferiority may indicate hamstring shortness or pelvic/pubic dysfunction.

Test C: standing flexion (iliosacral) test (Fig. 6.22A)

- With the patient still standing, and with any inequality of leg length having been compensated for by insertion of a pad under the foot on the short side, the practitioner's thumbs are placed firmly (a light contact is useless) on the inferior slope of the PSIS.

- The patient is asked to move into full flexion while the thumb contact is maintained (see Fig. 6.22A).

- The patient's knees should remain extended during lumbar flexion.

- The practitioner observes, especially near the end of the excursion of the bend, whether one or other thumb seems to start to travel with the PSIS on which it rests.

Interpretation. If one thumb moves superiorly during flexion it indicates that the ilium is 'fixed' to the sacrum on that side (or that the contralateral

hamstrings are short, or that the ipsilateral quadratus lumborum is short – therefore these muscles should have been assessed, and if necessary treated, prior to the standing flexion test). If muscle status is normal a positive standing flexion tests suggests an iliosacral dysfunction.

Test D: standing spinal rotation

- Before performing the seated flexion test, the practitioner moves to the front of the fully flexed patient.

- The practitioner looks down the spine for evidence of greater 'fullness' on one side or the other of the lumbar spine, indicating muscular mounding, possibly in association with spinal rotoscoliosis (or to excessive tension in quadratus lumborum, or hypertrophy of the erector spinae).

Test E: seated flexion (sacroiliac) test

- The seated flexion test involves exactly the same hand placement as in the standing flexion test (test C above) and observation of the thumb movement, if any, during full flexion, while the patient is seated on the table, legs over the side, knees in flexion (see Fig. 6.22B).

Interpretation. In this test, since the ischial tuberosities are being 'sat upon', the ilia cannot easily move, and if one thumb travels forward during flexion it means that the sacrum is fixed to the ilium, on that side, dragging the ilium with it in flexion. This suggests a sacroliac dysfunction.

Test F: seated spinal rotation

- With the seated patient still fully flexed, the practitioner moves to the front and looks down the spine for fullness in the paravertebral muscles, in the lumbar area.

- If greater fullness exists in one paraspinal area of the lumbar spine with the patient standing as opposed to seated, then this suggests a compensatory process, involving the postural muscles of the lower limbs and pelvic area, as a prime cause.

- If, however, fullness in the lumbar paraspinal region is the same when seated, or greater

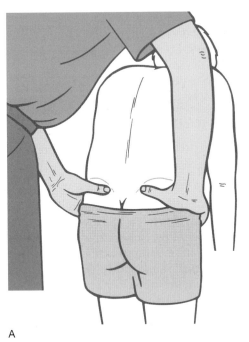

Figure 6.22A Standing flexion test for iliosacral restriction. The dysfunctional side is that on which the thumb moves during flexion.

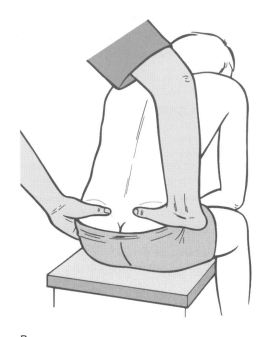

Figure 6.22B Seated flexion test for sacroiliac restriction. The dysfunctional side is that on which the thumb moves during flexion.

when seated, compared with standing, this suggests some primary spinal dysfunction and not a compensation for postural muscle imbalances.

Test G: confirmation of iliosacral restriction test

- The patient stands and the practitioner is behind, kneeling, with thumbs placed so that on the side being assessed the contact is on the PSIS, while the other hand palpates the median sacral crest directly parallel to the PSIS.

- The patient is asked to slowly and fully flex the ipsilateral hip to waist level.

- A normal response is for the thumb on the ipsilateral PSIS to move caudally, in relation to the thumb on the sacral base, as the hip and knee are flexed.

- If on the flexing of the hip there is a movement of the PSIS and the median sacral crest 'as a unit', together with a compensating adaptation in the lumbar spine, this indicates *iliosacral* restriction on the side being palpated.

- If this combined (PSIS and sacral thumb contact) movement occurred when the contralateral hip is flexed, it suggests a *sacroiliac* restriction on the side being palpated.

What type of iliosacral dysfunction exists?

Once an iliosacral restriction has been identified, it is necessary to define as far as possible what type of restriction exists. In this text only anterior rotation, posterior rotation, inflare and outflare will be considered. This part of the evaluation process depends upon observation of landmarks.

Test H: landmarks The patient lies supine and straight, while the practitioner locates the inferior slopes of the two ASISs, with thumbs, and views these contacts from directly above the pelvis with the dominant eye over the centre line (bird's eye view – see Fig. 6.23A):

- Which thumb is nearer the head and which nearer the feet?
- Is one side superior or is the other inferior?

In other words, has one ilium rotated posteriorly or the other anteriorly? This is determined by referring back to the standing flexion test (test C above).

The side of dysfunction – as determined by the standing flexion test 'travelling thumb' (test C above) and/or the standing hip flexion test (test G above) – defines which observed anterior landmark is taken into consideration (see Fig. 6.23Bi–iv).

The practitioner's eyes should be directly over the pelvis with the thumbs resting on the ASISs.

Rotations:

1. The side of the positive standing flexion, or hip flexion test, is the dysfunctional side, and if that is the side which appears inferior (compared with its pair) it is assumed that the ilium on the inferior side has rotated *anteriorly* on the sacrum on that side.

2. The side of the positive standing flexion, or hip flexion test, is the dysfunctional side, and if the ASIS appears superior to its pair on that side, then the ilium has rotated *posteriorly* on the sacrum on that side.

Flares: While in the same position observing the ASIS positions, note is made of the relative positions of these landmarks in relation to the midline of the patient's abdomen, using either the linea alba or the umbilicus as a guide:

- If one thumb is closer to the umbilicus than the other, it is necessary at this stage to once again refer to which side is dysfunctional.

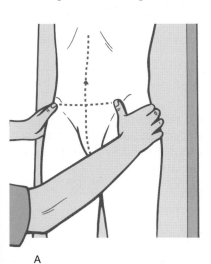

A

Figure 6.23   **A** Practitioner adopts a position providing a bird's-eye view of ASIS prominences on which rest the thumbs. **Bi** The ASISs are level and there is no rotational dysfunction involving the iliosacral joints. **Bii** The right ASIS is higher than the left ASIS. If a thumb 'travelled' on the right side during the standing flexion test this would represent a posterior right iliosacral rotation dysfunction. If a thumb 'travelled' on the left side during the test this would represent an anterior left iliosacral rotation dysfunction. **Biii** The ASISs are equidistant from the umbilicus and the midline, and there is no iliosacral flare dysfunction. **Biv** The ASIS on the right is closer to the umbilicus/midline, which indicates that either there is a right-side iliosacral inflare (if the right thumb moved during the standing flexion test), or there is a left-side iliosacral outflare (if the left thumb moved during the standing flexion test).

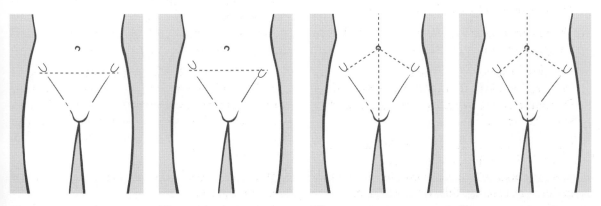

Bi   Bii   Biii   Biv

- Is the ASIS on the side which is further from the umbilicus outflared, or is the ASIS which is closer to the umbilicus indicative of that side being inflared?

The ASIS associated with the side on which the thumb travelled during the standing flexion test is the dysfunctional side, and the decision as to whether there is an inflare (ASIS closer to umbilicus) or an outflare (ASIS further from umbilicus) is therefore obvious. Flare dysfunctions are usually treated prior to rotation dysfunctions.

MET treatment of iliac inflare (Fig. 6.24A, B)

- The patient is supine and the practitioner stands on the dysfunctional side, with the cephalad hand stabilising the non-affected-side ASIS, and the caudad hand holding the ankle of the affected side (Fig. 6.24A).

- The affected-side hip is flexed and abducted and full external rotation is introduced to the hip.

- The practitioner's forearm aligns with the lower leg, elbow stabilising the medial aspect of the knee.

- The patient is asked to lightly adduct the hip against the resistance offered by the restraining arm for 10 seconds.

- On complete relaxation, and on an exhalation, with the pelvis held stable by the cephalad hand, the flexed leg is taken into increased abduction and external rotation, as new 'slack' should now be available.

- This process is repeated once or twice, at which time the leg is slowly straightened while abduction and external rotation of the hip are maintained.

- The leg is then returned to the table.

NOTE: Care should be taken not to use the powerful leverage available from the flexed and abducted leg; its own weight and gravity provide adequate leverage, and the 'release' of tone achieved via isometric contractions will do the rest. It is very easy to turn an inflare into an outflare by overenthusiastic use of force. The degree of flare should be re-evaluated and any rotation then treated (see below).

MET treatment of iliac outflare (Fig. 6.25)

- The patient is supine and the practitioner is on the same side as the dysfunctional ilium, supinated cephalad hand under the patient's buttocks with fingertips hooked into the sacral sulcus on the same side.

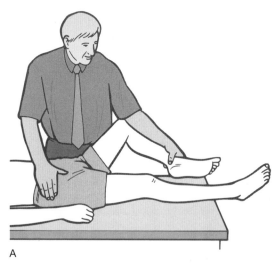

A

Figure 6.24A   An MET treatment position for left-side iliosacral inflare dysfunction. Note the stabilising hand on the right ASIS.

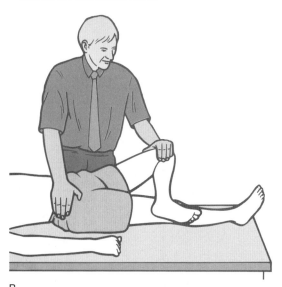

B

Figure 6.24B   An alternative MET treatment position for left-side iliosacral inflare dysfunction. Note the stabilising hand on the right ASIS.

- The caudad hand holds the patient's foot on the treated side, with the forearm resting along the medial calf/shin area as the hand grasps the foot.

- The hip on the treated side is fully flexed and adducted and internally rotated, at which time the patient is asked to abduct the hip against resistance, using up to 50% of strength, for 10 seconds.

- Following this, and complete relaxation, slack is taken out and the exercise repeated once more.

- As the leg is taken into greater adduction and internal rotation, to take advantage of the release of muscular tone following the isometric contraction, the fingers in the sacral sulcus exert a traction towards the practitioner, effectively guiding the ilium into a more inflared position.

- After the final contraction, adduction and internal rotation are maintained as the leg is slowly returned to the table.

- The evaluation for flare dysfunction is then repeated, and if relative normality has been restored, any rotational dysfunction is then treated, using the methods described below.

MET treatment of anterior iliac rotation (Fig. 6.26)

- The patient is prone. The practitioner stands at the side to be treated, at waist level.

- The affected leg and hip are flexed and brought over the edge of the table.

- The foot/ankle area is grasped between the practitioner's legs.

- The table-side hand stabilises the sacral area while the other hand supports the flexed knee and guides it into greater flexion, inducing posterior iliac rotation, until the restriction barrier is sensed:
  - By the palpating 'sacral contact' hand, or
  - By virtue of a sense of greater effort in guiding the flexed leg, and/or
  - By observation of pelvic movement as the barrier of resistance is passed.

- Once the barrier is engaged the patient is asked to attempt to straighten the leg against unyielding resistance, for 10 seconds using no more than 20% of available strength.

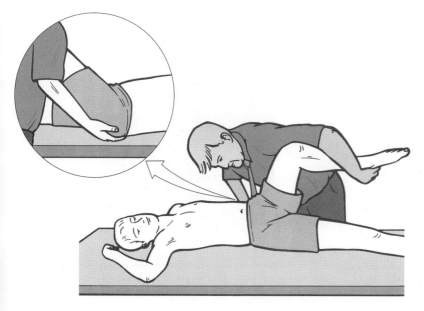

Figure 6.25 MET treatment of iliosacral outflare on the left.

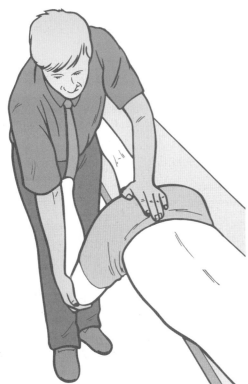

Figure 6.26   MET treatment of an anterior iliosacral restriction.

- On releasing the effort, and on complete relaxation, and on an exhalation, the leg/innominate is guided to its new barrier.

- Subsequent contractions can involve different directions of effort ('try to push your knee sideways', or 'try to bend your knee towards your shoulder', etc.) in order to bring into operation a variety of muscular factors to encourage release of the joint.[1]

- The standing flexion test as described above should be performed again to establish whether the joint is now free.

---

[1] A supine position may also be used, or the same mechanics precisely can be incorporated into a side-lying position. The only disadvantage of side-lying is the relative instability of the pelvic region compared with that achieved in the prone and supine positions.

MET for treatment of posterior iliac rotation (Fig. 6.27)

- The patient is prone and the practitioner stands on the side opposite the dysfunctional iliosacral joint.

- The table-side hand supports the anterior aspect of the patient's knee while the other rests on the SIJ of the affected side to evaluate bind.

- The affected leg is extended until free movement ceases, as evidenced by the following observations:
  - Bind is noted under the palpating hand, or
  - Sacral and pelvic motion are observed as the barrier is passed, or
  - A sense of effort is increased in the arm extending the leg.

- With the practitioner holding the joint at its restriction barrier, the patient is asked, with no more than 20% of strength, to flex the hip against resistance for 10 seconds.

- After cessation of the effort, and completely relaxing, on an exhalation, the leg is extended further to its new barrier.

- No force should be used; the movement after the contraction simply takes advantage of whatever slack is then available.

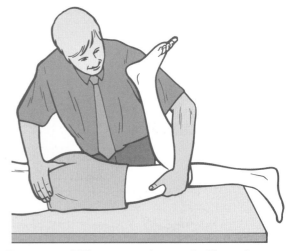

Figure 6.27   MET treatment of a posterior iliosacral restriction.

- Variations in the direction of the contraction (perhaps involving abduction or adduction, or even attempted extension) are sometimes useful if no appreciable gain is achieved using hip and knee flexion.

- The standing flexion test is performed again to establish whether iliosacral movement is now free, once a sense of 'release' has been noted following one of the contractions.

MET treatment for temporomandibular joint (TMJ) dysfunction

Dysfunction of the TMJ is a vast subject, and the implications of such problems have been related to a variety of other areas of dysfunction, ranging from cranial lesions to spinal and general somatic alterations and endocrine imbalance (Gelb 1977). The reader is referred to Janda's observations on postural influences on TMJ problems (Ch. 2).

Diagnosis of the particular pattern of dysfunction is, of course, essential before safe therapeutic intervention is possible. There are many possible causes of TMJ dysfunction, and a cooperative relationship with a skilled dentist is an advantage in treating such problems, since many aspects relate to the presence of faults in the bite of the patient.

A knowledge of cranial mechanics is useful, and a history of trauma should be sought in those patients presenting with TMJ involvement. One common source of injury is the equipment used in applying spinal traction, in which a head halter with a chinstrap is used. This can cause the mandible to be forced into the fossae, impacting the temporal bones into internal rotation. A strap causing pressure on the occipital region could jam the occipitomastoid and lambdoid sutures upwards and forwards, also resulting in internal rotation of the temporals. This can cause major dysfunction of cranial articulation and function which would be further exaggerated if imbalances were present in these structures prior to the trauma.

Inept manipulative measures can also traumatise the area, especially thrusting forces exerted onto the occiput while the head and neck are in extreme rotation.

Any situation in which the patient is required to maintain the mouth opened for lengthy periods, such as during dental work, or when a laryngoscope is being used, may induce strain, especially if the neck is extended at the time.

All, or any, such patterns of injury should be sought when TMJ pain, or limitation of mouth opening is observed. Apart from correction of cranial dysfunction via skilled cranial osteopathic work, the muscular component invites attention, using MET methods and other appropriate measures. Gelb suggests a form of MET which he terms 'stretch against resistance' exercises.

MET TMJ method 1 (Fig. 6.28A)

- Reciprocal inhibition is the objective when the patient is asked to open the mouth against resistance applied by the practitioner's, or the patient's own, hand (patient places elbow on table, chin in hand, and attempts to open mouth against resistance for 10 seconds or so).

- The jaw would have been opened to a comfortable limit before attempting this, and after the attempt it would be taken to its new barrier before repeating.

- This MET method would have a relaxing effect on the muscles which are shortened or tight.

MET TMJ method 2 (Fig. 6.28B)

- To relax the short tight muscles using postisometric relaxation, counterpressure would be required in order to prevent the open jaw from closing (using minimal force).

- This would require the thumbs (suitably protected) to be placed along the superior surface of the lower back teeth while an isometric contraction was performed by the patient.

- In this exercise the practitioner is directing force through the barrier (practitioner-direct method) rather than the patient (patient-direct) as in the first method (above).

MET TMJ method 3 (Fig. 6.28C)

Lewit (1991), maintaining that laterolateral movements are important, suggests the following method of treating TMJ problems using postisometric relaxation:

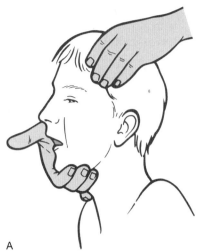

A

Figure 6.28A   MET treatment of TMJ restriction, involving limited ability to open the mouth. The isometric contraction phase of treatment is illustrated as the patient attempts to open against resistance.

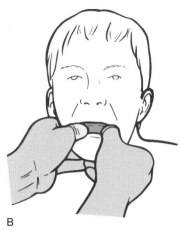

B

Figure 6.28B   MET treatment of TMJ restriction, involving an isometric contraction in which the patient attempts to close the mouth against resistance. Following both these procedures (A and B), the patient would be encouraged to gently stretch the muscles by opening the mouth widely. This can be assisted by the practitioner.

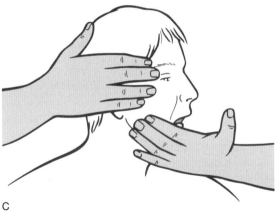

C

Figure 6.28C   MET treatment of lateral restrictions of the TMJ. Following the isometric contraction as described, the lateral excursion is increased.

- The patient sits with the head turned to one side (say the left in this example).
- The practitioner stands behind and stabilises the patient's head against his chest.
- The patient opens his mouth, allowing the chin to drop, and the practitioner cradles the mandible with his left hand, so that the fingers are curled under the jaw, away from him.

- The practitioner draws the jaw gently towards his chest, and when the slack has been taken up, the patient offers a degree of resistance to its being taken further, laterally.
- After a few seconds of gentle isometric contraction, the practitioner and patient relax simultaneously, and the jaw will usually have an increased lateral excursion.
- This is repeated several times.
- This procedure should be performed so that the lateral pull is away from the side to which the jaw deviates, on opening.

TMJ self-treatment exercise 1

Gelb (1977) suggests a retrusive exercise be used in conjunction with the above, both methods being useful in eliminating 'clicks' on opening the mouth.

- The patient curls the tongue upwards, placing the tip as far back on the roof of the mouth as possible.
- While this is maintained in position, the patient is asked to slowly open and close the

mouth (gently), to reactivate the suprahyoid, posterior temporalis and posterior digastric muscles (the retrusive group).

- This exercise should be repeated numerous times daily.

TMJ self-treatment exercise 2

- The patient places an elbow on a table, jaw resting on the clenched fist.

- This offers some resistance to the slow opening of the mouth.

- This is done five times with hand pressure, and then five times without, ensuring that the lower jaw does not come forward.

- The lower teeth should always remain behind the upper teeth on closing.

- A total of 25 such movements are performed, morning and evening.

In the next chapter the integrated use of MET with other soft tissue approaches are described, particularly in relation to treatment of myofascial (trigger-point) pain and dysfunction.

References

Bandy W, Irion J, Briggler M 1997 The effect of time and frequency of static stretching on flexibility of the hamstring muscles. Physical Therapy 77: 1090–1096

Barker P, Briggs C, Bogeski G 2004 Tensile transmission across the lumbar fasciae in unembalmed cadavers: effects of tension to various muscular attachments. Spine 29(2): 129–138

Brodin H 1982 Lumbar treatment using MET. Osteopathic Annals 10: 23–24

Brodin H 1987 Inhibition-facilitation technique for lumbar pain treatment. Manual Medicine 3: 24–26

Chaitow L 2001 Muscle energy techniques, 2nd edn. Churchill Livingstone, Edinburgh

Chaitow L 2002 Positional release techniques. Churchill Livingstone, Edinburgh

Chaitow L, Bradley D, Gilbert C 2002 Multidisciplinary approaches to breathing pattern disorders. Churchill Livingstone, Edinburgh

Cibulka M, Koldehoff R 1999 Clinical usefulness of a cluster of SIJ tests in patients with and without low back pain. Journal of Orthopaedic and Sports Physical Therapy 29(2): 83–92

Dreyfuss P, Dreyer S, Griffen J et al 1994 Positive SI screening tests in asymptomatic patients. Spine 19(10): 1138–1143

Evjenth O, Hamberg J 1984 Muscle stretching in manual therapy. Alfta Rehab, Alfta, Sweden

Feland J, Myrer J, Schulthies S et al 2001 The effect of duration of stretching of the hamstring muscle group for increasing range of motion in people aged 65 years or older. Physical Therapy 81: 1100–1117

Fryer G, Ruskowski W 2004 Influence of contraction duration in MET applied to atlanto-axial joint. Journal of Osteopathic Medicine 7(2): 79–84

Fryette H 1954 Principals of osteopathic technique. American Academy of Osteopathy, Newark, Ohio

Gelb H 1977 Clinical management of head, neck and TMJ pain and dysfunction. W B Saunders, Philadelphia

Gibbons P, Tehan P 1998 Muscle energy concepts and coupled motion of the spine. Manual Therapy 3(2): 95–101

Goodridge J 1981 Muscle energy technique. Journal of the American Osteopathic Association 81: 249

Goodridge J, Kuchera W 1997 Muscle energy techniques for specific areas. In: Ward R (ed) Foundations of osteopathic medicine. Williams and Wilkins, Baltimore

Greenman P 1996 Principles of manual medicine, 2nd edn. Williams and Wilkins, Baltimore

Grieve G 1984 Mobilisation of the spine. Churchill Livingstone, Edinburgh

Harakal J 1975 An osteopathically integrated approach to whiplash complex. Journal of the American Osteopathic Association 74: 941–956

Hartman L 1985 Handbook of osteopathic technique. Hutchinson, London

Janda V 1988 In: Grant R (ed) Physical therapy of the cervical and thoracic spine. Churchill Livingstone, New York

Jones L 1981 Strain and counterstrain. Academy of Applied Osteopathy, Colorado Springs

Kaltenborn F 1985 Mobilisation of extremity joints. Olaf Norlis Boekhandel, Norway

Knebl J 2002 The Spencer sequence. Journal of the American Osteopathic Association 102(7): 387–400

Kokmeyer D, van der Wurff P 2002 The reliability of multitest regimens with specific SI pain provocation tests. Journal of Manipulative and Physiological Therapeutics 25(1): 42–48

Kwolek A 1989 Rehabilitation treatment with post-isometric muscle relaxation for haemophilia patients. Journal of Manual Medicine 4: 55–57

Lardner R 2001 Stretching and flexibility: its importance in rehabilitation. Journal of Bodywork and Movement Therapies 5(4): 254–263

Lee D 1997 Treatment of pelvic instability. In: Vleeming A, Mooney V, Dorman T, Snijders C, Stoekart R (eds) Movement, stability and low back pain. Churchill Livingstone, New York

Lee D 2000 The pelvic girdle. An approach to the examination and treatment of the lumbo-pelvic-hip region, 2nd edn. Churchill Livingstone, Edinburgh

Lenehan K et al 2003 The effect of MET on gross trunk range of motion. Journal of Osteopathic Medicine 6(1): 13–18

Levangie P 1999 Four clinical tests of SI joint dysfunction. Physical Therapy 79(11): 1043–1057

Lewit K 1985 The muscular and articular factor in movement restriction. Manual Medicine 1: 83–85

Lewit K 1991 Manipulative therapy in rehabilitation of the motor system. Butterworths, London

Lewit K, Rosina A 1999 Why yet another sign of SI joint restriction. Journal of Manipulative and Physiological Therapeutics 22(3): 154–160

McAtee R, Charland J 1999 Facilitated stretching, 2nd edn. Human Kinetics, Champaign, Ilinois

Meijne W, van Neerbos K 1999 Intraexaminer and interexaminer reliability of the Gillet test. Journal of Manipulative and Physiological Therapeutics 22(1): 4–9

Mimura M, Moriya H, Watanabe T et al 1989 Three-dimensional motion analysis of the cervical spine with special reference to the axial rotation. Spine 14(11): 1135–1139

Mitchell F, Moran P, Pruzzo N 1979 An evaluation and treatment manual of osteopathic muscle energy procedures. MET Press, East Lansing, Michigan

Patriquin D 1992 Evolution of osteopathic manipulative technique: the Spencer technique. Journal of the American Osteopathic Association 92: 1134–1146

Peace S, Fryer G 2004 Methods used by members of the Australian osteopathic profession to assess the sacroliac joint. Journal of Osteopathic Medicine 7(1): 25–32

Ruddy T J 1962 Osteopathic rhythmic resistive technic. Academy of Applied Osteopathy Yearbook 1962, pp 23–31

Schenk RJ, Adelman K, Rousselle J 1994 The effects of muscle energy technique on cervical range of motion. Journal of Manual and Manipulative Therapy 2(4): 149–155

Scott-Dawkins C 1997 Comparative effectiveness of adjustments versus mobilizations in chronic mechanical neck pain. Proceedings of the Scientific Symposium. World Chiropractic Congress, June 1997

Shrier I, Gossal K 2000 Myths and truths of stretching. Individualised recommendations for healthy muscles. The Physician Sports Medicine 28(8): 1–7

Spencer H 1976 Shoulder technique. Journal of the American Osteopathic Association 15: 2118–2220

Steiner C 1994 Osteopathic manipulative treatment – what does it really do? Journal of the American Osteopathic Association 94(1): 85–87

Stiles E 1984a Manipulation – a tool for your practice? Patient Care 18: 16–42

Stiles E 1984b Manipulation – a tool for your practice. Patient Care 45: 699–704

Vleeming A, Pool-Goudzwaard A, Stoeckart R et al 1995 The posterior layer of the thoracolumbar fascia. Its function in load transfer from spine to legs. Spine 20(7):753–758

Vleeming A, Pool-Goudzwaard A, Hammudoghlu D, Stoeckart R, Snijders C, Mens J 1996 The function of the long dorsal sacroiliac ligament: Its implication for understanding low back pain. Spine 21(5): 556–562

Vleeming A, Snijders C, Stoeckart R, Mens J 1997 The role of the sacroiliac joints in coupling between spine, pelvis, legs and arms. In: Vleeming A, Mooney V, Dorman T, Snijders C, Stoekart R (eds) Movement, stability and low back pain. Churchill Livingstone, New York

Ward R (ed) 1997 Foundations of osteopathic medicine. Williams and Wilkins, Baltimore

Wilson E, Payton O 2003 Muscle energy technique in patients with acute low back pain: Pilot study. Journal of Orthopaedic and Sports Physical Therapy 33(9): 502–511

Yates S 1991 Muscle energy techniques. In: DiGiovanna E (ed) Principles of osteopathic manipulative techniques. Lippincott, Philadelphia

Integrated neuromuscular inhibition technique (INIT)

7

CHAPTER CONTENTS

Local facilitation	**248**
Locating trigger points	**248**
STAR palpation	248
Drag palpation	249
Trigger point treatment methods	249
Hypothesis	250
Selye's concepts	250
Ischaemic compression validation	250
Ischaemic compression in trigger point deactivation	251
An alternative methodology	252
Associated methods	252
Strain/counterstrain (SCS) briefly explained	252
INIT method	253
Summary	**254**
References	**254**

It is clear from the work of Travell and Simons (1983, 1992), in particular, that myofascial trigger points are a primary cause of pain, dysfunction and distress of the sympathetic nervous system. Melzack & Wall (1988), in their pain research, have shown that there are few chronic pain problems where myofascial trigger point activity is not a key feature maintaining or causing chronic pain.

Central sensitisation and consequent widespread pain (Mense 1997, Butler 2000) is a process that may be regarded as inevitable where a combination stress factors are operating. Stressors may include (in combination, or acting independently):

- Biomechanical stress overuse, misuse, disuse, hypermobility, and/or trauma factors (Buskila & Neumann 1997, McPartland et al 1997, Koelbaek Johansen et al 1999)

- Biochemical features such as hypothyroidism or use of particular pharmaceutical drugs such as statins (Black et al 1998); nutritional deficiencies, particularly involving ferritin and vitamin B12 (Simons et al 1999, Dommerholt 2001)

- Psychosocial distress (Schneider-Helmert et al 2001).

These stressors and the adaptation effects they cause can promote the evolution of localised peripheral painful areas, almost always involving localised oxygen deficit – reduced to around 5% of normal (Brückle et al 1990, Shah et al 2003), that sensitise the neural pathways, creating a background of frequent and sometimes constant, pain (Mense & Hoheisel 1999).

As noted in Ch. 2, there can be numerous biomechanical background causes for the production and maintenance of myofascial trigger points, including:

- Postural imbalances (Goldthwaite 1949, Barlow 1959, Lewit 1999)

- Congenital factors – such as warping of fascia via cranial distortions (Upledger 1983), short leg problems, small hemipelvis, etc.

- Occupational or leisure overuse patterns (Rolf 1977, Simons et al 1999)

- Referred/reflex involvement of the viscera that have produced facilitated segments paraspinally (Korr 1976, Beal 1983).

Additional contributory factors may involve emotional states reflecting into the soft tissues (Latey 1986).

Local facilitation

According to Korr, a trigger point is a localised, commonly peripheral, area of somatic dysfunction which behaves in a facilitated (i.e. sensitised) manner, that will amplify and be affected by any form of stress imposed on the individual, whether this is physical, chemical or emotional (Korr 1976).

A trigger point is palpable as an indurated, localised, painful entity, with a reference (target) area to which pain or other symptoms are referred (Chaitow 1991a).

Trigger points in muscles are located either close to the centre of the muscle, near the motor end point, or close to attachments. Simons et al (1999) have suggested that care is needed in treating attachment points as these tissues are prone to inflammatory responses (enthesitis), and that deactivation of centrally located points (by means of treatment – see below – or by elimination or modification of aggravating factors) tends to halt the activity of attachment points.

Management of trigger points by manual means (neuromuscular approaches) has been fully described elsewhere (Chaitow & DeLany 2000, 2002, Chaitow 2003).

Muscles housing trigger points can frequently be identified as being unable to achieve their normal resting length using standard muscle evaluation procedures (Janda 1983), as described in Ch. 5. The trigger point itself always lies in hypertonic tissue, and not uncommonly in fibrotic or scar tissue, which has evolved as the result of exposure of the tissues to diverse forms of stress, as outlined above.

Locating trigger points

STAR palpation

In osteopathic medicine an acronym 'STAR' is used as a reminder of the characteristics of somatic dysfunction, such as myofascial trigger points. STAR stands for:

- **S**ensitivity (or 'Tenderness')[1] – this is the one feature that is almost always present when there is soft tissue dysfunction.

- **T**issue texture change – the tissues usually 'feel' different (for example they may be tense, fibrous, swollen, hot, cold or have other 'differences' from normal; and/or the skin overlying dysfunctional tissues usually palpates as different from surrounding tissues) (Lewit 1999).

- **A**symmetry – there will commonly be an imbalance on one side, compared with the other, but this is not always the case.

- **R**ange of motion reduced – muscles will probably not be able to reach their normal resting length, or joints may have a restricted range.

If two or three of these features are present this is sufficient to confirm that there is a problem, a dysfunction.

Research by Fryer et al (2004) has confirmed that this traditional osteopathic palpation method is valid. When tissues in the thoracic paraspinal muscles were found to be 'abnormal' (tense,

---

[1] The acronym STAR is modified in some texts to 'TART' (**T**enderness – **A**symmetry – **R**ange of movement modified – **T**issue texture change).

dense, indurated) the same tissues (using an algometer) were also found to have a lowered pain threshold.

While the 'tenderness', altered texture and range of motion characteristics, as listed in the STAR (or TART) acronym, are *always* true for trigger points, additional trigger point changes have been listed by Simons et al (1999):

- The soft tissues housing the trigger point will demonstrate a painful limit to stretch range of motion – whether the stretching is active, or passive (i.e. the patient is stretching the muscle, or you are stretching the muscle).

- In such muscles there is usually pain or discomfort when it is contracted against resistance, with no movement taking place (i.e. an isometric contraction).

- The amount of force the muscle can generate is reduced when it contains active trigger points (or latent ones, i.e. trigger points that do not produce symptoms with which the patient is familiar) – and will usually test as being weaker than a normal muscle.

- There is a taut band, housing an exquisitely tender nodule, commonly located by palpation unless the trigger lies in very deep muscle and is therefore inaccessible to palpation.

- Pressure on an active trigger point produces pain familiar to the patient, and often a painful response ('jump sign').

Drag palpation

It is possible to assess the skin for variations in skin friction, by lightly running a fingertip across the skin surface (no lubricant should be used). This palpation method can be used to compare areas that are palpated as 'different' from surrounding tissues, or to rapidly investigate any local area for trigger point activity.

- The degree of pressure required is minimal – skin touching skin is all that is necessary – a 'feather-light touch'.

- Movement of a single palpating digit (pad of the index or middle finger is best) should be

purposeful, not too slow and certainly not very rapid. Around 3–5 cm (1–2 inches) per second is a satisfactory speed. (If movement is too slow it will not easily pick up differences, and if too fast information may be missed.)

- What is being sought is any sense of 'drag', suggesting a resistance to the easy, smooth passage of the finger across the skin surface.

- A sense of 'dryness', 'sandpaper', a slightly harsh or rough texture, may all indicate increased presence of hydrosis (sweat) on, or increased fluid in, the tissues.

The method of drag palpation is extremely accurate and speedy. It is thought to indicate a localised area of increased sympathetic activity, manifested by sweat. Lewit (1999) describes such regions as hyperalgesic skin zones'. A trigger point will commonly be found in such zones.

Trigger point treatment methods

A wide variety of treatment methods have been advocated in treating trigger points, including:

- Inhibitory (ischaemic compression) pressure methods (Nimmo 1966, Lief 1982/1989)
- Acupuncture and/or ultrasound (Kleyhans 1974)
- Chilling and stretching of the muscle in which the trigger lies (Travell & Simons 1986)
- Dry needling (Gerwin & Dommerholt 2002)
- Procaine or Xylocaine injections (Slocumb 1984)
- Active or passive stretching (Lewit 1999)
- Surgical excision (Dittrich 1954).

Clinical experience has shown that while all or any of these methods can successfully inhibit trigger point activity short-term, in order to completely eliminate the noxious activity of the structure, more is often needed.

Travell and Simons have shown that whatever initial treatment is offered to inhibit the neurological overactivity of the trigger point, the muscle in which it lies has to be made capable of reaching its normal resting length following such treatment or else the trigger point will rapidly reactivate.

In treating trigger points the method of chilling the offending muscle (housing the trigger), while holding it at stretch in order to achieve this end, was advocated by Simons et al (1999), while Lewit (1999) recommends muscle energy techniques in which a physiologically induced postisometric relaxation (or reciprocal inhibition) response is created, prior to passive stretching. Both methods are commonly successful, although a sufficient degree of failure occurs (trigger rapidly reactivating or failing to completely 'switch off') to require investigation of more successful approaches. One reason for failure may relate to the possibility that the tissues being stretched were not the precise structures housing the trigger point.

Hypothesis

The principal author hypothesises that partial contraction (using no more than 20–30% of patient strength, as is the norm in MET procedures, see Chs 3 and 4) may sometimes fail to achieve activation of the fibres housing the trigger point being treated, since the light contractions used in MET of this sort fail to recruit more than a percentage of the muscle's potential. Subsequent stretching of the muscle may therefore only marginally involve the critical tissues surrounding, and enveloping, the myofascial trigger point.

It is also suggested that when a muscle, such as hamstrings or upper trapezius, is stretched as a whole, the tissues in which the trigger point is embedded may not lengthen specifically, and that localised stretches would seem to offer a more certain way of achieving lengthening of the taut, short, myofascial tissues surrounding the trigger point.

Failure to actively stretch the muscle fibres in which the trigger is housed – for whatever reason – may account for the not infrequent recurrence of trigger point activity in the same site following treatment. Repetition of the same stress factors that produced it in the first place could undoubtedly also be a factor in such recurrence – emphasising the need for re-education in rehabilitation. Indeed, it has been suggested that removal of the irritating stress factors (such as excessive use of particular muscle groups), that result in, and maintain, the painful and other influences of active trigger points, is often all that is required. Nevertheless, because trigger points can create so much distress it is frequently important to deactivate them manually, or by other means (injection, dry needling, etc.).

A method that achieves precise targeting of the target tissues (in terms of tonus release and subsequent stretching) is clearly desirable, and such an approach will be described below.

Selye's concepts

Selye has described the progression of changes in tissue which is being locally stressed (see Ch. 2 for more detail). There is an initial alarm (acute inflammatory) stage, followed by a stage of adaptation or resistance when stress factors are continuous or repetitive, at which time muscular tissue becomes progressively fibrotic, and as we have seen in earlier chapters (Ch. 2 in particular), if this change is taking place in muscle which has a predominantly postural rather than a phasic function, the entire muscle structure will shorten (Selye 1984, Janda 1985).

Such hypertonic, and possibly fibrotic tissue, lying in altered (shortened) muscle, may not be easily able to 'release' itself in order to allow the muscle to achieve its normal resting length which, as has been noted, is a prerequisite of normalisation of trigger point activity.

Along with various forms of stretch (passive, active, MET, PNF, etc.), it has been noted above that inhibitory pressure is commonly employed in treatment of trigger points. Such pressure technique methods (analogous to acupressure or shiatsu methodology) are often successful in achieving at least short-term reduction in trigger point activity, and have variously been dubbed 'neuromuscular techniques' (Chaitow 1991b).

Ischaemic compression validation

Researchers at the Department of Physical Medicine and Rehabilitation, University of California, Irvine, evaluated the immediate benefits of treating an active trigger point in the upper trapezius muscle by comparing four commonly used approaches, as well as a placebo treatment (Hong et al 1993). The methods used included:

1. Ice spray and stretch (Simons et al (1999) approach)
2. Superficial heat applied by a hydrocolator pack (20–30 minutes)
3. Deep heat applied by ultrasound (1.2–1.5 watt/cm^2 for 5 minutes)
4. Dummy ultrasound (0.0 watt/cm^2)
5. Deep inhibitory pressure soft tissue massage (10–15 minutes of modified connective tissue massage and shiatsu/ischaemic compression).[2]

For the study 24 patients were selected who had active triggers in the upper trapezius which had been present for not less than 3 months and who had had no previous treatment for these for at least 1 month prior to the study (as well as no cervical radiculopathy or myelopathy, disc or degenerative disease). The following measurements were carried out:

- The pain threshold of the trigger point area was measured using a pressure algometer three times pre-treatment and within 2 minutes of treatment.

- The average was recorded on each occasion.

- A control group were similarly measured twice (30 minutes apart); this group received no treatment until after the second measurement.

The results showed that:

- All methods (but not the placebo ultrasound) produced a significant increase in pain threshold following treatment, with the greatest change being demonstrated by those receiving deep pressure treatment.

- The spray and stretch method was the next most efficient in achieving reduction in pain threshold.

Why is deep pressure technique more effective than other methods? The researchers suggest that:

---

[2] Application of inhibitory pressure may involve elbow, thumb, finger or mechanical pressure (a wooden rubber-tipped T-bar is commonly employed in the USA), or cross-fibre friction. Such methods are described in detail in a further text in this series (Chaitow 2003).

'Perhaps deep pressure massage, if done appropriately, can offer better stretching of the taut bands of muscle fibers than manual stretching because it applies stronger pressure to a relatively small area compared to the gross stretching of the whole muscle. Deep pressure may also offer ischemic compression which [has been shown to be] effective for myofascial pain therapy' (Simons 1989).

Ischaemic compression in trigger point deactivation

There is an apparent contradiction in applying deep pressure to already ischaemic tissues, as originally suggested by Travell & Simons (1983), since the effect of this would seem to be to reduce blood flow even more (McPartland 2004). Indeed, in the second edition of that 1983 text, Simons et al (1999) modified their suggested digital pressure approach (which they now describe as 'trigger point pressure release'), recommending a lighter compression, meeting tissue tension, engaging the restriction barrier and allowing gentle stretching of the affected tissues.

Australian research has validated Simons et al's (1999) suggested methodology (Fryer & Hodgson 2005). The pressure pain threshold (PPT) of latent trigger points in upper trapezius of 37 individuals was recorded pre and post intervention, using a digital algometer (see Box 7.1). It was found that there was a significant increase in the mean PPT of trigger points following use of ischaemic compression ($p > 0.001$). The researchers report that pressure was monitored and maintained during the application of treatment and a reduction in perceived pain and significant increase in tolerance to treatment pressure ($p > 0.001$) appeared to be caused by a change in tissue sensitivity, rather than any unintentional reduction of pressure by the examiner.

Spanish research (de las Penas et al 2005) has also confirmed that PPTs reduced significantly (measured by an algometer and also using a visual analogue scale) when active and latent trigger points in upper trapezius were treated using either ischaemic compression, or cross-fibre friction massage methods.

'The results showed a significant improvement in the PPT ($p = 0.03$), and a significant decrease in the visual analogue scale ($p = 0.04$) within each group. No differences were found between the improvements noted in both groups.'

An alternative methodology

In the application of INIT (below) an alternative method of ischaemic compression is suggested, in which firm pressure is applied to the trigger point, but not sustained. Rather an on-and-off pressure application is suggested, 5 seconds of pressure, 2–3 seconds release, followed by a further 5 seconds of pressure, and so on, repeated until a perceptible change is palpated, or the patient reports a change in the reported pain sensation.

The alternating pressure allows a pumping effect, a flushing, as the ischaemic compression is released.

Box 7.1 The use of algometrics in treating trigger points

An area of concern in trigger point evaluation lies in the non-standard degree of pressure being applied to tissues when they are being tested manually. In order to establish the 'type' and behaviour of trigger points, various researchers have evaluated the usefulness of an algometer in the process (Fryer & Hodgson 2005).

A basic algometer is a hand-held, spring-loaded, rubber-tipped, pressure-measuring device, which offers a means of achieving standardised pressure application. Using an algometer, sufficient pressure to produce pain is applied to preselected points. The measurement is taken when pain is reported. When the point is retested at a subsequent visit, if the same amount of pressure activates the patients pain then the trigger point was not successfully deactivated previously. Ideally there should be a measurable increase in the pain threshold, requiring greater pressure to produce the characteristic pain.

Baldry (1993) suggests that algometers should be used to measure the degree of pressure required to produce symptoms, 'before and after deactivation of a trigger point, because when treatment is successful, the pressure threshold over the trigger point increases'.

A variety of algometer designs exist, including sophisticated versions that are attached to the thumb or finger, with a lead running to an electronic sensor that is itself connected to a computer. This gives very precise readouts of the amount of pressure being applied by the finger or thumb during treatment.

This allows a circulatory influence on the previously ischaemic tissues, alongside the other obvious effects of pressure, including release of pain relieving opioid peptides (endorphin and enkephalin) (Baldry 1993, 2001, Thompson 1984), mechanoreceptor stimulation, and hence an influence on pain perception (Wall & Melzack 1990), as well as myofascial stretching of the tissues (Barnes 1997).

Associated methods

It is worth recalling that the stretching methods advocated by Travell & Simons, subsequent to applied pressure on trigger points, were derived from muscle energy procedures, something they acknowledged in Volume 2 of their text (1992), having earlier (1983) ascribed the methods to Lewit, who had in fact studied with the original developers of MET, including Fred L Mitchell (McPartland 2004). MET can therefore be seen to offer benefits in trigger point treatment. It forms a major element of the INIT approach described below, as does intermittent compression.

By combining the methods of direct inhibition (pressure mildly applied, continuously or in a make-and-break pattern), along with the concept of strain/counterstrain (see below) and MET, a specific targeting of dysfunctional soft tissues can be achieved (Chaitow 1994).

Strain/counterstrain (SCS) briefly explained

Jones (1981) has shown that particular painful 'points' relating to joint or muscular strain, chronic or acute, can be used as 'monitors' – pressure being applied to them as the body or body part is carefully positioned in such a way as to remove or reduce the pain felt in the palpated point.[3]

When the position of ease is attained (using what is known in SCS terminology as 'fine tuning') in which pain vanishes from the palpated monitoring

---

[3] These tender points, as described by Jones, are found in tissues which are short rather than being stretched at the time of injury (acute or chronic) and are usually areas in which the patient is unaware of pain previous to their being palpated. They seem to equate in most particulars with 'Ah shi' points in traditional Chinese medicine.

tender point, the stressed tissues are felt to be at their most relaxed – and clinical experience indicates that this is so, since they palpate as 'easy' rather than having a sense of being 'bound' or tense (see Ch. 3 for more detailed discussion of this phenomenon).

SCS is thought to achieve its benefits by means of an automatic resetting of muscle spindles, which help to dictate the length and tone in the tissues. This resetting apparently occurs only when the muscle housing the spindle is at ease, and usually results in a reduction in excessive tone and release of spasm. When positioning the body (part) in strain/counterstrain methodology, a sense of 'ease' is noted as the tissues reach the position in which pain vanishes from the palpated point.

INIT method (Fig. 7.1A–C)

1. Locate the trigger point, by means of palpation, using methods as described in relation to 'STAR' or 'drag'.

2. Apply ischaemic compression (sustained or intermittent) until the pain changes or until a significant 'release' is noted in the palpated tissues.

3. Positionally release trigger point tissues. Pressure is applied and the patient is asked to ascribe this a value of '10', and then tissues are repositioned (fine-tuned) until the patient reports a score of '2' or less.

4. With the tissues held in this 'folded' ease position a local focused isometric contraction of these tissues is created.

5. This is followed by a local stretch of the tissues housing the trigger point, in the direction of the muscle fibres.

6. The whole muscle is then contracted isometrically as in all MET procedures (see Ch. 5).

7. This is followed by a stretch of the whole muscle, as in all MET procedures for muscles.

8. Facilitation of the antagonists may then be considered, as a means of having the patient perform home exercises to encourage

inhibition of the muscle housing the trigger point (see below).

Discussion

It is reasonable to assume, and palpation confirms, that when a trigger point is being palpated by direct finger or thumb pressure, and when the

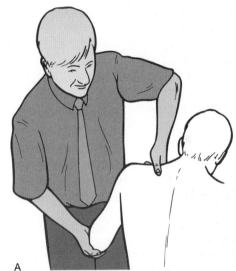

A

Figure 7.1A First stage of INIT in which a tender/pain/trigger point in supraspinatus is located and ischaemically compressed, either intermittently or persistently.

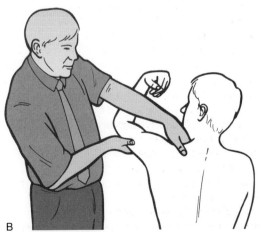

B

Figure 7.1B The pain is removed from the tender/pain/trigger point by finding a position of ease, which is held for at least 20 seconds, following which an isometric contraction is achieved involving the tissues which house the tender/pain/trigger point.

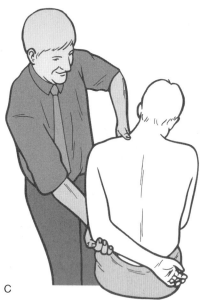

C

Figure 7.1C   Following the holding of the isometric contraction for an appropriate period, the muscle housing the point of local soft tissue dysfunction is stretched. This completes the INIT sequence.

very tissues in which the trigger point lies are positioned in such a way as to take away the pain (entirely or at least to a great extent), that the most (dis)stressed fibres in which the trigger point is housed will be in a position of relative ease.

The trigger point would by then have received direct inhibitory pressure (mild or perhaps inter-mittent – see discussion earlier in this chapter) and (using positional release/SCS methods) would have been positioned so that the tissues housing it are relaxed (relatively or completely).

Following a period of 10–15 seconds in this 'position of ease' – accompanied by palpatory pressure – the patient would be asked to introduce

an isometric contraction into the tissues housing the trigger (currently resting 'at ease') and to hold this for 7 seconds or so, so contracting the very fibres that had been repositioned to obtain the strain/counterstrain release. The palpating finger(s) would determine that the contraction was focused precisely in the tissues around the trigger point.

Following the isometric contraction there would be a reduction in tone in these tissues and they could then be gently stretched locally.

Subsequently, after a more general, whole muscle, isometric contraction – as in any MET procedure (as described in previous chapters) – the entire muscle would be stretched (see Fig. 7.1C).

To complete the sequence

Ruddy's pulsed MET can be used to facilitate weak antagonists to complete the INIT sequence. The methods of pulsed MET as developed by Ruddy (1961) were discussed in earlier chapters (see Ch. 5 for examples). To complete the INIT sequence, pulsating contractions of the weak antagonists to muscles housing trigger points would further inhibit these muscles, as well as helping to tone and proprioceptively re-educate the antagonists.

Summary

The integrated use of inhibitory pressure and strain/counterstrain together with muscle energy technique, applied to a trigger point or other area of soft tissue dysfunction involving pain or restriction of range of motion (of soft tissue origin), is a logical approach since it has the advantage of allowing precise targeting of the culprit tissues.

References

Baldry P 1993 Acupuncture, trigger points and musculoskeletal pain. Churchill Livingstone, Edinburgh

Baldry P 2001 Myofascial pain and fibromyalgia syndromes. Churchill Livingstone, Edinburgh

Barlow W 1959 Anxiety and muscle tension pain. British Journal of Clinical Practice 13: 5

Barnes M 1997 The basic science of myofascial release. Journal of Bodywork and Movement Therapies 1(4): 231–238

Beal M 1983 Journal of the American Osteopathic Association (July)

Black D M, Bakker-Arkema R G, Nawrocki J W 1998 An overview of the clinical safety profile of atorvastatin (lipitor), a new HMG-CoA reductase inhibitor. Archives of Internal Medicine 158(6): 577–584

Brückle W, Sückfull M, Fleckenstein W et al 1990 Gewebe-pO₂-Messung in der verspannten Rückenmuskulatur (m. erector spinae). Zeitschrift Rheumatologie 49: 208–216

Buskila D, Neumann L 1997 Increased rates of fibromyalgia following cervical spine injury. Arthritis and Rheumatism 40(3): 446–452

Butler D 2000 The sensitive nervous system. Noigroup, Adelaide, pp 72–95

Chaitow 1991a Palpatory literacy. Harper Collins, London

Chaitow L 1991b Soft tissue manipulation. Healing Arts Press, Rochester, Vermont

Chaitow L 1994 INIT in treatment of pain and trigger points. British Journal of Osteopathy 13: 17–21

Chaitow L 2003 Modern neuromuscular techniques, 2nd edn. Churchill Livingstone, Edinburgh

Chaitow L, DeLany J 2000 Clinical applications of neuromuscular techniques: vol 1, Upper body. Churchill Livingstone, Edinburgh

Chaitow L, DeLany J 2002 Clinical applications of neuromuscular techniques: vol 2, Lower body. Churchill Livingstone, Edinburgh

de las Penas C F, Alonso-Blanco C et al 2005 Immediate effects of ischemic compression technique and transverse friction massage on tenderness of active and latent myofascial trigger points: a pilot study. Journal of Bodywork and Movement Therapies (accepted for publication 2005)

Dittrich R 1954 Somatic pain and autonomic concomitants. American Journal of Surgery

Dommerholt J 2001 Muscle pain syndromes. In: Cantu R I, Grodin A J (eds) Myofascial manipulation. Aspen, Gaithersburg, pp 93–140

Fryer G, Hodgson L 2005 The effect of manual pressure release on myofascial trigger points in the upper trapezius muscle. Journal Bodywork and Movement Therapies (accepted for publication 2005)

Fryer G, Morris T, Gibbons P 2004 Relation between thoracic paraspinal tissues and pressure sensitivity measured by digital algometer. J Osteopathic Medicine 7(2): 64–69

Gerwin R, Dommerholt J 2002 Treatment of myofascial pain syndromes. In: Weiner R (ed) Pain management; a practical guide for clinicians. CRC Press, Boca Raton, pp 235–249

Goldthwaite J 1949 Essentials of body mechanics. Lippincott, Philadelphia

Hong C-Z, Chen Y-C, Pon C, Yu J 1993 Immediate effects of various physical medicine modalities on pain threshold of an active myofascial trigger point. Journal of Musculoskeletal Pain 1(2)

Janda V 1983 Muscle function testing. Butterworths, London

Janda V 1985 Pain in the locomotor system. In: Glasgow E (ed) Aspects of manipulative therapy. Churchill Livingstone, London

Jones L 1981 Strain/counterstrain. Academy of Applied Osteopathy, Colorado Springs

Kleyhans A 1974 Digest of Chiropractic Economics (September)

Koelbaek Johansen M, Graven-Nielsen T, Schou Olesen A et al 1999 Generalised muscular hyperalgesia in chronic whiplash syndrome. Pain 83(2): 229–234

Korr I 1976 Spinal cord as organiser of the disease process. Yearbook of the Academy of Applied Osteopathy, Newark, Ohio

Latey P 1986 Muscular manifesto. Latey, London

Lewit K 1999 Manipulation in rehabilitation of the locomotor system, 3rd edn. Butterworths, London

Lief S 1982/9 Described in: Chaitow L Neuromuscular technique, 1982, revised as Soft tissue manipulation, 1989 (further revised in 1991). Thorsons, Wellingborough

McPartland J M et al 1997 Chronic neck pain, standing balance, and suboccipital muscle atrophy. J Manipulative and Physiological Therapeutics 21(1): 24–29

McPartland J 2004 Travell trigger points – molecular and osteopathic perspectives. Journal of the American Osteopathic Association 104(6): 244–249

Melzack R, Wall P 1988 The challenge of pain. Penguin, New York

Mense S 1997 Pathophysiologic basis of muscle pain syndromes. In: Fischer A A (ed) Myofascial pain; update in diagnosis and treatment. Philadelphia: W B Saunders Company, pp 23–53

Mense S, Hoheisel U 1999 New developments in the understanding of the pathophysiology of muscle pain. J Musculoskeletal Pain 7(1/2): 13–24

Nimmo R 1966 Receptor tonus technique. Lecture notes

Ruddy T 1961 Osteopathic rhythmic resistive duction therapy. In: Yearbook of Academy of Applied Osteopathy 1961, Indianapolis

Schneider-Helmert D, Whitehouse I, Kumar A et al 2001 Insomnia and alpha sleep in chronic non-organic pain as compared to primary insomnia. Neuropsychobiology 43(1): 54–58

Selye H 1984 The stress of life. McGraw Hill, New York

Shah J, Phillips T et al 2003 A novel microanalytical technique for assaying soft tissue demonstrates significant quantitative biochemical differences in 3 clinically distinct groups: normal, latent, and active. Archives of Physical Medicine and Research 84(9): Abstracts

Simons D 1989 Myofascial pain syndromes. Current therapy of pain. B C Decker, pp 251–266

Simons D, Travell J, Simons L 1999 Myofascial pain and dysfunction: The trigger point manual, vol 1, Upper half of the body, 2nd edn. Williams and Wilkins, Baltimore

Slocumb J 1984 Neurological factors in chronic pelvic pain. American Journal of Obstetrics and Gynaecology 49: 536

Thompson J 1984 Opioid peptides. British Medical Journal 288(6413): 259–260

Travell J, Simons D 1983 Myofascial pain and dysfunction: The trigger point manual, vol 1, Upper half of the body, 1st edn. Williams & Wilkins, Baltimore

Travell J, Simons D 1992 Myofascial pain and dysfunction: The trigger point manual, vol 2, Lower extremities. Williams & Wilkins, Baltimore

Upledger J 1983 Craniosacral therapy. Eastland Press, Seattle

Wall P, Melzack R 1990 Textbook of pain, 2nd edn. Churchill Livingstone, Edinburgh

Manual resistance techniques in rehabilitation

8

Craig Liebenson

CHAPTER CONTENTS

Clinical progression of care 257
Postisometric relaxation (PIR) techniques 258
Proprioceptive neuromuscular facilitation 259
The neurodevelopmental basis for muscle
imbalance 260
Experiment in postural correction 261
Developmental influences 262
The key role of coactivation of antagonists in
producing and maintaining upright posture 263
Functional screening tests 264
Experiment in facilitation of an inhibited
muscle chain 265
Brügger's facilitation method for inhibited muscle
chains in the extremities 267
Conclusion 268
References 272

The goal of rehabilitation is to restore function in the locomotor system. Manual resistance techniques (MRTs) – of which muscle energy technique variations form a major part – are excellent bridges between passive and active care. When applying MRTs/METs the practitioner, or health care provider, is able to control the direction, magnitude, velocity and time of each force generated by the patient. MRTs can be used to inhibit overactive muscles and to facilitate underactive muscles or to mobilise joints; they are also ideal for self-treatment.

Clinical progression of care

Once diagnosis of the site of tissue injury or pain generation has been made, treatment matched to the goals of acute care – namely pain relief – can be initiated. As the patient's acute pain subsides, the recovery phase starts. During this phase the health care provider should attempt to identify the potential sources of biomechanical overload that may have led to tissue injury or pain in the first place. When these sources are identified and linked to the pain generator, rehabilitation efforts can be used to improve function in the relevant kinetic chain.

MRTs can be used during both the acute and recovery phases. For example, gentle isometric contractions or hold–relax (HR) methods are ideal during acute care, while facilitation methods, such as the diagonal patterns of proprioceptive neuromuscular facilitation (PNF), described later in this chapter, are more applicable in the recovery phase.

Postisometric relaxation (PIR) techniques

The use of isometric contractions is an excellent technique for treating the neuromuscular component of a stiff, shortened or tight muscle (Lewit 1986, Liebenson 1989, 1990, Liebenson & Murphy 1998). In particular, if trigger points are present, PIR is clinically very effective as a major part of their deactivation (for more on trigger points and MET methodology, see also Ch. 7) (Lewit & Simons 1984).

As discussed in Ch. 4, the physiological influence of isometric contractions may not explain the clinical benefits, to the extent previously considered. Enhanced stretch tolerance, following the isometric contraction, is now thought to offer a more likely explanation (Sterling et al 2001, Wilson et al 2003).

Method

- The clinician's first priority is to identify the pathological barrier (Fig. 8.1).

- This is noted the moment resistance starts when taking out the slack.

- The location of the barrier is confirmed by a sense of a lack of normal resilience, or 'spring', at the end of range.

- Tension is held at the barrier without letting go of the slack while waiting for a release of tissue tension.

- There should be no stretch or bounce.

- If, after a brief latency, no release phenomenon occurs, the patient can be requested to gently push away from the barrier against matched resistance – using approximately 10% of maximum effort – so as to create an isometric contraction.

- Once the isometric contraction is achieved, the patient can be requested to take a deep breath in and to hold this for 5–8 seconds.

- The patient then releases both the breath and the effort, and the clinician waits to feel a sense of 'release' of the tissue tension.

- Only after feeling the release should slack be taken up and the tissues eased to the new barrier.

- This process is repeated up to three times.

- At the conclusion a reciprocal inhibition contraction can be usefully introduced, by having the patient contract the antagonist muscles, attempting to move away from the barrier, against resistance.

If, however, no release occurs using the above method, the following may be attempted:

1. Utilise respiratory synkinesis (e.g. breathe in during most contractions and exhale during release).

2. Have the patient increase the contraction phase.

3. Have the patient use more force (i.e. 'as little as possible or as much as necessary').

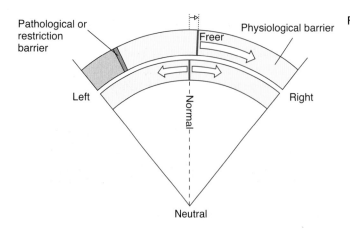

Figure 8.1 The barrier phenomenon.

4. Add visual synkinesis if appropriate (look in the direction of contraction and then the direction of release – see also Chs 3 and 5).

5. It may be useful to vary how the muscle is isolated. For example, when lengthening the anterior fibres of upper trapezius, slack is taken out with the upper cervical spine in flexion, together with contralateral lateral flexion of the neck, ipsilateral rotation of the neck, and shoulder depression. The order in which the slack is taken out can be altered in order to isolate tension to the part of the muscle that needs to be targeted.

6. Other related tissues may need to be treated before use of MET (for example joint mobilisation or facilitation of antagonists, using reciprocal inhibition).

According to Lewit (personal communication 1999), muscle is contractile tissue; if a muscle has decreased in length, 90% of the time this is due to it being contracted. The treatment in these cases is therefore relaxation. He estimates that in approximately 10% of cases it is due to connective tissue changes, and the treatment is therefore stretching. It is not, however, wise to stretch a muscle containing an active trigger point until it has been inhibited.

Proprioceptive neuromuscular facilitation

Proprioceptive neuromuscular facilitation (PNF) was originally utilised for neuromuscular re-education in stroke victims (Kabot 1950). Later it was discovered that it was clinically useful in rehabilitating children with cerebral palsy (CP) (Levine et al 1954). This led to its use for a wide range of orthopaedic conditions.

PNF is associated with a philosophy of care that treats the whole body by stimulation of basic movement patterns (Adler et al 1993). These patterns are of neurodevelopmental origin and are incorporated in functional activities such as swimming, running, climbing, throwing, etc. Therefore, in contrast to most isotonic training approaches that are uniplanar, PNF methods resist movement in multiple planes simultaneously. For instance, a diagonal pattern of movement will be resisted at the same time as a flexion/extension and abduction/adduction of an extremity (see Fig. 6.6A, B).

The shoulder girdle is a good example of the clinical utility of PNF principles in rehabilitation of physical performance capacity. Once pain and inflammation begin to subside, PNF patterns can be utilised to restore function in the shoulder (Figs 8.4, 8.5). Such exercises can be combined with muscle balancing approaches, joint mobili-

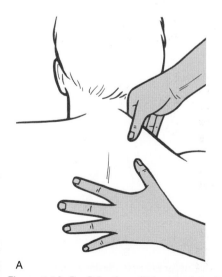
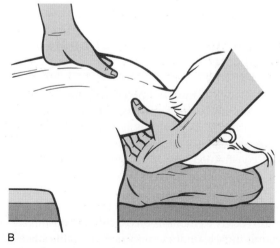

A   B

Figure 8.2A, B   Palpation of trigger point with local twitch response in upper trapezius.

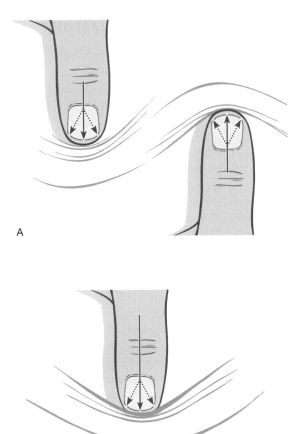

A

B

Figure 8.3A, B   Myofascial release technique for the pectoralis major muscle.

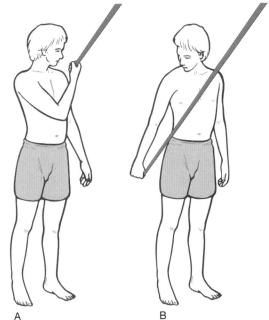

A   B

Figure 8.4A, B   D1 upper extremity extension technique ('seatbelt').

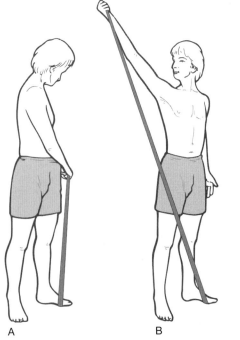

A   B

Figure 8.5A, B   D2 upper extremity flexion technique ('drawing a sword').

sation/manipulation and closed chain stabilisation procedures.

The neurodevelopmental basis for muscle imbalance

Janda's model of muscle imbalance drives much of our clinical decision making. Certain muscles active during static postures have a tendency to become overactive or even shorten due to prolonged use of constrained postures (Lewit 1999a). Other muscles active during dynamic activities tend to become inhibited or even weak from disuse. Static postural muscle overactivity is a natural result of modern society's emphasis on constrained postures. Dynamic muscle underactivity is predictable since modern lifestyles are predominantly sedentary.

- The static muscle system typically involves superficial muscles such as upper trapezius, sternocleidomastoid, erector spinae and the hamstrings.

- In contrast, the dynamic muscle system utilises more the deep stabilisers such as transverse abdominus, quadratus lumborum, multifidus and the deep neck flexors.

The development of these predictable muscle imbalances is further spurred by the diminished afferent flow of sensory information from the periphery, in particular the sole of the foot, due to sedentarism and a lack of variety of movements. Naturally, movement patterns are altered and fatigue ability increased, rendering the motor control system less able to adapt to various biomechanical sources of repetitive strain.

The goal of neurodevelopment of the locomotor system is to achieve the upright posture. Brügger and Janda have shown how deleterious sedentarism is (Lewit 1999a). Brügger describes the typical sedentary posture of man via a linkage system. He has shown how approximation of the sternum and symphysis increases both end-

range loading, and muscular tension (Lewit 1999a, Liebenson 1999). It is possible, however, to demonstrate that postural correction can immediately improve joint function and muscle tone.

Experiment in postural correction (Figs 8.6, 8.7)

- Check upper trapezius tension/trigger points in slump position.

- Perform the Brügger relief position and then recheck (see Fig. 8.7).

- Check cervical rotation in the slump position; perform the Brügger relief position and recheck.

- Check arm abduction in slump; perform the Brügger relief position and recheck.

Brügger's relief position facilitates phasic muscles (muscles which tend to inhibition) and reciprocally inhibits postural muscles (muscles which tend to shortening). His advice is very effective in improving patient compliance with home exercises. It is also an excellent way to increase awareness of postural corrections (Lewit 1999a).

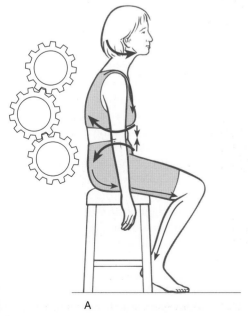

A

Figure 8.6A Sternosymphyseal syndrome.

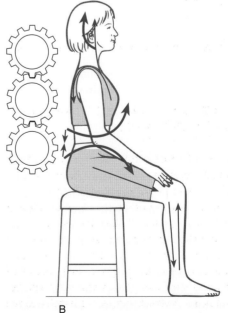

B

Figure 8.6B Brügger relief position.

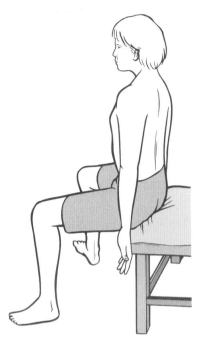

Figure 8.7
Brügger relief position.

Brugger's relief position

To perform Brugger's postural exercise:

- The individual is asked to sit or stand tall (see Figs 8.6B and 8.7).

- Forearm supination and finger abduction are performed, along with lengthening of the cervical spine (carefully avoiding chin-poking).

- When in this position active exhalation is performed using the abdominal wall muscles.

Developmental influences

It is worth pointing out that the muscles that Janda has suggested tend to hypertonicity include most of the muscles shortened in the foetal position. These are, in the upper quarter, the finger, hand and wrist flexors, the shoulder internal rotators and adductors, and the shoulder girdle elevators (Kolár 1999). In the lower quarter they are the ankle plantar flexors and invertors, the hip flexors, internal rotators and adductors. As the infant's motor control system develops, the antagonists of these muscles become facilitated and the muscles become inhibited. Muscles inhibited in the upper extremity include:

- finger, wrist elbow and shoulder extensors
- forearm supinators
- shoulder external rotators and abductors.

Those in the lower extremity include:

- toe extensors
- ankle dorsiflexors and pronators
- hip abductors and external rotators.

The parallel between the postural muscles that tend to overactivity in adults as a result of sedentarism, and the muscles that are used to maintain the foetal position is obvious. Similarly, Janda's phasic muscles are almost identical to the muscles whose activation during neurodevelopment brings about an upright posture. That there is a central neurological programme for these different types of muscles is further reinforced by noting which muscles become spastic in children with cerebral palsy, and which muscles are paralysed in people who have suffered a stroke. It becomes clear that balance between agonist and antagonist muscles is essential for a proper functional motor control system (Cholewicki & McGill 1996, Kolár 1999).

Certain landmark stages exist in the transition from a tonic, reflex motor system (brain stem control) to a balanced postural control system, capable of volitional control locomotion (supraspinal control). Each stage of the neurodevelopment of posture depends upon a set of specific conditions being met. Specific points of body support, centration of key joints, and agonist–antagonist muscular coactivation, are all necessary for development of each landmark of neurodevelopment of the postural control system (Kolár 1999).

Kolár (1999) points out that agonist–antagonist coactivation patterns evolve as neurodevelopment progresses to take the infant from a foetal position at birth, to a stable upright posture at approximately 3 years of age. In the first month of life the infant's muscles (maintaining the foetal position) are in a state of tonic contraction. At the end of the first month, in response to visual and auditory stimuli from the mother, the child begins to orient its head. This is not a reflex movement, but under higher motor control (Kolár 1999).

As posture develops, the tonic contractions, which are reflexly based, begin to relax, thus reducing reciprocal inhibition and facilitating the coactivation patterns necessary for joint centration and load bearing. For instance, at the end of the first month, coactivation of anatagonists at the cervicocranial junction centrates C0–C1:

- Deep neck flexors are facilitated.
- Short cervical extensors are no longer tonically active.

If the tonic contraction of the upper cervical extensors does not relax, then joint centration of C0–C1 is not possible, and the infant will not be able to control its head movements for successful orientation.

Coactivation of antagonists occurs proximally at the shoulder and hip by the third month as a prerequisite for weight bearing on all fours (i.e. creeping and crawling):

- Activation of lower scapular fixators, shoulder external rotators, trunk extensors, hip abductors external rotators

- Reduction in tonic activity of scapular elevators, shoulder internal rotators, trunk hip adductors and internal rotators.

Failure of coactivation due to persistent tonic activity results in faulty neurodevelopment of the motor system. This allows a persistence of trunk flexion, eventually promoting both the upper crossed and lower crossed syndromes (see Figs 8.8, 8.9).

Kolár utilises treatments including stimulation of reflex trigger zones at key areas of postural support in the infant such as the symphysis pubis, sternum or occiput to facilitate coactivation patterns (Kolár 1999).

The key role of coactivation of antagonists in producing and maintaining upright posture

Equilibrium is a result of co-contraction of antagonists. This co-activation develops in the first three months of infancy. During the first 3–4 weeks of life the muscles are tonic under reflex control (brain stem). At 4–6 weeks orientation to the mother begins visually with turning of the head. This is

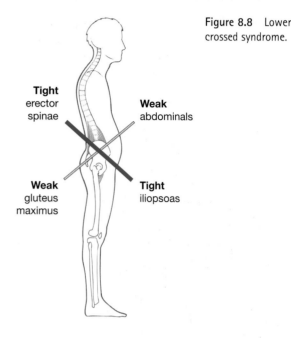

Figure 8.8 Lower crossed syndrome.

Tight erector spinae

Weak abdominals

Weak gluteus maximus

Tight iliopsoas

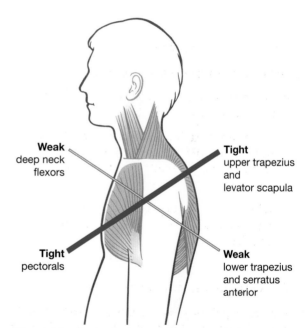

Weak deep neck flexors

Tight upper trapezius and levator scapula

Tight pectorals

Weak lower trapezius and serratus anterior

Figure 8.9 Upper crossed syndrome.

the birth of posture and motor control. Postural reactions are supraspinal. The coactivation of antagonists creates maximum congruence of joints, thus promoting equilibrium and joint loading (Kolár 1999).

During development of upright posture, the upper extremity tonic activity (flexion, internal rotation, adduction and pronation) is joined with phasic activity (extension, external rotation, abduction and supination). In the lower extremity tonic activity (ankle plantar flexion and inversion, hip flexion, internal rotation and adduction) is joined with phasic activity (ankle dorsiflexion and eversion, hip external rotation and abduction).

Development from one stage to another requires that balanced muscle contraction of antagonists replaces dominance of tonic muscular activity. This coactivation centrates or aligns joints in maximum congruence. Such coactivation is not reflex (brain stem), but supraspinal, and is the beginning point of postural-motor activity in the human (Kolár 1999).

Sedentarism reduces afferent input – particularly from the sole of the foot – and promotes tension in postural (anti-gravity) muscles while leading to inhibition in dynamic phasic muscles. Janda's muscle imbalances are a predictable result of this with their typical associated faulty movement patterns and repetitive microtrauma to joints. Brügger has developed a systematic approach to improving posture complementing that evolved by Janda (Lewit 1999a).

Functional screening tests

Certain screening tests have been developed by Janda for identifying agonist–antagonist–synergist relationships during stereotypical movement patterns (Janda 1996, Liebenson & Chapman 1998, Liebenson

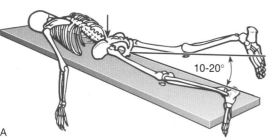

A

Figure 8.10A Abnormal hip extension movement pattern associated with shortened psoas. Leg raising is initiated with an anterior pelvic tilt.

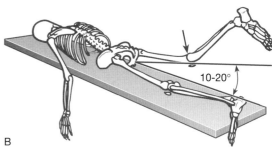

B

Figure 8.10B Abnormal hip extension movement pattern associated with excessive substitution of the hamstrings. Leg raising is initiated with knee flexion.

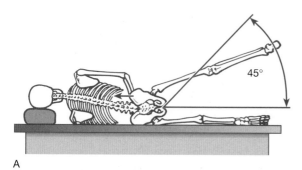

A

Figure 8.11A Abnormal hip abduction movement pattern associated with excessive substitution of the quadratus lumborum. Leg raising is initiated with a cephalad shift of the pelvis.

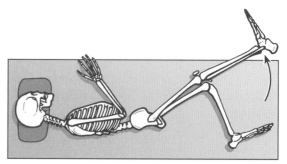

B

Figure 8.11B Abnormal hip abduction movement pattern associated with excessive substitution of the tensor fascia lata. Leg raising is initiated with flexion of the hip joint.

et al 1998, Lewit 1999a). These kinesiological relationships – called muscle imbalances – alter joint stress by changing movement patterns, or the axis of rotation, during movement. The screening tests illustrated in Figs 8.10–8.16 include hip extension, hip abduction, trunk flexion, scapular fixation during arm abduction, upper cervical flexion, trunk lowering from a push-up, and respiration.

When faulty movement patterns are present they are a key perpetuating factor of myofascial or joint pain (Watson & Trott 1993, Treleaven et al 1994, Babyar 1996, Barton & Hayes 1996, Edgerton et al 1996). Unless movement patterns are improved during performance of activities of daily life, so that joint stability is maintained, then soft tissue or

mobilisation/manipulation treatments will fail to achieve lasting results. In fact, exercises performed without proper form only reinforce such muscle imbalances because 'trick' movement patterns are used, due to synergist substitution for inhibited agonists (Paarnianpour et al 1988, Grabiner et al 1992, Arendt-Nielson et al 1995, Edgerton et al 1996, Hodges & Richardson 1996, O'Sullivan et al 1997, Sparto et al 1997, Hodges & Richardson 1998, 1999).

Experiment in facilitation of an inhibited muscle chain

Eccentric facilitation of a chain of inhibited muscles brings about reciprocal inhibition of the tonic muscle

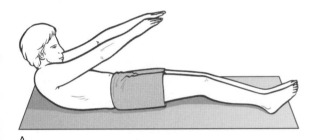

A

Figure 8.12A   Normal trunk flexion movement pattern.

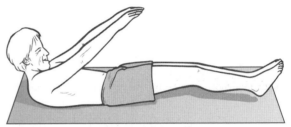

B

Figure 8.12B   Abnormal trunk flexion movement pattern associated with excessive substitution of the psoas. Heels rise up off the table before the shoulder blades are lifted.

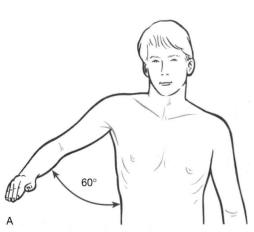

60°

A

Figure 8.13A   Normal scapular fixation during arm abduction movement pattern.

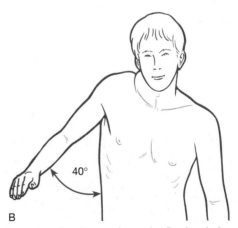

40°

B

Figure 8.13B   Abnormal scapular fixation during arm abduction movement pattern associated with excessive substitution of the upper trapezius and levator scapulae. Scapulae or shoulder girdle elevate before the arm has abducted 45°.

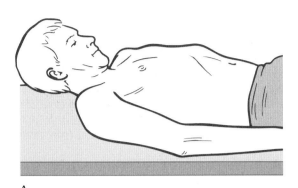

A

Figure 8.14A Normal upper cervical flexion movement pattern.

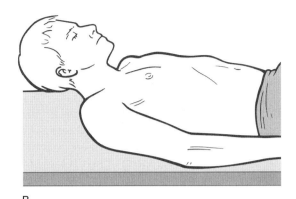

B

Figure 8.14B Abnormal upper cervical flexion movement pattern associated with excessive substitution of the sternocleidomastoid and/or shortening of the suboccipitals. Head is raised towards the chest with chin poking (i.e. upper cervical extension) occurring.

chain. The tonic muscle chain is typically over-activated in individuals with sternosymphyseal syndrome (Lewit 1999a, 1999b).

The muscle imbalance is typical in that it involves overactivity in the muscles described by Kolár as tonic together with inhibition of those responsible for coactivation during development from a kyphotic to upright posture (Kolár 1999). Such hypertonic muscle chains often involve trigger or tender points in both inhibited and overactive muscle groups (Lewit 1999b). They are expected in chronic pain states as a result of the body's attempt to immobilise the region (Lewit 1999b).

Investigation

To identify a hypertonic muscle chain in the upper extremity look for one-sided predominance of the following dysfunctions:

- Restricted wrist extension mobility

- Trigger points in upper trapezius, pectoralis major

- Tender attachment points in upper ribs 1–3 and the lateral or medial epicondyle.

In the lower extremity look for one-sided predominance of the following dysfunctions:

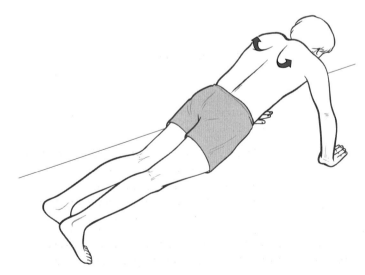

Figure 8.15 Abnormal trunk lowering from a push-up movement pattern associated with inhibition/weakness of the serratus anterior. Winging of the right scapula.

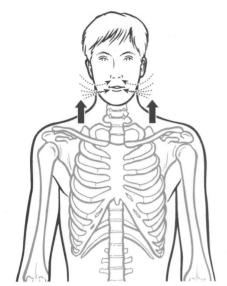

Figure 8.16A Abnormal respiration associated with elevation of the clavicle(s) during relaxed inhalation.

- Restricted hamstring length
- Trigger points in adductor longus and magnus, pectineus, gluteus medius, gluteus maximus and the longitudinal arch of the foot.

Brügger's facilitation method for inhibited muscle chains in the extremities

Indications:

- Any time it is appropriate to release tension in multiple muscles simultaneously
- When a one-sided chain is present, especially in chronic pain patients.

Once a predominately one-sided chain has been found, in either the upper or the lower extremity, then treatment with a strong (40–80% of maximum effort) contraction of a sequence of movements, involving a chain of inhibited muscles, can be used to bring about reciprocal inhibition of the chain of hypertonic muscles. An eccentric muscle energy technique is used to maximise reciprocal inhibition of the hypertonic muscle chain. Each of the following movements is

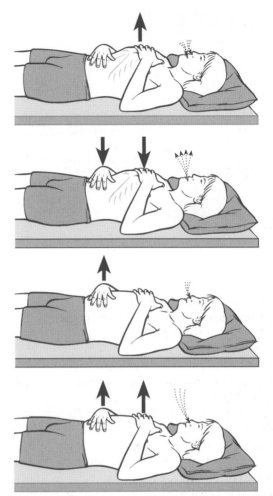

Figure 8.16B The most severe dysfunction occurs when the belly moves inwards during inhalation ('paradoxical breathing').

resisted individually, one after the other. Approximately three repetitions of each movement is performed.

- The patient contracts against the clinician's resistance.

- The clinician then slowly stretches the muscle while the patient maintains resistance, thus achieving an eccentric contraction (see discussion of slow eccentric contractions in Ch. 3).

The purpose is to facilitate these muscles and reciprocally inhibit the antagonistic muscles.

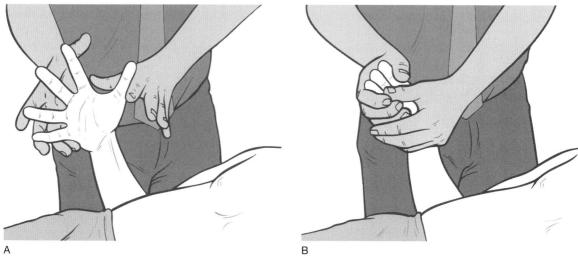

A   B

Figure 8.17A, B   Eccentric resistance of finger and thumb abduction.

In the upper quarter eccentrically resist:

- Finger and thumb abduction (Fig. 8.17A, B)
- Wrist and finger extension and thumb abduction (Fig. 8.18A, B)
- Forearm supination (Fig. 8.19A, B)
- Shoulder external rotation (Fig. 8.20A, B)
- Shoulder abduction and external rotation (Fig. 8.21A, B).

In the lower quarter eccentrically resist:

- Toe extension, ankle dorsiflexion and eversion (Fig. 8.22A, B)

- Hip abduction (Fig. 8.23A, B)
- Hip external rotation (Fig. 8.24A, B).

It is notable that the resistance to shoulder abduction and external rotation is almost identical to the final position of the PNF D2 upper extremity flexion – 'drawing a sword' position (see Fig. 8.5).

Conclusion

What has been presented in this chapter is an exciting new approach to rehabilitation of the motor

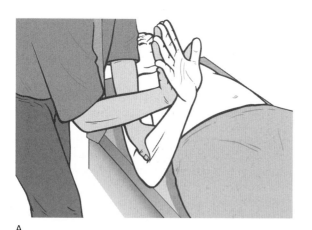

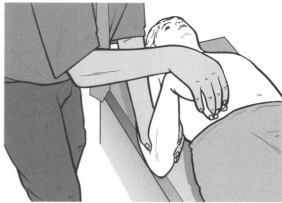

A   B

Figure 8.18A, B   Eccentric resistance of wrist and finger extension and thumb abduction.

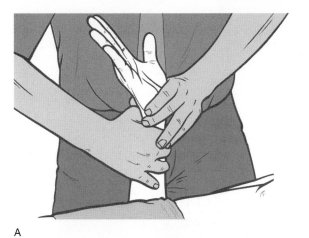

A

B

Figure 8.19A, B   Eccentric resistance of forearm supination.

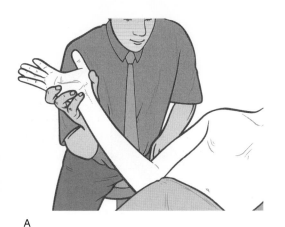

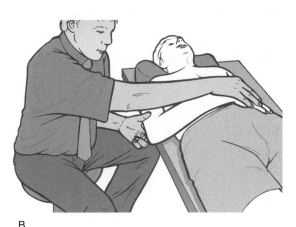

A

B

Figure 8.20A, B   Eccentric resistance of shoulder external rotation.

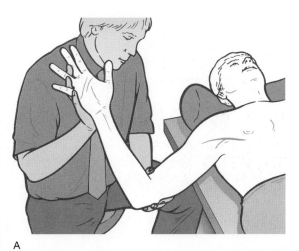

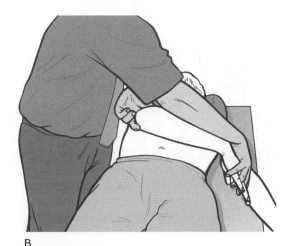

A

B

Figure 8.21A, B   Eccentric resistance of shoulder abduction and external rotation.

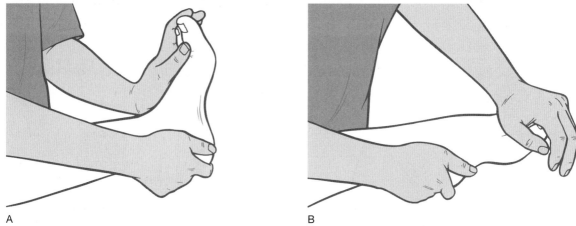

A

B

Figure 8.22A, B Eccentric resistance of toe extension, ankle dorsiflexion and eversion.

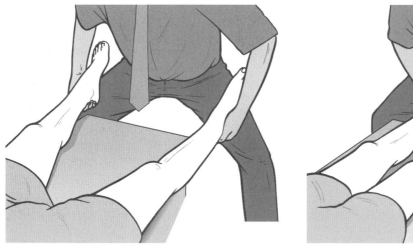

A

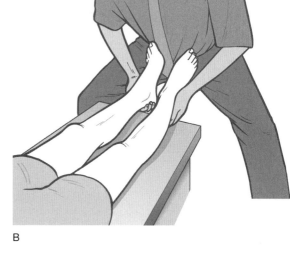

B

Figure 8.23A, B Eccentric resistance of hip abduction.

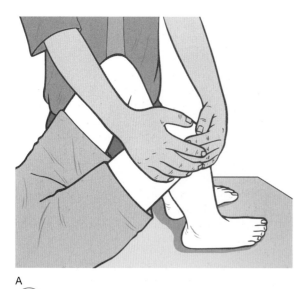

A

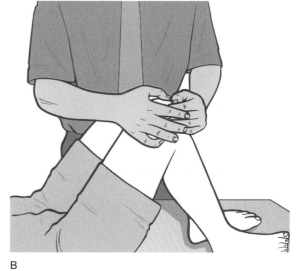

B

Figure 8.24A, B Eccentric resistance of hip external rotation.

system. The identification of a nociceptive chain involving agonist/antagonist trigger points enhances our ability to restore muscle balance and improve joint stability. The concept of muscle imbalance is reinforced by knowledge of neurodevelopment of the upright posture.

Chains form in our patients which are invaluable aids in troubleshooting. It is not enough simply to identify a muscle imbalance and treat those muscles. The chain which is dysfunctional must also be identified, and treatment of a key link given. Supraspinal control, which begins after 3 weeks of life, is the beginning of voluntary motor control. If chains of agonist–antagonist muscle incoordination, hypothetically related to various stages of neurodevelopment of the upright posture, are improved, this may be a significant advance in treatment of motor system problems. Research into agonist–antagonist coactivation, joint congruence, equilibrium, maximisation of joint load handling ability, and neurological programmes in the adult, representative of neurodevelopmental stages, is eagerly anticipated.

Box 8.1 Common questions about manual resistance techniques (MRTs)

Q1. Should the muscle be lengthened gently or firmly?
A: Gently.

Q2. Is the 'barrier phenomenon' similar in MRTs and in thrust techniques?
A: Yes.

Q3. How long does it take to perform MRT on a muscle?
A: Less than a minute.

Q4. If MRT is unsuccessful, what does that suggest?
A: The problem is in the connective tissue.

Q5. Are these techniques arduous for the health care provider to perform?
A: Not typically.

Q6. Besides relaxing a muscle, MRT can be used for what other purposes?
A: To mobilise joints or prepare a muscle for more aggressive stretching techniques.

Q7. What are the indications for MRT?
A: Increased muscle tension, trigger points and joint restriction.

Box 8.2 Common clinical applications of manual resistance techniques

A. Trigger point (semi–active)
Indication: palpation of taut band in muscle, with twitch sign and referred pain phenomenon.
Treatment: this is primarily a neuromuscular phenomenon, not a connective tissue problem. Treatment therefore requires a minimum of force. Use MRTs (isometric contractions). Light ischaemic compression can also be used, especially for trigger points on the surface. The pressure should be just enough to engage a barrier to resistance and, following a latency, should achieve a release phenomenon. Greater force risks facilitating a contraction in the muscle as it 'defends' the barrier (see also Ch. 7).
Experiment: try to find a trigger point in the upper trapezius (using a light pincer grip). Hold the taut band between your fingers. Then roll the taut band through your fingers as you search the length of the muscle for a motor response in the trigger point (i.e. local twitch response (LTR), see Fig. 8.2). Once you have found an LTR try to release the trigger point with MRTs (isometric contractions) and then repalpate.

B. Shortened muscle (passive or semi–active)
Indication: positive length test for decreased range of motion.
Treatment: start with MRTs. If MRT is unsuccessful, it is likely that there are connective tissue changes since mere relaxation alone did not result in a release of the muscle to a new resting length. There are two options:
1. Perform myofascial release by folding the muscle perpendicularly against itself and hold until release is 'sensed' (see Fig. 8.3). Then take out slack. This avoids the stretch reflex and is ideal for superficial muscles such as the pectoralis major.
2. If muscle is deep (e.g. iliopsoas), treat with a more forceful technique such as contract–relax antagonist contract (CRAC) or postfacilitation stretch (PFS). PFS is similar to MRT as described earlier except that a greater contraction force (25–100% of a patient's maximum) is used, after which a fast stretch is applied (Liebenson 1996). Note: if you are using PFS certain safety rules should be observed. These include the following: stretch over the largest, most stable, least painful joint; joints should be 'loose packed'; avoid uncoupled movements; and do not stretch nerves if they are irritated.
Experiment: Test the length of the iliopsoas and adductors (see Figs 8.10A, B and 8.11A, B) and then perform a muscle energy procedure and re-evaluate.

References

Adler S S, Beckers D, Buck M 1993 PNF in practice – an illustrated guide. Springer-Verlag, Berlin

Arendt-Nielson L, Graven-Nielson T, Svarrer H, Svensson P 1995 The influence of low back pain on muscle activity and coordination during gait. Pain 64: 231–240

Babyar S R 1996 Excessive scapular motion in individuals recovering from painful and stiff shoulders: causes and treatment strategies. Physical Therapy 76: 226–238

Barton P M, Hayes K C 1996 Neck flexor muscle strength, and relaxation times in normal subjects and subjects with unilateral neck pain and headache. Archives of Physical Medicine and Rehabilitation 77: 680–687

Cholewicki J, McGill S M 1996 Mechanical stability of the in vivo lumbar spine: implications for injury and chronic low back pain. Clinical Biomechanics 11(1): 1–15

Edgerton V R, Wolf S L, Levendowski D J, Roy R R 1996 Theoretical basis for patterning EMG amplitudes to assess muscle dysfunction. Medical Science Sports and Exercise 28: 744–751

Grabiner M D, Koh T J, Ghazawi A E 1992 Decoupling of bilateral paraspinal excitation in subjects with low back pain. Spine 17: 1219

Hodges P W, Richardson C A 1996 Inefficient muscular stabilization of the lumbar spine associated with low back pain. Spine 21: 2640–2650

Hodges P W, Richardson C A 1998 Delayed postural contraction of the transverse abdominus associated with movement of the lower limb in people with low back pain. Journal of Spinal Disorders 11: 46–56

Hodges P W, Richardson C A 1999 Altered trunk muscle recruitment in people with low back pain with upper limb movements at different speeds. Archives of Physical Medicine and Rehabilitation 80: 1005–1012

Janda V 1996 Evaluation of muscle imbalances. In: Liebenson C (ed) Rehabilitation of the spine: a practitioner's manual. Williams and Wilkins, Baltimore

Kabot H 1950 Studies on neuromuscular dysfunction XIII: new concepts and techniques of neuromuscular reeducation for paralysis. Permanente Foundation Medical Bulletin 8: 121–143

Koár P 1999 The sensomotor nature of postural functions, its fundamental role in rehabilitation. Journal of Orthopaedic Medicine 21(2): 40–45

Levine M G, Kabat H, Knott M et al 1954 Relaxation of spasticity by physiological techniques. Archives of Physical Medicine and Rehabilitation 35: 214–223

Lewit K 1986 Postisometric relaxation in combination with other methods of muscular facilitation and inhibition. Manual Medicine 2: 101–104

Lewit K 1999a Manipulative therapy in rehabilitation of the motor system, 3rd edn. Butterworths, London

Lewit K 1999b Chain reactions in the locomotor system in the light of coactivation patterns based on

developmental neurology. Journal of Orthopaedic Medicine 21(2): 52–58

Lewit K, Simons D G 1984 Myofascial pain: relief by post-isometric relaxation. Archives of Physical Medicine and Rehabilitation 65: 452–456

Liebenson C S 1989 Active muscular relaxation techniques, part one. Basic principles and methods. Journal of Manipulative and Physiological Therapeutics 12: 6

Liebenson C S 1990 Active muscular relaxation techniques, part two. Clinical application. Journal of Manipulative and Physiological Therapeutics 13: 1

Liebenson C 1996 Manual resistance techniques. In Liebenson C (ed) Rehabilitation of the spine: a practitioner's manual. Williams and Wilkins, Baltimore

Liebenson C 1999 Advice for the clinician. Journal of Bodywork and Movement Therapies 3: 147–149

Liebenson C, Chapman S 1998 Rehabilitation of the spine: functional evaluation of the lumbar spine. Williams and Wilkins, Baltimore [videotape]

Liebenson C, Murphy D 1998 Rehabilitation of the spine: post-isometric relaxation techniques –low back and lower extremities. Williams and Wilkins, Baltimore [videotape]

Liebenson C, DeFranca C, Lefebvre R 1998 Rehabilitation of the spine: functional evaluation of the cervical spine. Williams and Wilkins, Baltimore [videotape]

O'Sullivan P, Twomey L, Allison G et al 1997 Altered patterns of abdominal muscle activation in patients with chronic low back pain. Australian Journal of Physiotherapy 43: 91–98

Paarnianpour M, Nordin M, Kahanovitz N, Frank V 1998 The triaxial coupling of torque generation of trunk muscles during isometric exertions and the effect of fatiguing isoinertial movements on the motor output and movement patterns. Spine 13: 982–992

Sparto P J, Paarnianpour M, Massa W S, Granata K P, Reinsel T E, Simon S 1997 Neuromuscular trunk performance and spinal loading during a fatiguing isometric trunk extension with varying torque requirements. Spine 10: 145–156

Sterling M, Jull G A, Wright A 2001 Cervical mobilisation: concurrent effects on pain, sympathetic nervous system activity and motor activity. Manual Therapy 6(2): 72–81

Treleaven J, Jull G, Atkinson L 1994 Cervical musculoskeletal dysfunction in post-concussional headache. Cephalgia 14: 273–279

Watson D H, Trott P H 1993 Cervical headache: an investigation of natural head posture and upper cervical flexor muscle performance. Cephalgia 13: 272–284

Wilson E, Payton O, Donegan-Shoaf L et al 2003 Muscle energy technique in patients with acute low back pain: a pilot clinical trial. Journal of Orthopaedic and Sports Physical Therapy 33: 502–512

MET in the physical therapy setting

9

Eric Wilson

CHAPTER CONTENTS

Classification models	**274**
Further refinement of classification	275
Misconceptions in the literature	**277**
Clinical utilisation of muscle energy technique	**280**
Staging	281
Addressing impairments: segmental-specific strengthening	283
Summary	**291**
References	**295**

Low-back pain (LBP) is managed with a diverse assortment of treatments that run the spectrum from well-constructed theories to ridiculous gadgets, and all points in between. Perhaps the reason there are so many different 'treatments' for low-back pain is that none of them seems to work all of the time. This is an unsettling thought. Instead, it may be that 'low-back pain' is not a single entity but a vast array of impairments that can be summed up with 3 letters – LBP. One of the problems inherent in treating patients with LBP is the difficulty determining which interventions to apply to which patients. Why does *manipulation* work for some patients but not others? Why does *traction* resolve some patients' symptoms but exacerbate others?

The medical model tells us that 'diagnosis drives treatment'. This is true in most cases: a patient with 'knee pain', for example, would receive a different course of treatment if the source of the pain was diagnosed as a patella tendonopathy versus an iliotibial band syndrome. Unfortunately, trying to apply this medical model to low-back pain is akin to attempting to force a square peg into a round hole because low-back pain is not homogenous. While often portrayed as homogenous, a pathoanatomical diagnosis is only available in approximately 20% of all LBP cases. Therefore, the identification of subgroups of patients with low-back pain who respond favourably to specific interventions has been deemed a research priority (Borkan et al 1998).

Classification models

This mandate has produced numerous classification models, most of which have not withstood the attentions of repeated testing via randomised controlled trials. One classification model, originally reported by Delitto et al (1995) has weathered the rigours of repeated testing and as a result, has been refined over the past decade into a valid and clinically useful tool. Some people may confuse the term *classification model* with that of *cookbook therapy*. A cookbook approach requires all patients receive the same treatment, regardless of their clinical presentation. This would be akin to providing McKenzie's extension exercises to all patients with low-back pain regardless of their signs and symptoms. While some patients would improve from this treatment, most would not. A classification model attempts to group patients into categories based upon the treatment that will provide them the most benefit. Consider a cookbook approach to be like a hammer – everything gets treated like a nail regardless of its individual characteristics, whereas a classification model makes the hammer more efficient (by finding it more nails and fewer screws to hit).

A classification model also allows the physical therapist to work outside of the often limiting confines of a diagnosis. The difference between a *diagnosis* and a *classification* is striking. Diagnosis can be defined as *the means of establishing the source of a patient's impairment or symptoms,* while classification is *a method of arranging clinical data into predetermined categories of impairments or diagnoses in order to make informed decisions regarding treatment.* Classification systems are beneficial in the treatment of low-back pain because the majority of patients with low-back pain have no attributable pathology, the population comprises numerous heterogenous subgroups, and the use of a classification-based scheme may allow clinicians to treat their patients more effectively (Riddle 1998).

An additional benefit of using a classification-based model is that it does not rely on the acuity of a patient's symptoms to drive the treatment process. A symptom acuity or time model often relies on time since injury, or time since onset of symptoms. If the time model was adequate, physical therapists would rarely treat patients with severe symptoms and/or inflammation, months or years after an injury occurred. Using the time model, all patients should be completely healed within 12 weeks of the initial injury, barring the effects of infection, etc. The vast majority of patients who present for physical therapy do not fit into this category.

Instead, the classification-based model uses 'staging' (Delitto et al 1995) in an attempt to classify patients into one of several categories during the initial evaluation. Staging also advocates the continuous reassessment of patients in order to determine if they warrant reclassification. This component of a classification-based model is ideal since patients typically see their physical therapist more frequently than they do their physician.

Staging is based on patient symptoms and functional disability (measured with disability indexes) in order to 'classify' patients. The use of patient-reported measures of disability (disability indexes) is a key component of the classification model and as such warrants further discussion. While there are numerous disability indexes available to clinicians, we will focus on two of the more clinician-friendly in classifying and treating patients with low-back pain – the Oswestry (ODI) and the FABQ.

The Oswestry Disability Index (Fairbank et al 1980) is one of the best-known disability indexes for use with patients with low-back pain. The ODI is a 10-item, 100-point index in which higher scores equate to more disability. It has been reported as reliable, valid and sensitive to change, and is universally accepted as the gold standard for low-back pain research (Kopec et al 1996, Deyo et al 1998). Moreover, it has a reported minimal clinically important difference (MCID) of 6 points (Fritz & Irrgang 2001), which allows the clinician to measure true change in a patient's status. Research has demonstrated that patients with a score of 12% or less are capable of returning to full occupational or recreational activities. The ODI takes approximately 3–5 minutes for a patient to complete and requires less than 30 seconds to score.

The Fear Avoidance Belief Questionnaire (FABQ) was originally described by Waddell et al (1993) and measures a patient's fear avoidance using two subscales: physical activity and work. The FABQ has been shown to predict disability and work loss, as well as future disability (Waddell et al 1993,

Hadijistavropoulos & Craig 1994, Klenerman et al 1995, Crombez et al 1999). The FABQ has also been shown to be a key component of a clinical prediction rule for low-back pain (Flynn et al 2002).

Both the ODI and FABQ are powerful tools that are appropriate for use in almost all orthopaedic physical therapy settings.

The treatment-based classification approach for the treatment of low-back pain (Delitto et al 1995) demonstrated that matching treatments to classifications resulted in faster, more efficient, and cost-effective care. The classification system is divided into three distinct stages:

1. Patients in Stage 1 are unable to perform basic functions (walk <1/4 mile, stand <15 minutes, sit <30 minutes) and typically have an ODI score between 40–60%. The primary goal of physical therapy during this stage is *pain modulation*.

2. Patients in Stage 2 are able to accomplish basic functions but are limited in their activities of daily living (ADLs). Their ODI scores typically fall between 20–40%. Physical therapy goals are to *continue to modulate pain and to begin addressing impairments*.

3. The third and final stage pertains to a patient's *inability to return to high-demand activity* such as manual labour or athletic competition. The ODI scores for patients in this stage are typically below 20% and the goal of physical

therapy should be to facilitate their return to their previous activity level. Muscle energy technique is a very effective intervention for patients in both Stages 1 and 2.

Further refinement of classification

Fritz et al (2003) modified the classification scheme originally described by Delitto and compared it with the Agency for Healthcare Research and Quality (AHCPR) guidelines. The authors randomised 76 subjects with work-related low-back pain of less than 3 weeks' duration into either the AHCPR group or the Classification group. Patients in the Classification group were placed into one of four categories: mobilisation, specific exercise, stabilisation, or traction (Fig. 9.1) based upon the most current physical examination criteria in the peer-reviewed literature (Table 9.1). Criteria for the mobilisation category included unilateral symptoms without signs of nerve root compression, asymmetrical lumbar side-bending restrictions, lumbar hypomobility and sacroiliac dysfunction. Patients in the AHCPR group received treatment based upon AHCPR guidelines (staying active, reassurance, low-stress aerobics, general muscle conditioning). ODI measures taken at intake and at 4 weeks demonstrated a statistically significant difference ($p = 0.031$) in favour of the Classification group. Return to work status was also measured at the 4-week mark demonstrating a statistically significant difference ($p = 0.017$) in favour of the Classification group.

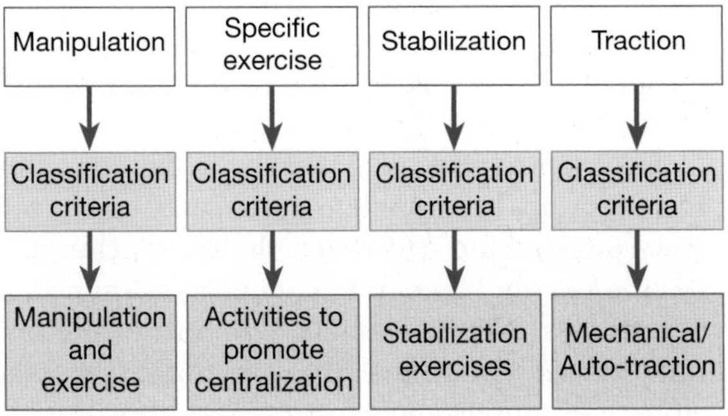

Figure 9.1   Modified treatment-based classification system for patients with LBP. (Adapted from Fritz et al 2003.)

Table 9.1   Classification criteria for mobilization category

Mobilization category	Examination findings
	Unilateral symptoms without signs of nerve root compression
Sacroiliac joint pattern	Positive findings for SI joint dysfunction using pelvic symmetry and standing and seated forward flexion tests
	Unilateral symptoms without signs of nerve root compression
Lumbar pattern	Assessment of lumbar side-bending asymmetry
	Lumbar hypomobility

Adapted from Fritz et al (2003)

In order for this treatment-based classification scheme to be successful the classification criteria for each of the four categories must be valid. Flynn et al (2002) investigated the factors that favoured success with SI joint manipulation in 75 patients with low-back pain. The authors developed a clinical prediction rule (CPR) based upon five factors:

- Duration of symptoms less than 16 days
- FABQ work subscale less than 19 points
- Symptoms not distal to the knee
- At least one hip with internal rotation greater than 35°
- Hypomobility and pain at one or more lumbar levels with posterior–anterior spring testing.

Flynn reported that the more factors present, the greater the chance of success with manipulation. For example, a patient with four out of five factors present would have 95% chance of success as opposed to 68% for a patient with only three factors present. While the CPR holds true regardless of which factors are present, the authors reported the most important factor for success was 'duration of symptoms less than 16 days' with a positive likelihood ratio of 4.3. Note these criteria differ significantly from the physical examination criteria used by Fritz et al (2003). This CPR was a critical step in establishing valid examination findings in order to subclassify patients with low-back pain into the mobilisation category.

The next step in confirming this CPR was performed by Childs et al (2004). The authors randomised 131 patients into either a manipulation and exercise group or an exercise only group. Each group received five treatments and follow-ups at 1 week, 4 weeks and 6 months. The manipulation/exercise group ($n = 70$) received manipulation and

range of motion exercises for the first two treatments and then stabilisation exercises for the last three treatments. The exercise group received stabilisation exercises only. Childs reported that a patient with four of the five factors reported by Flynn et al had a 92% chance of success with manipulation. Moreover, the authors reported an amazing 91% chance of success if the following two factors were present: no symptoms distal to the knee and pain duration of less than 16 days. The authors also reported that a patient presenting with symptoms distal to the knee only had a 12% chance of success with manipulation.

The authors also assessed the impact on health care utilisation during the 6-month follow-up. Missed time from work was reported by 9.6% of the manipulation/exercise group and by 25% of the exercise only group, and 11.5% of the manipulation/exercise group reported they were currently seeking care for their low-back pain as opposed to 42.5% of the exercise only group. By utilising these classification criteria, physical therapists can finally predict, with a large degree of certainty, which of our patients will and will not respond favourably to manual therapy.

The efficacy of manual therapy in the preceding research can be readily extrapolated to muscle energy technique. However, the direct effects of muscle energy technique have been examined in few studies. Wilson et al (2003) published the first randomised controlled trial to investigate the efficacy of muscle energy technique at the lumbar spine in symptomatic populations. Sixteen subjects (8 male, 8 female; ages 19–44) with low-back pain (duration 2–9 weeks) were randomised with stratification (age, gender, ODI score) into the control group ($n = 8$) or the experimental group

(n = 8). Each group received identical supervised neuromuscular re-education and strengthening exercises with the experimental group receiving the independent variable (muscle energy technique, four isometric repetitions). Each group received physical therapy twice a week for 4 weeks for a total of eight visits. ODI scores were obtained at the first and eighth visits. A two-tailed t-test revealed a statistically significant difference ($p > 0.05$) in favour of the experimental group. The mean number of muscle energy interventions required for the experimental group was 3.3 (range 2–4). This data supports what many clinicians have known for years: muscle energy technique is a reliable means to return patients to full activity in a quick and efficient manner.

The recent literature clearly demonstrates the efficacy of manual therapy, to include muscle energy technique, in the physical therapy setting. However, the literature demonstrates that not receiving physical therapy for acute low-back pain may increase the likelihood of the condition becoming chronic in nature (Hides et al 1994, 1996, 2001, Danneels et al 2001).

Danneels et al (2001) demonstrated that multifidus atrophy occurred in patients with chronic low-back pain, compared with asymptomatic controls. Patients with acute, unilateral low-back pain have multifidus atrophy correlated to the segment and side of their lumbar pain (Hides et al 1994, 1996). The authors also reported that the multifidus muscle's recovery is not 'automatic' after acute low-back pain. A longitudinal study conducted by Hides et al (2001) investigated the difference between patients with acute low-back pain who received standard medical management versus instruction on exercises focused on retraining the multifidus muscle. One- and three-year follow-ups demonstrated that the patients who received standard medical management had an 84% and 75% chance of an insidious recurrence of their pain at 1 and 3 years, respectively. Compare this to the 30% and 35% chance of recurrence (1- and 3-year follow-up) with the exercise group, and it is clear that multifidus muscle re-education is an important component in the successful long-term management of low-back pain. Muscle energy technique offers physical therapists a unique tool for the initial treatment of this problem.

Misconceptions in the literature

Physical therapists treat appendicular musculoskeletal impairments with a diverse and vast array of interventions and techniques. However, some clinicians treat spinal dysfunction as if it were an entity separate from the rest of the body. However, not all fault lies with the individual practitioners. Several prominent articles in the peer-reviewed literature have perpetuated the belief that the treatment of 'low-back pain' has its own set of rules, regardless of their contradictions to basic rehabilitative science. Some have even gone as far as to discredit the efficacy of physical therapy for patients with spinal pain. Therefore a brief discussion of articles that have been detrimental to the use of physical therapy to combat LBP is warranted. An understanding of each article's limitations is important for educating referral sources and patients alike.

The primary concern with the following two articles is that they perpetuate the belief that physical therapy is either not indicated for patients with low-back pain, or that it should only be tried after standard care by a general practitioner has failed. There is evidence in the literature supporting manual therapy and other physical therapy interventions in the treatment of low-back pain (Hadler et al 1987, MacDonald et al 1990, Spratt et al 1993, Stankovic & Johnell 1995, O'Sullivan et al 1997, Wilson et al 2003).

Unfortunately, clinical trials investigating their efficacy have not sought to determine which patients might benefit from a specific treatment (Dettori et al 1995, Faas et al 1995, Cherkin et al 1998). As one might expect, the results of these trials are usually not strong enough to advocate one intervention over another. This has led to the argument that physical therapy offers no advantage above standard care provided by general practitioners. This line of thought may skew the referral practice of general practitioners who would otherwise refer their patients with spinal pain to physical therapy. This causes two problems. First, delaying physical therapy care can impede the patients' recovery (Wilson et al 2003, Childs et al 2004). As is true of most medical conditions, whether a bacterial infection or an acute onset of low-back pain, the sooner the patient receives appropriate treatment the better the likelihood of that treatment's success. Finally, recent findings in the literature suggest that the impetus of chronic low-back pain can be linked to improperly managed acute low-back pain (Hides et al 1994, 1996, 2001).

Several authors have reported that 80–90% of patients with low-back pain will 'spontaneously' recover within 3 months (Faas et al 1993, Malanga & Nadler 1999). In light of this statement, one must question the odds of the 'spontaneous' recovery of a ruptured anterior cruciate ligament or of a flexor tendon tear in the same time period. While the overgeneralisation is obvious, one must question the validity of such statements instead of accepting them at face value.

Faas et al (1993) randomised 473 patients with acute, nonspecific low-back pain of less than 3 weeks' duration into one of three treatment groups: placebo, usual care by a general practitioner, and physical therapy. The authors concluded that 'patients who are referred to a physiotherapist for exercise therapy or to a back school in this way receive a lot of needless, expensive attention for complaints that in most cases would have disappeared spontaneously anyway'. A critical review of this study identified limitations in the use of the Nottingham Health Profile Questionnaire as an outcome measure, assessment of patient compliance, and in the authors' rationale for their choice of physical therapy intervention – Williams' flexion exercises. The results of this study are limited to the lack of demonstrated efficacy of Williams' flexion exercises and should not be extrapolated to the profession of physical therapy in the treatment of low-back pain. Unfortunately, this article has made many

health care providers sceptical regarding physical therapy's efficacy in treating this impairment. A comprehensive review of this article can be found in Appendix A.

Cherkin et al (1998) compared the efficacy of physical therapy, chiropractic care, and an educational booklet in patients with acute low-back pain. Three hundred and twenty-one patients were randomised without stratification into three treatment groups as follows: McKenzie treatment by physical therapists, high-velocity/low-amplitude (HVLA) thrust spinal manipulation by chiropractors, and an educational booklet provided by general practitioners. Patients who sought care from a primary care physician who continued to have pain 7 days after consultation were eligible for inclusion in this study. These potential subjects were screened by research assistants utilising the SF-36 health survey questionnaire and a list of exclusion criteria that included sciatica. The authors reported that patients receiving physical therapy and chiropractic care had only slightly better outcomes than patients in the booklet group that only neared significance ($p = 0.05$) at the 1-year follow-up. A critical review of this study revealed limitations in the use of a 'bothersome' scale as an outcome measure, discrepancies between the number of treatments in the McKenzie and chiropractic groups and the lack of control for exercise in the chiropractic and booklet groups. The limitations in this study's design weaken the authors' conclusions that physical therapy and spinal manipulation are no better than an educational booklet for patients with acute low-back pain. A comprehensive review of this article can be found in Appendix A.

Appendix A: REVIEWS OF STUDIES

Faas et al (1993)

The subjects in Faas' study were randomly divided into one of three groups. The placebo group ($n = 162$) received pulsed, non-thermal ultrasound at 0.1 W/cm^2 for 20 minutes per session, two times a week for 5 weeks. No other information or counselling was provided to the patients in this group. The general practitioner group ($n = 155$) was provided analgesics on demand as well as information pertaining to low-back pain. This consisted primarily of the importance of heat, physical activity and the need for consistent follow-up

visits. The general practitioners participating in this study were trained in the course of low-back pain. The physical therapy group ($n = 156$) met twice a week for 5 weeks. Each session lasted 20 minutes and consisted of individual instruction by a physical therapist involving Williams' flexion exercises.

The authors selected the Nottingham Health Profile Questionnaire (NHQ) and an 85 cm visual analogue scale (VAS) for pain as their dependent variables. The use of the NHQ as an outcome measure is questionable based on

Appendix A: Continued

research comparisons with other tools. The NHQ measures perceived health (Jenkinson & Fitzpatrick 1990) and has been compared with the General Health Questionnaire (GHQ), which measures non-psychotic psychiatric disturbances, in two studies (McKenna & Payne 1989, Jenkinson & Fitzpatrick 1990). The NHQ and GHQ have been used to determine the health of unemployed and re-employed workers (McKenna & Payne 1989) and more recently to determine the perceived health of rheumatoid arthritis and migraine headache sufferers (Jenkinson & Fitzpatrick 1990) at which time the authors reported that the NHQ had difficulty in accurately measuring pain.

The NHQ did not correlate well with the SF-36 for emotional and mental health issues when compared on elderly subjects with chronic airways limitation (Crockett et al 1996) and demonstrated less sensitivity to change than the SF-36 on long-term myocardial infarction survivors (Brown et al 2000). A Medline search from 1980 to present revealed no studies that attempted to establish the reliability or validity of the NHQ for patients with low-back pain by comparing it with the Oswestry or Roland-Morris disability indices. Moreover, the literature has clearly demonstrated that generic functional status questionnaires are not as sensitive to change as region-specific questionnaires such as the Oswestry or the Roland-Morris. Finally, according to the systematic review on LBP published by van Tulder et al (2000) the NHQ was specifically listed as a secondary outcome measure while the authors considered region-specific questionnaires, such as the Oswestry, to be primary outcome measures. The use of the NHQ as the dependent variable for this study weakens the design and brings into question the study's conclusions.

Faas et al chose Williams' flexion exercises as their independent variable for physical therapy intervention. The authors chose flexion exercises over extension exercises because 'it is questionable whether extension exercises should have a place in the treatment of acute low back pain' (Faas et al 1993). The authors cited a 1990 study (Stankovic & Johnell 1990) as the only research that demonstrated the positive results of extension exercise. The authors pointed to several design flaws in this study such as the absence of a placebo group and discrepancies between treatment durations.

However, Faas et al do not report the 1984 study comparing Williams' flexion and McKenzie's extension protocols (Ponte et al 1984). Ponte and colleagues found that patients who received the McKenzie protocol had a significant improvement ($p > 0.001$) in outcome measures in a significantly ($p > 0.01$) shorter amount of time. Comparing the studies by Faas and Ponte revealed similar patient inclusion and exclusion criteria resulting in patient populations that were almost identical in regard to symptom location and duration, history of previous symptoms, and age range. Patients also received a similar number of treatments prior to post-treatment evaluation. After reviewing the study by Ponte, it would seem inappropriate for Faas to discount the positive effects of extension exercises for patients in this specific population.

A further concern in the choice of flexion exercises was the lack of specific diagnostic criteria. Faas made no report of the evaluative process the patients underwent. Instead, they were diagnosed with nonspecific low-back pain and provided with flexion exercises. The authors also did not report the parameters of the physical therapy interventions. Information such as number of repetitions performed, duration and intensity of each exercise and increases in range of motion or strength would have been beneficial and necessary if replication of the study was desired.

Compliance with a home-based exercise programme was also an issue in this study. The authors determined that patients who had performed at least one exercise within 4 weeks were compliant with their home programme. One dosage of any intervention within a 4-week period, whether exercise-based or pharmacological, is a minimal definition of compliant.

Faas stated that the outcome measures demonstrated that there were no positive effects of physical therapy, and concluded that physical therapy was not recommended for patients with nonspecific low-back pain. However, given the limitations identified in regard to outcome measure and physical therapy intervention selection, it is not reasonable to conclude that physical therapy for acute low-back pain is contraindicated based upon the results of this study.

Cherkin et al (1998)

In Cherkin's study, the physical therapy group received McKenzie extension exercises from 13 physical therapists with a median of 14 years' experience. All but one had successfully completed the advanced McKenzie credentialing examination and all were trained by faculty from the McKenzie Institute prior to the study. Ninety-two percent of the patients were treated for 'derangement syndrome'. Treatment for derangement syndrome attempts to teach patients positions and postures that centralise their symptoms and emphasises self-care. Physical therapists were asked to refrain from using adjunct modalities; however, no control for this was mentioned. Patients were allowed a maximum of nine treatments in a 4-week period. The frequency of these treatments was left to the discretion of the therapist.

Appendix A: Continued

Chiropractic care was provided by four chiropractors. HVLA was the only chiropractic intervention authorised, although the chiropractors were allowed to make recommendations regarding activity and prescribe both clinic and home-based flexibility and strengthening exercises. Like the patients in the physical therapy group, the patients were allowed a maximum of nine treatments in a 4-week period with frequency left to the discretion of the chiropractor.

Patients in the booklet group received an educational booklet that addressed the causes of back pain and recommended activities to facilitate healing and to prevent re-injury. The authors do not report on specific activities recommended to the patients in this group. Cherkin stated that patient-reported use of exercise was approximately equal between the three groups at baseline (57%) as well as at 1 month (81%). However, the authors did not report any control used to prevent patients in the booklet group from exercising prior to the completion of the study. Better reporting of this information would assist the reader in evaluating the differences between the control and treatment groups.

Much like the study by Faas, the study by Cherkin et al had some significant limitations in design. Ninety-two percent of the patients in the physical therapy group were treated for 'derangement syndrome' as defined by McKenzie. This treatment attempts to centralise a patient's symptoms. This centralisation only occurs in patients with derangement syndromes (Riddle & Rothstein 1993) and not in patients classified in McKenzie's other two syndromes: postural and dysfunctional. Of the seven sub-categories of derangement syndrome, buttock and/or thigh pain can be present in six categories, pain below the knee in two categories and neurologic deficits are seen in one category (Riddle & Rothstein 1993). However, patients with a diagnosis of 'sciatica' were excluded from participating in this study.

The authors used a modified Roland-Morris Disability Questionnaire and an 11-point 'bothersome' scale as their dependent variables. The 'bothersome' scale ranged from zero to 10 with scores of zero reflecting symptoms that were 'not bothersome at all' and scores of 10 reflecting symptoms that were 'extremely bothersome'. The authors cited a study conducted by Patrick et al (1995) that used a 'similar scale' with 'substantial construct validity' (Cherkin et al 1998). Given the previous research on the bothersome scale, it does not appear to be an appropriate outcome measure for this study.

A careful review of the study by Patrick et al revealed several discrepancies between the scale used by Patrick and the one referenced and described by Cherkin. First and foremost, the scale used by Patrick was designed to assess the frequency and 'bothersomeness' of back and lower extremity symptoms in patients with sciatica. The authors' inclusion criterion was a diagnosis of sciatica made by a surgeon and they defined sciatica as 'symptoms and findings considered to be secondary to herniation of a lumbar intervertebral disc' (Patrick et al 1995). As previously stated, patients with sciatica or with 'severe neurologic signs' were excluded from participating in the study performed by Cherkin.

The original 'bothersome' scale as described by Patrick was a seven-point rating scale that was used at 3 months follow-up, whereas Cherikin used an 11-point scale at follow-up times of 3 months, 1 year and 2 years. The generalisability of Patrick's bothersomeness scale to Cherkin's population is questionable.

Cherkin reported that patients receiving physical therapy and chiropractic care had only slightly better outcomes than patients in the booklet group that only neared significance ($p = 0.05$) at the 1-year follow-up. Based upon a critical review of this article and the articles cited in this study, the authors' conclusions do not appear to be a valid reflection of the use of physical therapy or spinal manipulative therapy in the treatment of acute low-back pain.

Clinical utilisation of muscle energy technique

Traditionally, muscle energy technique has been utilised to break the pain/spasm cycle as described by Roland (1986), restore normal structure and function to a joint or motion segment (often overlapping with breaking the pain/spasm cycle), and strengthen previously inhibited and/or weakened muscles. This paradigm can be easily shifted to follow the classification model previously reported by Delitto and colleagues. Recall that the stages of the classification system involve pain modulation (Stage 1), pain modulation and addressing impairments (Stage 2) and facilitating return to high-demand activities (Stage 3). Muscle energy technique is an exceptional intervention for patients in the first two of these stages.

Staging

Clinical correlation: LBP and ankle sprains

Most physical therapists who work in an outpatient orthopaedic setting feel comfortable treating a patient with an ankle sprain. The same principles used to treat an ankle sprain can be used to treat a patient with a spinal dysfunction. Let's quickly compare the two injuries and their treatments. When a patient sustains an acute ankle injury, the physical therapist will typically utilise the PRICE mnemonic (protect, rest, ice, compression, elevation) during the initial treatment in order to limit the effects of the injury and to reduce pain. This coincides with Stage 1 of Delitto's classification model.

Stage 1: Pain modulation

We typically modulate pain at the injured ankle by placing the patient on a partial or non-weight-bearing status, as well as the use of either tape or a brace. These treatments serve to keep stresses off of the injured tissues, primarily the ligaments and joint capsule. When a patient injures their back we can use muscle energy technique to protect the area by restoring normal structure and function to the joint (taking the stresses off of the soft tissues) and by decreasing pain. Muscle energy technique is an excellent intervention for breaking the pain/spasm cycle. Passive manual therapy techniques (e.g. joint mobilisations, high-velocity/low-amplitude (HVLA) thrust techniques) assist in breaking the pain/spasm cycle by inhibiting alpha motor-neuron activity via a stretch reflex (Indahl et al 1997, Dishman & Bulbulian 2000). This inhibition has been shown to last from 2 seconds to 6 minutes (Dishman & Bulbulian 2000). Muscle energy technique not only inhibits the alpha motor neuron, but the technique's gentle stretching also inhibits Ia afferent nerves via post-activation depression. This is due to muscle energy technique's ability to decrease the sensitivity of muscle spindles to stretch. This effect has been shown to last for more than 2 days (Avela et al 1999a, 1999b). This evidence fortifies the argument for the use of MET over other techniques in that the effects are not only longer lasting, but also in that MET resolves the pain/spasm cycle by acting on both the efferent and afferent nerves. This is particularly true at the lumbar spine where

afferents from nocioceptors synapse with alpha motor neurons of the spinal extensors.

One of the concerns many practitioners have regarding muscle energy technique is that it can be time consuming to apply to a patient with multiple segmental levels of dysfunction. During the pain modulation stage, muscle energy technique can be viewed as the follow-on treatment of choice after utilising a general/non-specific HVLA manipulation technique at the spinal region of interest. An example would be a patient with right-sided low-back pain without symptoms distal to the knee. The practitioner could perform a right sacroiliac joint gapping HVLA in order to clear up the compensatory spinal and/or SI joint dysfunctions and upon reassessment, discover the location of the primary dysfunction and treat it with muscle energy technique. A point should be made that the muscle energy technique is not the ancillary intervention in this scenario. The non-specific HVLA is being used to 'clean up' the clinical picture so the physical therapist can more quickly identify the location of the primary dysfunction. Once identified, the segment can be more effectively treated with muscle energy technique because the adjacent spinal segments will not act as a 'dirty lever' throughout the treatment. Also, recall that the HVLA can attenuate the alpha motor-neuron activity for up to 6 minutes. The practitioner can use this small window of analgesia to their advantage in the application of muscle energy technique.

Other interventions can be applied beforehand to 'clean up' or 'set up' the muscle energy technique instead of HVLA. Grade 1 or 2 posterior–anterior (PA) joint mobilisations can be applied over the spinous processes or the facet joints of the spinal region. These reduce alpha motor-neuron activity via the stretch reflex as previously discussed. The practitioner can also use several modalities as a pre-treatment such as ice packs, ice massage or brief/intense transcutaneous electrical nerve stimulation (TENS). Ice massage is one of the favoured pre-treatments in the sports medicine setting since it can decrease Type C afferent nerve fibre activity, decrease local inflammation and modulate pain via the gate control theory, and the time to maximum effect is considerably less than that of an ice pack.

For these reasons, an ice massage is also an excellent choice for a post-muscle energy technique intervention (if it was not used during the pre-treatment). Post-treatment interventions allow the practitioner to obtain longer-lasting results from the primary intervention, especially if a patient must return to occupational activities immediately following the treatment session. Particular focus should be paid to interventions that inhibit pain and/or spasm. Examples include TENS, ice, and analgesic balms. Finally, the benefits of muscle energy technique can be prolonged by prescribing a specific home exercise programme (HEP). A HEP specific to the patient's dysfunction can decrease the number of muscle energy technique sessions required to return the patient to full activity (Wilson et al 2003).

Stage 2: Pain modulation and addressing impairments

Returning to the analogy of the ankle sprain, most physical therapists will attempt to promote and facilitate the proliferation phase of tissue healing by applying gentle, controlled forces to the soft tissues in a pain-free range once the inflammation has subsided. The practitioner can provide the same treatment to a patient with spinal dysfunction by utilising muscle energy technique in a segment-specific strengthening role. It is important to consider that most patients with an ankle sprain will continue to report slight to moderate pain during this time and we should expect the same from our patients with spinal pain at the onset of this stage.

Muscle energy technique is highly effective in treating spinal impairments by restoring normal structure and function to a joint and/or motion segment. There are numerous theories on how these 'joint dysfunctions' occur. The two more credible theories pertain to either a dysfunction of the spine's intersegmental muscles or the facet joint/capsule. These two theories overlap in numerous ways thus creating a 'chicken or the egg' question. Understanding the basics of these theories and their underlying biomechanical and neurological principles can be a major advantage in the treatment of patients with spinal pain.

Intersegmental muscles   An alteration in the length and/or tone of the intersegmental muscles (e.g. intertransversarii, rotatores and multifidi) can cause numerous compounding problems. These 'short restrictors' can act as a biomechanical tether (Greenman 1996) at a motion segment. This shifts the motion segment's axis of rotation posteriorly from the vertebral body to the facet joint. Therefore, the means by which the motion segment attenuates and distributes forces across the joint surfaces becomes altered. This 'tethering' also places prolonged strain on the static restraints of the motion segment. These structures are richly innervated, primarily by the major and lesser descending branches of the sinovertebral nerve, and thus can become a major contributor to the patient's pain. The primary role of the intersegmental muscles is proprioception, as they lack both the size and the biomechanical advantage of the prime movers of the spine. A dysfunction of these muscles can lead to incorrect afferent input to the central nervous system, resulting in a distorted view of the spatial relationships of the motion segments. This can lead to an ineffective use and/or disuse of the primary dynamic stabilisers of the spine (Hides et al 2001).

Facet joint   The facet joint and its capsule can cause significant pain and dysfunction. When the axis of rotation of a dysfunctional segment moves posteriorly to the facet joint, the entire motion segment must pivot upon the now-engaged facet joint surfaces. In the lumbar spine, the facet joints are accustomed to accepting only 15% (Porterfield & DeRosa 1998a) of the axial load placed upon the motion segment. When the axis of rotation shifts, the facet joint surfaces become maximally engaged. As loads continue to increase, shear forces develop across the joint surfaces. This shearing can cause damage to the hyaline cartilage of these synovial joints, thus creating another pain mechanism. This continued loading can also lead to stresses at the facet joint capsule which can cause altered afferent input to the central nervous system from the type 1 mechanoreceptors within the capsule. The effects of this mechanism are similar to that of the intersegmental muscles.

The application of muscle energy techniques can reverse the effects of both of these theoretical causes of joint dysfunction. The contract–relax mechanism of muscle energy technique on intersegmental muscles unbinds the motion segment, thus relieving the stresses on the joint capsule and other static restraints. The ability of muscle energy technique to mobilise a motion segment within a pain-free range causes a stretch reflex to occur at the facet joint capsule. This results in an inhibition of alpha motor-neuron activity which effectively relaxes the dynamic 'tetherers' of the motion segment. Muscle energy technique effectively utilises the biomechanical and neurological components of the motion segment to reverse the effects of joint dysfunction by treating the cause, not the symptoms, of the impairment.

Muscle energy technique is the intervention of choice to continue to modulate pain during Stage 2. Patients will typically present with only a few dysfunctions, so the treatment is not as time consuming as it would have been in Stage 1. The use of muscle energy technique will also allow the patient to be more active, since its effects typically last longer than passive treatments. This is an important consideration. As patients increase their activity levels, they also increase the loading and the stress to the injured tissues. Muscle energy technique can often keep an active (or even an overactive) patient in Stage 2, whereas they might regress to Stage 1 if a passive technique was used instead.

Addressing impairments: segmental-specific strengthening

There are numerous ways in which strength training can be incorporated into the rehabilitation of patients with joint and/or motion segment dysfunctions. While many practitioners view strength training as a separate entity, many clinicians and researchers alike, advocate the importance of a seamless transition from manual therapy interventions to resistance exercise prescription (Hides et al 1996, 2001, O'Sullivan et al 1997, Wilson 2001, Wilson et al 2003, Childs et al 2004) as well as the use of precision strength training exercises focused at specific levels of spinal segment dysfunction (Hides 2004).

Utilising muscle energy technique as an initial means of strength training is a vital bridge between manual therapy and resistance exercise prescription. The technique should be used only after the patient

has progressed from Stage 1 to Stage 2 and the corrective muscle energy technique (or other manual therapy intervention) has successfully broken the pain/spasm cycle and/or restored normal structure and function to the motion segment. Wilson (2003) reported that patients with acute low-back pain required an average of only three muscle energy technique sessions for normal structure to be restored to the motion segments of the lumbar spine.

The need for segmental-specific strengthening is based on the neurological process of reciprocal innervation. Reciprocal innervation is a process, controlled at the spinal cord level, in which the activation of an agonist muscle causes immediate inhibition of its antagonist muscle(s). As previously stated, a dysfunction at a spinal motion segment can be explained by several theories. However, a common underlying component of these theories involves the inhibition of muscles due to either a tethering/tightening effect on their antagonists or via inhibition from the stretch reflex at a facet capsule or both (Gordon 1991, Greenman 1996, Indahl et al 1997).

Recent research has demonstrated a need for segmental specific re-education in order for the lumbar multifidus musculature to recover from an acute injury (Hides 2004). Using muscle energy technique provides an excellent, albeit time-consuming, method of selectively targeting and strengthening previously inhibited muscles. The physical therapy setting is the ideal environment to utilise this intervention, especially in areas where physicians are hit hard by managed care and third-party payer restrictions. Performing segmental-specific strength training requires the same skills needed to perform the corrective manual therapy technique. Therefore, it should not be delegated to an assistant or a technician, nor should it be provided as a home exercise programme.

To reduce confusion, the quadrant method is a simple and effective technique for remembering how to treat a patient with segmental-specific strengthening exercises. An example of the quadrant method can be found in Fig. 9.2. By using this technique, the patient is placed in the opposite position to that in which they received the corrective muscle energy technique procedure. Therefore, if a patient had an extended, right-rotated, right side-bent (ERS right) restriction at L4 and was treated in right side-

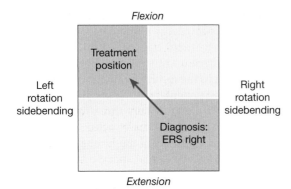

Figure 9.2 Quadrant method for segment-specific strength training.

lying to correct the dysfunction (Fig. 9.3), he/she would be placed in left side-lying, as if being treated for a flexed, left-rotated, left side-bent (FRS left) restriction at L4 (Fig. 9.4B–9.4E). The rationale for this is simple. A patient with an ERS right at L4 has a tightness or hypertonicity of the extensors, right rotators and right side-benders at the L4 motion segment. This hypertonicity causes an inhibition (via the reciprocal inhibition mechanism) of the flexors, left rotators and left side-benders at L4. If allowed to persist, this inhibition can quickly lead to disuse atrophy. By placing the patient in left side-lying as if treating an FRS left allows the practitioner to isolate the flexors, left rotators and left side-benders with the muscle energy technique. The only difference between the

corrective technique and the *strengthening* technique is that the practitioner does not take the slack out of the motion segment after each contraction.

Positioning for segmental-specific strengthening

Patient positioning is an important consideration during this procedure. While muscle energy technique can be performed in numerous positions, it is advantageous to have the patient lie on the same side as the inhibited muscles (left side-lying for an 'FRS left'). This position will require the clinician to hold the patient's lower extremity against gravity. If the technique were performed with the patient on the right side, the patient would have to assist the clinician in holding the leg against gravity and an over-riding contraction of the prime mover muscles would be elicited.

Isolation of effort: three-finger stacking

It is very important to isolate the motion segment in question while performing this technique. To do this, the practitioner should incorporate a three-finger 'stacked' palpation method (Fig. 9.4). This is done by placing the pad of the 3rd digit over the spinous process of the segment in question and the pads of the 2nd and 4th digits over the spinous processes of the segments above and below. This will allow the practitioner to quickly determine

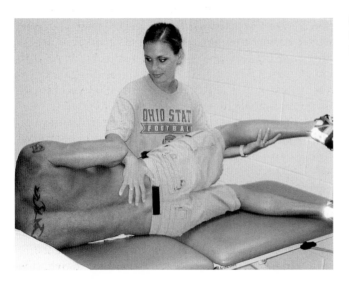

Figure 9.3 Segmental-specific strengthening of ERS right dysfunction at L4. Patient being treated in left side-lying for FRS left.

whether the motion has been isolated to the motion segment. This principle is based on Fryette's third law of spinal motion: the more motion you introduce into a motion segment from one plane, the less motion you will be able to introduce from other planes. The three-finger stacked method allows the clinician to feel the motion coming to the segment with the first finger, feel the motion at the segment of interest with the middle finger, and determine if any motion has 'spilled over' with the third finger.

For example, using the above illustration of an FRS left at L4, the patient lies on the left side facing the practitioner.

Finger placement The practitioner would place the pad of the right 3rd finger over the spinous process of L4 with the 2nd finger over the spinous process of L5 and the 4th finger over the spinous process of L3 (Fig. 9.4A).

Introduction of extension The practitioner would then fully flex the patient's hips and then slowly move them into extension (Fig. 9.4B). Since motion (extension) is being introduced from the 'bottom up', the examiner's 2nd finger (over the spinous process of L5) would be the first to palpate the motion, followed by the 3rd finger at L4. When the examiner begins to palpate the initial motion at L3 (4th finger), the process is stopped and a slight amount of flexion at the hips is introduced until the motion is felt moving inferior to L3 and back into the L4 motion segment. The examiner would then begin to introduce motion from the 'top down' by flexing the patient's trunk. Some practitioners will continue to palpate with the right hand and reach across with the left arm in order to extend the patient's trunk. This is bad tradecraft as the position does not allow the practitioner the degree of fine control required to isolate the motion segment, especially in a highly symptomatic patient.

The examiner should switch hands, placing the 3rd finger of the left hand over the spinous process of L4 and the 4th and 2nd fingers over the spinous processes of L5 and L3 respectively. The examiner would then extend the patient's trunk until motion was palpated under the 2nd finger at L3 and continue as described above until L4 was isolated (Fig. 9.4C).

Introduction of right rotation The examiner can now use the right hand to introduce right rotation down to L4 by rotating the patient at the shoulder (Fig. 9.4D). The examiner would first palpate the motion under the 2nd finger of the left hand (L3) and then under the 3rd finger as the motion entered the L4 motion segment. Many practitioners advocate introducing rotation prior to introducing the sagittal plane motion; however, it is much more difficult to isolate the motion segment this way. The sagittal plane motion (extension in this example) provides a natural stopping point for the rotation, making the isolation of the motion segment easier.

Introduction of right side-bending The practitioner will switch hands once again and place the right hand over the spinous processes of interest as described above. The patient's right leg should be grasped at the knee and hip abduction (right side-bending) will be introduced (Fig. 9.4E). Recall that Fryette's third law stipulates that very little motion will be required to finish isolating the motion segment since two planes of motion have already been introduced into the motion segment. As the right leg is abducted, the examiner will feel the motion (coming from 'bottom up') first under the 2nd finger (L5) as it moves up to L4. The motion segment is now isolated and is ready for the first muscle contraction.

Muscle activation It is important for the patient to provide a very small contraction. The focus is to strengthen the small intersegmental muscles. These will quickly become overpowered by the larger prime mover muscles if too great a contraction is elicited. The clinician should bear in mind that the core musculature will activate before the periphery, therefore the muscle contraction should be measured in 'ounces' (grams) instead of 'pounds' (kilos). The following are some examples of useful instructions to give to the patient:

- 'Meet my force as I pull your leg towards the ceiling, but do not overpower me.'
- 'Push into my hand as if you were pushing on an egg you did not want to break.'

The practitioner should be careful to note the location of the muscle contraction in relation to the

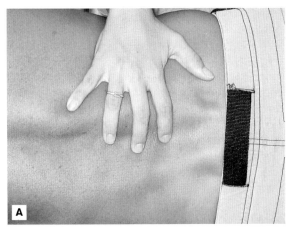

Figure 9.4 Three-finger stacked palpation technique. **A** Right hand on spine, 3rd digit on L4. **B** Right hand on spine, introduce extension at hips. **C** Left hand on spine, introduce extension at trunk. **D** Left hand on spine, introduce right rotation at right shoulder. **E** Right hand on spine, introduce right side-bending at hip (right LE abducted).

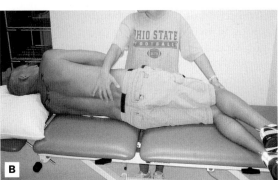

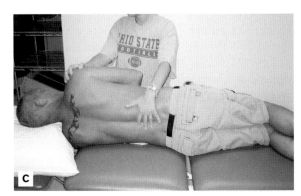

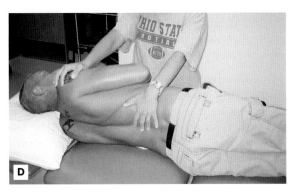

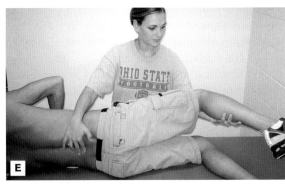

spinal segment. Any contraction felt along the paraspinal musculature is indicative of too strong a contraction. It is important that the clinician observe for compensatory movements or muscle activation during these exercises. Typically, patients will attempt to compensate at a region other than their back (legs, chest, neck, shoulders). A patient that is unable to cease this compensatory activity is no longer receiving a benefit, and the exercise set should be concluded.

Progressing the process

There are numerous ways to progress this exercise programme. While individual tastes will vary, it is important to keep several factors in mind. Segmental-specific strengthening should have three distinct focuses or phases:

1. Neuromuscular re-education
2. Hypertrophy
3. Endurance.

The focus of the exercise can be changed by manipulating some basic parameters of exercise prescription: number of sets, duration of each set, total time of each contraction, type of contraction, rest intervals between sets (Table 9.2). It should be noted that sets are measured in time and not repetitions. This will allow the clinician to focus on training energy systems within the muscle while allowing the patient to focus on the quality of each repetition instead of the quantity. The clinician should focus on training the fast glycolysis and oxidative energy systems since these muscles need to be active in all anti-gravity positions. (Porterfield & DeRosa 1998b) The following contains an overview of the process. An example with detailed step-by-step instructions can be found in Appendix B.

Rest intervals are easily overlooked, but their importance is critical, especially during the neuromuscular re-education focus when a work:rest ratio of 1:12 to 1:20 between sets is advocated. These prolonged rest periods will allow an almost, if not a complete, recovery of the muscles' energy system before the next set is performed (Komi 1986, Stone & Conley 1994). It is imperative to avoid overworking these muscles during the neuromuscular re-education phase of this programme. The intersegmental muscles will fatigue quickly and this may lessen their ability to prevent the dysfunction from returning. Appropriate follow-ups should be scheduled to ensure the patient does not have a reoccurrence of their dysfunction during this period. Progression criteria from neuromuscular re-education to the muscle hypertrophy phase should be based on the patient's ability to perform all contractions without pain or fatigue.

The muscle hypertrophy phase consists of isometric and/or concentric contractions held for 5 seconds. These should be performed for 3–6 sets with each set lasting between 15 and 30 seconds. A work:rest ratio of 1:3 to 1:5 is indicated to focus on the fast glycolytic system (Stone & Conley 1994). The patient should be encouraged to perform *active rest* between each set, such as walking on a treadmill or around the treatment area. It has been shown that light activity during the post-exercise period can enhance lactate clearance from the trained muscles (Stone & Conley 1994). This is of prime importance when training the fast glycolysis energy system. The three-finger stacked technique is useful when performing concentric contractions as it will let the clinician know when the motion has passed through the motion segment of interest. The endurance phase consists of isometric, concentric, and/or eccentric exercises with 4–8 sets lasting between 1 and 3 minutes each. This phase will focus on both the fast glycolytic and oxidative energy systems with a recommended work:rest ratio of 1:3 to 1:4 (Stone & Conley 1994).

Parameters

There are three independent parameters that should be included as well:

1. Patient position
2. Surface stability
3. Motion resisted.

These parameters (Fig. 9.5) are progressed independent of one another with the patient's desired return to activity as a primary determining force. *Patient positioning* progresses from long to short

Table 9.2 Segmental strengthening progression: basic exercise parameters

Phase	Contraction type	Contraction duration (seconds)	Duration of set (seconds)	Sets	Rest interval between sets (work:rest)
Re-education	Isometric	1–2	5–10	2–4	1:12–1:20
Hypertrophy	Isometric Concentric	5	15–30	3–6	1:3–1:5
Endurance	Isometric Concentric Eccentric	5	60–180	4–8	1:3–1:4

Appendix B: SEGMENTAL STRENGTHENING PROGRAMME

Part 1: Neuromuscular re-education

Patient treated with corrective technique for ERS right at L4.

Patient treated with segmental strengthening in FRS left (L4) position.

Isolate motion segment as previously described.

1st set (total time: 5–10 seconds):
Instruct the patient to perform a gentle, isometric contraction for 1–2 seconds.
Rest for 1 second and ask the patient to produce another contraction.
Continue for a total of 5–10 seconds.

Rest period:
Rest for approximately 1–3 minutes (work:rest ratio 1:12–1:20).

Additional sets (2–4 total):
Perform remaining sets and rest periods as described.

Criteria to progress to hypertrophy phase:
Perform all reps and sets without pain or fatigue.

Part 2: Hypertrophy

Isolate motion segment as described.

1st set (total time: 15–30 seconds):
Instruct patient to perform gentle isometric or concentric contraction (Box 9B.1) for 5 seconds.
Rest for 1 second and ask the patient to perform another contraction.
Continue for a total of 15–30 seconds.

Rest period:
Rest for approximately 45 seconds to 3 minutes depending on the length of the set.
Instruct the patient to walk around the clinic during the rest period in order to facilitate lactate clearance from the muscles.

Additional sets (3–6 total):
Perform remaining sets and rest periods as described.
Criteria to progress to endurance phase.
Perform six 30-second sets at 1:3 work:rest ratio without pain or fatigue.

Box 9B.1 Concentric and eccentric contractions

Concentric contractions
- Remember the muscles being trained are very small, therefore they do not require a lot of motion.
- Use the three-finger stacked technique to determine when the concentric contraction has left the motion segment. Stop at this time and use the brief interlude between repetitions to reposition the patient.

Eccentric contractions
- Begin with the motion segment isolated at the 'bottom' of the available motion.
- Instruct the patient to 'gently resist' your force: 'I am going to slowly raise your leg to the ceiling. I want you to gently resist this motion. I am going to slightly overpower your force.' This will produce an eccentric contraction.

Part 3: Endurance phase

Isolate motion segment:
Motion segment isolation for eccentric contraction.
Place motion segment at 'bottom' of available motion.

In the example of treating a patient in left side-lying (FRS left) position:
Feel for motion entering the L5 motion segment (2nd finger of right hand).
Slowly add motion until the initial motion is palpated at L4: do not continue past this point
1st set (total time: 1–3 minutes)
Instruct patient to perform gentle isometric, concentric or eccentric contraction (Box 9B.1) for 5 seconds.
Rest for 1 second and ask the patient to perform another contraction.
Continue for a total of 1–3 minutes.

Rest period:
Rest for approximately 3–12 minutes depending on the length of the set.
Instruct the patient to walk around the clinic during the rest period in order to facilitate lactate clearance from the muscles.

Additional sets (4–8 total):
Perform remaining sets and rest periods as described.

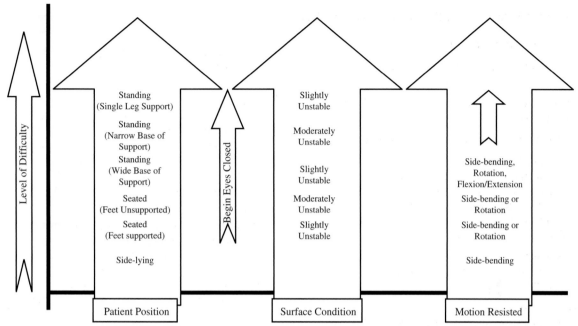

Figure 9.5 Three independent parameters for segmental strengthening programme. Slightly unstable: foam roll, bolster, Dyna-Disc, trampoline, etc. Moderately unstable: exercise ball, foam wedge, etc.

Appendix C: PATIENT POSITIONS

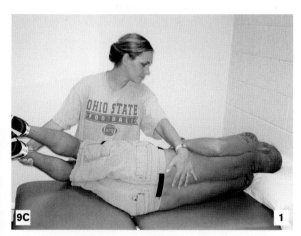

Figure 9C.1 ERS right side-lying.

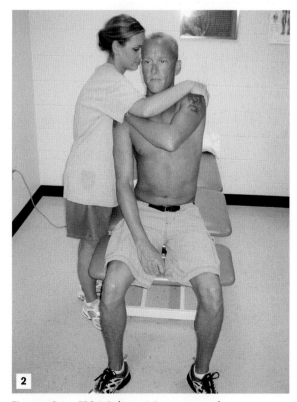

Figure 9C.2 FRS left (seated feet supported).

lever-arms and from an unloaded to a loaded spine. Utilising long lever-arms (legs) that the clinician supports against gravity makes it easier for weakened muscles to fire without fatigue. It is imperative the patient be trained with their spine in a loaded position in order to decrease the likelihood of their impairment becoming a chronic condition (Hides 2004). Examples of these positions can be found in Appendix C.

Patient surfaces should progress from stable to unstable once the patient is capable of performing the exercise in the seated position (Appendix D). Unstable surfaces should progress from uniplanar (foam rolls, bolsters) to multiplanar (trampoline, Dyna-Disc, exercise ball) and uniplanar surfaces

should be used in multiple axes, especially the oblique. Adding a change to the surface should be done on a set-by-set basis depending on the individual patient's tolerance.

Finally, the *motion being resisted* (side-bending, rotation, flexion, extension) can be manipulated. The programme should begin by resisting single-plane motions, primarily side-bending and rotation. The spinal flexors and extensors have an incredible mechanical advantage over the intersegmental muscles and they will most likely override any initial attempts to isolate the intersegmental muscles. For this reason, resisting the sagittal plane muscles should not be incorporated in the programme until the patient has progressed to the standing

Appendix C: Continued

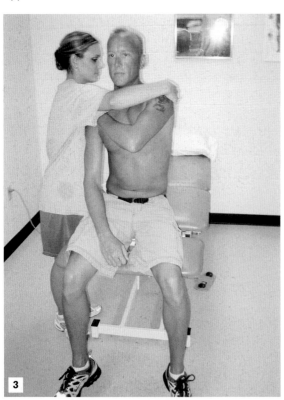

Figure 9C.3   FRS left (seated feet unsupported).

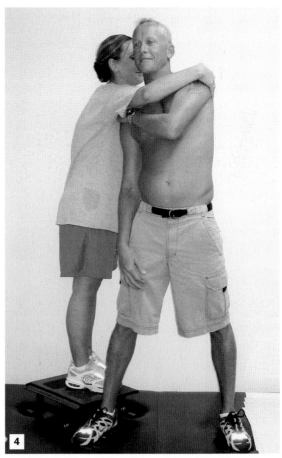

Figure 9C.4   FRS left standing (wide base of support) showing PT standing on box or treatment table.

Appendix C: Continued

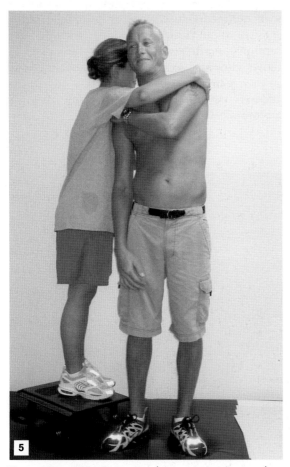

Figure 9C.5   FRS left standing (narrow base of support).

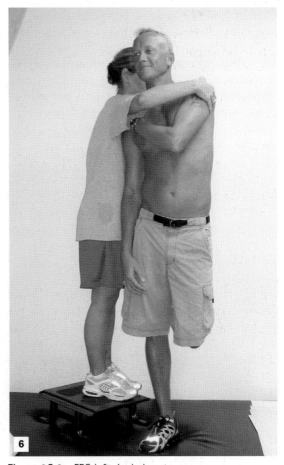

Figure 9C.6   FRS left single leg stance.

positions. As the patient advances through the seated progression the therapist can begin having the patient resist motions from two or more planes simultaneously.

Summary

Physical therapists and other appropriately trained manual therapy practitioners, as a general rule, are able to treat patients more frequently and for longer durations than many other medical practitioners. For that reason, PT's tend to have a larger array of treatment options at their disposal. This also affords PT's the opportunity to use multiple techniques and/or interventions in their treatments and to use specific interventions in multiple ways. This is especially true of muscle energy technique; it is extremely malleable to the environment and it can be adjusted to work with different types of therapists, patients, clinical settings, and stages of pain or dysfunction. A benefit of muscle energy technique is that once the underlying principles are learned, techniques can be immediately and easily modified by the practitioner.

This chapter has attempted to place muscle energy technique's role in the physical therapy clinic within the context of the current peer-reviewed literature (Delitto et al 1995, Flynn et al 2002, Fritz et al 2003, Wilson et al 2003, Childs et al 2004) in order to make a powerful clinical tool even more effective. To do this, a paradigm shift has been advocated to begin classifying patients into subgroups utilising a classification model (Delitto et al 1995) and clinical prediction rules (Flynn et al 2002, Childs et al 2004). A new role for muscle energy technique has been discussed in segment-specific strengthening programmes and appropriate exercise prescription principles have been outlined. Muscle energy technique is one of the most practical, safe, and user-friendly interventions available to physical therapists. It allows clinicians to make an immediate impact on their patients' pain and disability and can be utilised when other interventions may be contraindicated.

Appendix D: UNSTABLE SURFACES

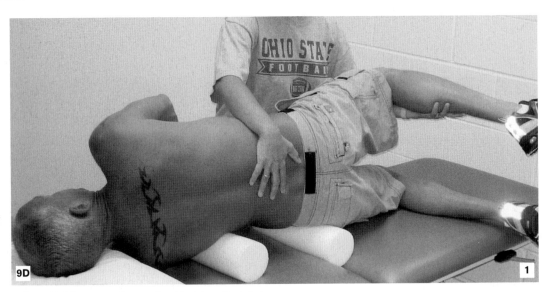

Figure 9D.1   Uniplanar, two foam rolls, side-lying, frontal plane.

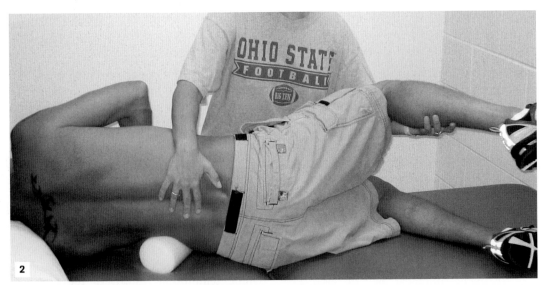

Figure 9D.2   Uniplanar, foam roll, side-lying, oblique plane.

Appendix D: Continued

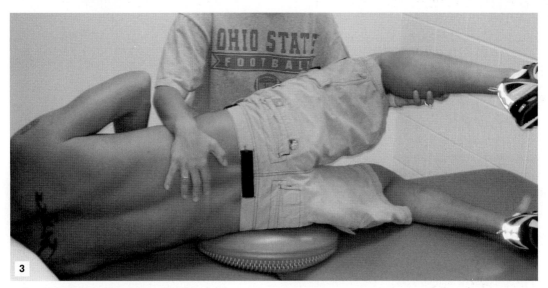

Figure 9D.3   Multiplanar, Dyna-Disc, side-lying.

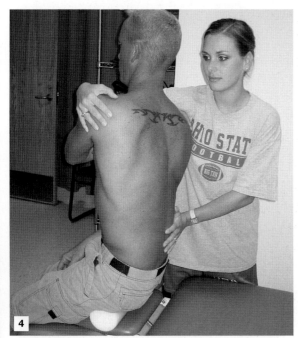

Figure 9D.4   Uniplanar, foam roll, seated, frontal plane.

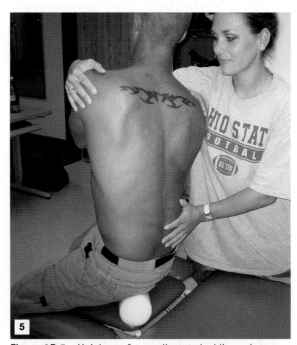

Figure 9D.5   Uniplanar, foam roll, seated, oblique plane.

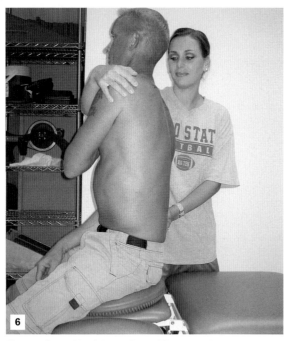

Figure 9D.6 Multiplanar, Dyna-Disc, seated.

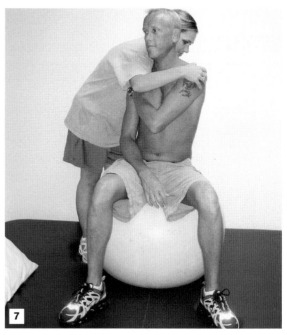

Figure 9D.7 Multiplanar, exercise ball, seated.

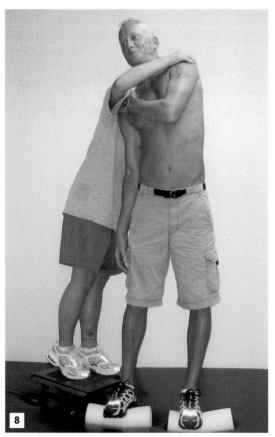

Figure 9D.8 Uniplanar, foam roll, standing, frontal plane (2 feet wide).

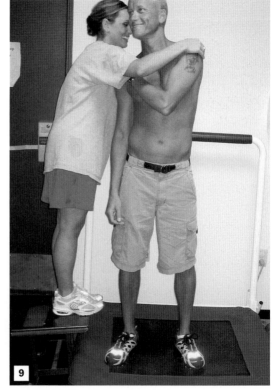

Figure 9D.9 Multiplanar, trampoline, standing (2 feet wide).

Appendix D: Continued

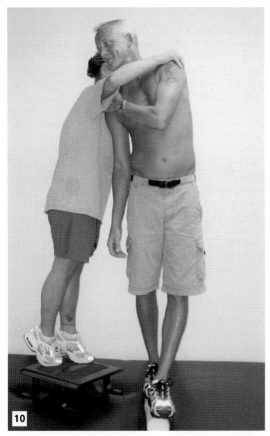

Figure 9D.10   Uniplanar, foam roll, standing, tandem stance (narrow).

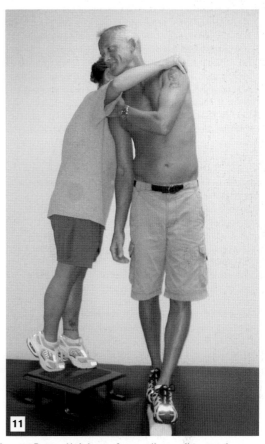

Figure 9D.11   Uniplanar, foam roll, standing, one leg.

References

Avela J, Kryolainen H, Komi P et al 1999a Reduced reflex sensitivity persists several days after long-lasting stretch-shortening cycle exercises. Journal of Applied Physiology 86: 1292–1300

Avela J, Kryolainen H, Komi P et al 1999b Reduced reflex sensitivity after repeated and prolonged passive muscle stretching. Journal of Applied Physiology 86: 1283–1291

Borkan J M, Koes B, Reis S et al 1998 A report from the second international forum for primary care research on low back pain: reexamining priorities. Spine 23: 1992–1996

Brown N, Melville M, Gray D et al 2000 Comparison of the SF-36 health survey questionnaire with the Nottingham health profile in long-term survivors of a myocardial infarction. Journal of Public Health Medicine 22(2): 167–175

Cherkin D C, Deyo R A, Battie M et al 1998 A comparison of physical therapy, chiropractic manipulation, and provision of an educational booklet for the treatment of patients with low back pain. New England Journal of Medicine 339(15): 1021–1029

Childs J D, Fritz J, Flynn T et al 2004 Validation of a clinical prediction rule to identify patients with low back pain likely to benefit from spinal manipulation: a randomized controlled trial. Annals of Internal Medicine 141: 920–928

Crockett A J, Cranston J M, Moss J R et al 1996 The MOS SF-36 health survey questionnaire in severe chronic airflow limitation: comparison with the Nottingham health profile. Quality of Life Research 5: 330–338

Crombez G, Vlaeyen J W, Heuts P H et al 1999 Pain-related fear is more disabling than fear itself: evidence on the role of pain-related fear in chronic back pain disability. Pain 80: 329–339

Danneels L, van der Straeten G, Cambier D et al 2001 The effects of three different training modalities on the cross-sectional area of the lumbar multifidus. British Journal of Sports Medicine 35: 186–194

Delitto A, Erhard R E, Bowling R W 1995 A treatment-based classification approach to low back syndrome: identifying and staging patients for conservative management. Physical Therapy 75: 470–479

Dettori J R, Bulock S H, Sutlive T G et al 1995 The effects of spinal flexion and extension exercises and their associated postures in patients with acute low back pain. Spine 20: 2303–2312

Deyo R A, Battie M, Beurskens A J et al 1998 Outcome measures for low back pain research. A proposal for standardized use. Spine 23: 2003–2013

Dishman J, Bulbulian R 2000 Spinal reflex attenuation associated with spinal manipulation. Spine 25: 2519–2525

Faas A, Chavannes A, Eijk J et al 1993 A randomized, placebo-controlled trial of exercise therapy in patients with acute low back pain. Spine 18: 1388–1395

Faas A, van E T, Chavannes A W et al 1995 A randomized trial of exercise therapy in patients with acute low back pain: efficacy on sickness absence. Spine 20: 941–947

Fairbank J C, Couper J, Davies J B et al 1980 The Oswestry low back pain disability questionnaire. Physiotherapy 66: 271–273

Fritz J M, Irrgang J J 2001 A comparison of a modified Oswestry low back pain disability questionnaire and the Quebec back pain disability scale. Physical Therapy 81: 766–788

Fritz J M, Delitto A, Erhard R E 2003 Comparison of classification-based physical therapy with therapy based on clinical practice guidelines for patients with acute low back pain: a randomized clinical trial. Spine 28: 1363–1372

Flynn T, Fritz J, Whitman J et al 2002 A clinical prediction rule for classifying patients with low back pain who demonstrate short-term improvement with spinal manipulation. Spine 27: 2835–2843

Gordon J 1991 Spinal mechanisms of motor coordination In: Kandel E, Schwartz J, Jessell T (eds) Principles of neural science, 3rd edn. Appleton & Lange, Norwalk, pp 581–595

Greenman P 1996 Principles of manual medicine, 2nd edn. Williams & Wilkins, Baltimore, pp 65–73

Hadijistavropoulos H D, Craig K D 1994 Acute and chronic low back pain: cognitive, affective, and behavioral dimensions. Journal of Consulting and Clinical Psychology 62: 341–349

Hadler N M, Curtis P, Gillings D B et al 1987 A benefit of spinal manipulation as an adjunctive therapy for acute low back pain: a stratified controlled study. Spine 12: 703–705

Hides J 2004 Paraspinal mechanism in low back pain. In: Richardson C, Hodges P, Hides J (eds) Therapeutic exercise for lumbopelvic stabilization: a motor control approach for the treatment and prevention of low back pain. Churchill Livingstone, Edinburgh, pp 149–161

Hides J, Stokes M J, Saide M et al 1994 Evidence of lumbar multifidus muscle wasting ipsilateral to symptoms in patients with acute/subacute low back pain. Spine 19: 165–172

Hides J, Richardson C, Jull G et al 1996 Multifidus muscle recovery is not automatic following resolution of acute first episode low back pain. Spine 21: 2763–2769

Hides J, Jull G, Richardson C 2001 Long-term effects of specific stabilising exercises for first-episode low back pain. Spine 26: E243–E248

Indahl A, Kaigle A, Reikeras O et al 1997 Interaction between the porcine lumbar intervertebral disc, zygapophysial joints and paraspinal musculature. Spine 22: 2834–2840

Jenkinson C, Fitzpatrick R 1990 Measurement of health status in patients with chronic illness: comparison of the Nottingham health profile and the general health questionnaire. Family Practice 7: 121–124

Klenerman L, Slade P D, Standly I M et al 1995 The prediction of chronicity in patients with an acute attack of low back pain in a general practice setting. Spine 20: 478–484

Komi P 1986 Training of muscle strength and power: interaction of neuromotoric, hypertrophic and mechanical factors. International Journal of Sports Medicine 7(suppl): 10–15

Kopec J A, Esdaile J M, Abrahamowicz M et al 1996 The Quebec back pain disability scale: conceptualization and development. Journal of Clinical Epidemiology 49: 151–161

MacDonald R S, Bell C M J 1990 An open controlled assessment of osteopathic manipulation in nonspecific low back pain. Spine 15: 364–370

Malanga G, Nadler S 1999 Nonoperative treatment of low back pain. Mayo Clinic Proceedings 74: 1135–1148

McKenna S P, Payne R L 1989 Comparison of the general health questionnaire and the Nottingham health profile in a study of unemployed and re-employed men. Family Practice 6: 3–8

O'Sullivan P B, Phyty G D, Twomey L T et al 1997 Evaluation of specific stabilizing exercise in the treatment of chronic low back pain with radiologic diagnosis of spondylolysis or spondylolisthesis. Spine 22: 2959–2967

Patrick D, Deyo R, Atlas S et al 1995 Assessing health-related quality of life in patients with sciatica. Spine 20: 1899–1909

Ponte D, Jensen G, Kent B 1984 A preliminary report on the use of the McKenzie protocol versus the Williams protocol in the treatment of low back pain. Journal of Orthopaedic and Sports Physical Therapy 6: 130–139

Porterfield J, DeRosa C 1998a Mechanical low back pain: perspectives in functional anatomy, 2nd edn, W B Saunders, Philadelphia, pp 121–168

Porterfield J, DeRosa C 1998b Mechanical low back pain: perspectives in functional anatomy, 2nd edn, W B Saunders, Philadelphia, p 81

Riddle D 1998 Classification and low back pain: a review of the literature and critical analysis of selected systems. Physical Therapy 78: 708–737

Riddle D, Rothstein J 1993 Intertester reliability of McKenzie's classifications of the syndrome types present in patients with low back pain. Spine 18: 1333–1344

Roland M 1986 A critical review of the evidence for a pain-spasm-pain cycle in spinal disorders. Clinical Biomechanics 1: 102–109

Spratt K F, Weinstein J N, Lehmann T R et al 1993 Efficacy of flexion and extension treatments incorporating braces for the low back pain patients with retrodisplacement, spondylolisthesis, or normal sagittal translation. Spine 18: 1839–1849

Stankovic R, Johnell O 1990 Conservative management of acute low-back pain. A prospective randomized trial. Spine 15: 120–123

Stankovic R, Johnell O 1995 Conservative management of acute low-back pain: a 5-year follow-up study of two methods of treatment. Spine 20: 469–472

Stone M H, Conley M S 1994 Bioenergetics. In: Baechle T (ed) Essentials of strength training and conditioning. Human Kinetics, Champaign, pp 67–85

van Tulder M W, Malmivaara A, Esmail R et al 2000 Exercise therapy for low back pain. Spine 25: 2784–2796

Waddell G, Newton M, Henderson I et al 1993 A fear-avoidance beliefs questionnaire (FABQ) and the role of fear-avoidance beliefs in chronic low back pain and disability. Pain 52: 157–168

Wilson E 2001 Neuromuscular re-education and strengthening of the lumbar stabilizers. Journal of Strength and Conditioning 24: 72–74

Wilson E, Payton O, Donegan-Shoaf L, Dec K 2003 Muscle energy technique in patients with acute low back pain: a pilot clinical trial. Journal of Orthopaedic and Sports Physical Therapy 33: 502–512

MET in a massage therapy setting

10

Sandy Fritz

CHAPTER CONTENTS

Marrying assessment and treatment 299
Soft tissues 300
Joints 300
Laxity 300
Summary 300
Integrating muscle energy methods into the
massage session 301
'Wellness' and therapeutic (clinical) modes
of massage 301
Example. Massage including MET to stretch
the quadriceps muscles 302
MET in a typical massage setting 303
MET as part of a general massage application 303
Case study 306
Summary 309
References 309

Therapeutic massage is often thought of as a method of stroking and kneading the tissues to promote relaxation, circulation and the general restorative properties of the body. A typical massage protocol involves gliding, kneading, compressing, pounding, tapping, slapping and oscillating (rocking, vibrating, shaking) of soft tissues.

This is a very simplistic view of therapeutic massage. A more accurate description of massage consists of various types of stimulus and force application to positively influence the entire body function, including neuro-endocrine control functions, fluid movement through the tissues, including blood and lymph, and pliability of connective tissue structures (DeDominico & Wood 1997, Cassar 1999, Lowe 2003).

Other than the typical gliding, kneading, compressing, oscillating and percussive methods used in therapeutic massage to affect the body, the approach also includes passive and active movement of the joints. The massage practitioner uses various joint movements as part of assessment and/or treatment, and muscle energy methods are easily integrated into the massage at this point to enhance the benefits of massage.

Marrying assessment and treatment

Most massage methods can be used for both assessment and treatment. Palpation assessment includes typical massage methods such as gliding, kneading and compressing to assess for temperature changes, tissue texture, tissue pliability, fluid balance, and tissue congestion. These same methods can then be used to introduce a variety of mechanical forces, including tension, shear, bend and torsion to affect the structure and function of the soft tissues being treated.

Various stimuli are also applied, again using the same methods to influence neural and endocrine functions that effect mood, pain perception and proprioceptive changes, to produce functional benefits (Lederman 1997).

Soft tissues

The movement of joints assesses for range of motion as well as relative length of attaching soft tissue structures. The lengthened or shortened areas identified during such assessment may be the result of modifications of neural control (e.g. increased motor tone), viscoelastic connective tissue changes, and/or fluid congestion that would modify the stiffness of the tissues (Lederman 1997, Simons & Mense 1998).

Joints

Alteration in joint structure can lead to changes in movement potential. The joint may be diseased (as in degenerative joint disease), or there may be alterations in joint play, or the joint may have effusion which influences its ability to move freely, so altering the firing sequences of attaching muscles. Joint stability may also be influenced by the relative tightness or laxity of ligaments, as well as by the tone and tightness of attaching musculature. Both form stability (shape and structure of the joint surfaces, capsule and ligaments) and force stability (action of muscles around the joint) may be affected, something particularly true of the sacroiliac joint (Neumann 2002). By influencing the muscles that form the force-couples at the joint, the stability and the movement potential of a joint can be altered (Neumann 2002).

When there is joint dysfunction there are almost always changes in the muscle function associated with the joint, as well as in adjacent areas, resulting in a combination of imbalance between agonist,

synergists, fixators and antagonists, some of which may be hypertonic and short, while others may be inhibited and possibly lengthened (Lederman 1997, Chaitow & DeLany 2002). It is in such situations that muscle energy methods become particularly useful to introduce changes in muscle function. Muscle energy techniques appear to be particularly effective in treatment of neurologically mediated shortened soft tissue dysfunction.

In general, therapeutic massage application is effective in addressing shortened and abnormally tight structures regardless of the reason. If the shortening is the result of proprioceptive dysfunction, resulting in reduction of muscle length, MET can be an effective addition to the massage protocol to address these changes.

Laxity

Experience indicates that massage is not particularly effective for addressing lax or inhibited soft tissue structures. Some form of therapeutic exercise is usually required to re-establish strength and tone in weakened or lax tissues. Muscle energy methods can be used to treat these conditions (see Chs 3 and 5). MET applied to over-shortened, hypertonic muscles will automatically result in improved tone and function in their weak/inhibited antagonists (Lewit 1999).

Additional exercise, possibly using isotonic forms of MET, can be introduced to enhance function in the inhibited structures. MET methods that are most effective for the stimulation of inhibited muscles include pulsed MET and isotonic eccentric methods (see Ch. 5).

Summary

- Massage consists of methods that affect the soft tissue and the joints.
- Enhancing joint movement is part of the massage system.
- Movement is a primary assessment tool.
- Movement dysfunction can be addressed during the application of massage using muscle energy methods.

Integrating muscle energy methods into the massage session

There seems to exist an opinion among massage practitioners that therapeutic massage needs to have a flowing rhythmic integrated quality that provides a relaxation experience (DeDominico & Wood 1997, Tappan & Benjamin 1998, Salvo & Anderson 2004). Because of this view, many who perform massage are hesitant to move the client around, to change the position of the client, or ask the client to participate in the massage session. While a passive rhythmic application of massage has value, it represents only one aspect of therapeutic massage. Massage therapy involves many outcome objectives, including those that result in increases in range of motion and more optimal neuromuscular function. MET is an appropriate addition to massage methodology to achieve these goals.

The question really is not if MET should be part of the massage system, but how to incorporate MET into the typical massage session so that the general impression of the massage as passive, rhythmic and soothing is not lost.

One can also ask whether it is necessary for massage to have a passive rhythmic soothing quality in order to be effective. The author of this chapter holds an opinion that this is not the case. How a massage is delivered should totally depend on the objectives and desired overall outcome.

'Wellness' and therapeutic (clinical) modes of massage

The typical massage application is often a general (constitutional, 'wellness') whole body approach, with the results being an increase in well-being and normalisation of nonspecific homeostatic body functioning. All massage, including relaxation, restorative or wellness massage (different names – similar outcomes), can be classified as therapeutic in the sense that the aim is to provide benefit to the client. The terms increasingly used to describe focused, outcome-based massage that is targeting a pathology or dysfunction, are medical or clinical massage. MET can be incorporated into both massage styles.

It is necessary to determine if the massage approach is wellness, restorative and pleasure based, or whether the massage is addressing a specific outcome, such as pain reduction or increased mobility. If a client's goal for the massage is to be pampered, to sleep, to be soothed, and other such goals, then any method, including MET, that requires active client participation, might be inappropriate. If the massage has an outcome objective of pain relief and increased mobility or the targeting of some other specific result, then adaptive methods – including MET – are appropriate, and indeed probably essential.

There are some myths about massage that need to be challenged in order to justify the inclusion of MET methods into the massage setting:

1. *The client should be passive during massage.*
   The client does not have to be passive during the massage. Unless the goal of the massage is sleep, the client should be actively involved, to at least some extent, to provide feedback during assessment and intervention processes.

2. *Massage must be provided with rhythmic flowing strokes.* Massage does not have to follow a set protocol where one stroke flows into the next. This is only one form of massage.

It is important to acknowledge that one of the strengths of full body massage is an interconnected approach to the body allowing all areas to be addressed. This 'interconnected approach' supports integration of the body to the stimuli and forces imposed upon it during massage. Therefore, massage provides an excellent platform for not only integration of MET methods into the session, but generally supports the body in adapting to the changes provided by the methods, be it strengthening weak muscles (by removing inhibitory influences from antagonists, as well as use of toning methods), or by lengthening shortened muscles.

The question arises as to whether it is possible to provide a soothing integrated rhythmic massage that also addresses a situation requiring adaptation where MET would be effective. The answer is yes, and the rest of this chapter will describe how this can be accomplished.

Earlier in the chapter an explanation of massage was offered that included gliding, kneading, compressing, oscillating and movement methods. In therapeutic massage, passive and active movement of the joints are included, and MET is easily integrated into massage at this point. An example follows as to how this may be achieved.

Example. Massage including MET to stretch the quadriceps muscles

Imagine that the client is in the prone position and the leg is being treated. The massage therapist might use passive joint movement to flex and extend the knee to assess the range and quality of movement. Let's assume that knee flexion is found to be limited as a result of soft tissue changes rather than joint restriction (a judgement based on the quality of end-feel as the knee is flexed) and that the quadriceps muscle is short (Fig. 10.1).

- The massage therapist uses passive joint movement to position the muscle just short of bind.

- The client is asked to move the heel gently towards the buttocks while an equal resistance force is applied by the massage therapist, and the hamstring isometrically contracts for about 7 seconds.

- After the contraction the massage therapist stretches the quadriceps by easing the foot towards the buttocks.

The contraction of the antagonists to the shortened quadriceps (hamstrings) would result in an improved ability to stretch the quadriceps (see Ch. 5).

An alternative to waiting until the contraction ceases before stretching quadriceps would be to introduce a stretch of the hamstrings while they were being contracted. This is accomplished by applying a resistance force to the leg greater than the contraction force created by the hamstrings and the knee would extend. This application is an eccentric isotonic stretch (Fig. 10.2), and the effect would be to simultaneously tone the hamstrings

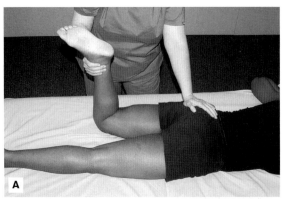

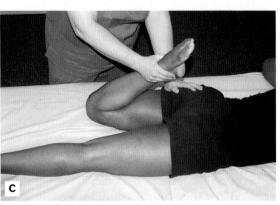

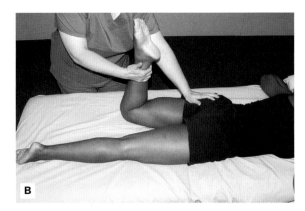

Figure 10.1 **A** Range of motion of the knee. **B** Isometric contraction of hamstrings. **C** Stretch of quadriceps.

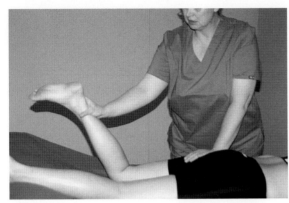

Figure 10.2   Eccentric isotonic stretch of hamstrings.

- *Passive:* Therapist performs the action, client does nothing.
- *Active:* Client performs the action.
- *Active assisted:* Client performs the action but is partially assisted by the therapist.
- *Active resisted:* Client performs the action but this is partially resisted by the therapist.

The total movement pattern of any jointed area is its range of motion. During all types of joint movement the soft tissue (i.e. muscle connective tissue unit) is being addressed.

MET as part of a general massage application

The client wishes to receive a full body restorative massage with specific focus on elbow discomfort. The following description targets the aspect of the full body massage relating to the upper limb on the affected side.

- The client is supine and the upper limb is being massaged. It is assumed that the posterior torso and shoulder have already been massaged.

- When beginning to massage an area, passive joint movement is used to identify the condition of the range of motion in the area. The massage practitioner gently and rhythmically moves the joints being assessed through the available ranges of motion.

- Let us assume that the initial assessment of the elbow and wrist using passive joint movement identifies a decreased range of motion in elbow extension of 15°, with wrist extension being slightly limited. There is moderate pain reported and apprehension exhibited, during elbow extension.

- Once the area has been assessed passively, and limits in motion identified, the client actively moves the area and the massage therapist compares the results with the passive assessment. In this example let us assume that during the active joint movement the wrist limitation was normal, but the elbow motion remained limited, as described above.

- Massage addresses the arm as the next area in the general massage application.

at the same time as inhibiting the quadriceps, so that they are more easily stretched.

This example describes how MET can be integrated into massage. Using other massage methods to gain the same degree of release that MET procedures can achieve could take far longer and would possibly be less effective.

The following section will provide sample protocols for effective integration of MET into massage treatment.

MET in a typical massage setting

Two scenarios are presented as examples of how to incorporate MET into the massage session. The first describes general inclusion of MET into massage of an area (arm). The second is a hypothetical case involving how massage, including MET, could be used to address low-back pain.

The description of the massage is as if the reader is watching the massage as it occurs. It would be helpful for the reader to visualise the examples or to actually perform them as they are described.

It is assumed that the reader understands the basic methods of gliding (effleurage), kneading (petrissage), compression, oscillation (rocking and shaking) and percussion (Fig. 10.3). These are the main methods of massage that introduce various stimuli and force into the soft tissue to elicit a beneficial response. It is necessary to clarify the meaning of the terms that describe various joint movements.

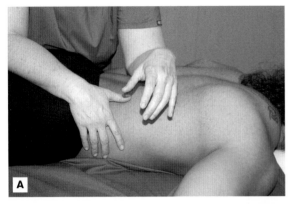

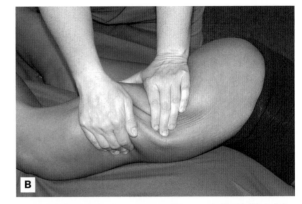

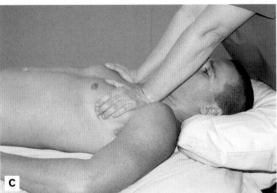

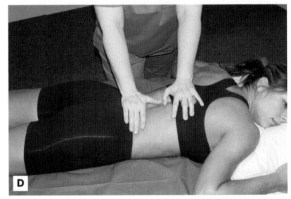

Figure 10.3   **A** Gliding. **B** Kneading. **C** Compression. **D** Oscillation (rocking). **E** Percussion.

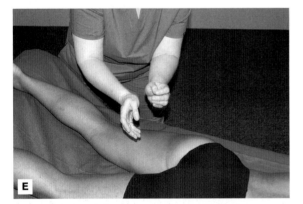

- Let us assume palpation assessment using massage methods identifies trigger point activity in the brachialis and brachioradialis that has resulted in increased muscle tension in the forearm.

- Compression is applied to the trigger point while passive joint movement positions the tissues so that the pain sensation is reduced

– an approach to treatment involving positional release (Fig. 10.4) (see Ch. 7).

- When the area is returned to the neutral position (i.e. the elbow is straightened), kneading is applied to the area of the trigger point with the intention of lengthening and stretching the local tissue (Fig. 10.5).

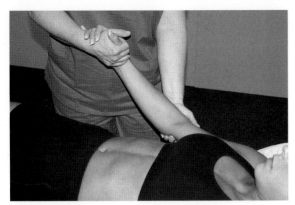

Figure 10.4   Positional release of brachialis.

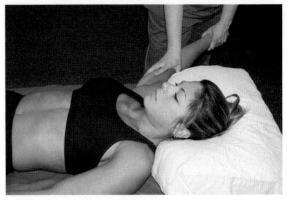

Figure 10.5   Stretching area of trigger point.

- At this time the elbow would be moved through passive ranges of motion, in order to identify any remaining restrictions.

- The area is again massaged and then positioned so that the elbow is slightly flexed. A muscle contraction is introduced to activate the flexors by having the client lightly push against the massage therapist's restraining hand for 5–7 seconds. Then the elbow is extended to stretch the tight soft tissues (Fig. 10.6).

- General massage and passive joint movement reassess the area.

- Attention then shifts to the forearm and the wrist and the forearm is massaged.

- The wrist flexors are positioned at slight tension, and the client resists against

counterpressure provided by the massage therapist, to assess for muscle strength.

- Then the wrist extensors are positioned at slight tension and again the client resists a counterpressure provided by the massage therapist, to assess for muscle strength.

- Let us assume that the flexor muscles test as strong, and the wrist extensors test weak.

- The wrist flexors are massaged to reduce muscle tension and then MET methods prepare the wrist flexors for stretching.

- It would be appropriate to use postisometric relaxation, reciprocal inhibition or some integrated combination of both. The massage therapist then stretches the wrist flexors.

- Next, the wrist extensors are isolated and the client is instructed to pulse rhythmically

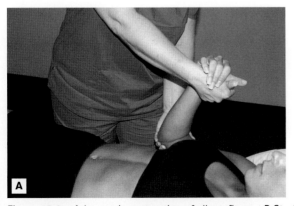

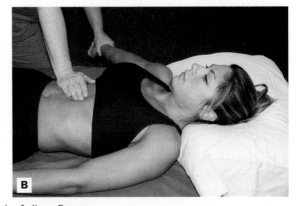

Figure 10.6   **A** Isometric contraction of elbow flexors. **B** Stretch of elbow flexors.

against the massage therapist's resisting hand, with the intention of activating (toning, facilitating) the weak extensor muscles (see notes on Ruddy pulsed MET in Ch. 3).

- After 20 pulses the client is asked to again contract the wrist extensors against a counterpressure applied by the massage therapist. In this example let us assume that the wrist extensors now test strong and the area is generally massaged again to integrate the response.

- The hand is next to be massaged.

- The entire area is again taken through passive joint movement to reassess the range of motion. Any changes would be noted and charted.

- The massage then continues in the typical full body massage style.

Case study

A 48-year-old female has been referred for massage as part of a management programme for low-back pain. The client has been diagnosed with reduced disc space at L345 with slight disc bulging at L5. Surgery is not indicated and conservative treatment has been prescribed. The main source of pain and disability appears to be muscular, both as a result of protective guarding and intermittent nerve impingement involving shortened soft tissue structures. The forms of treatment being received include: physical therapy, osteopathic care, massage, and muscle relaxing medication to be used as needed.

The treatment plan for the massage is to provide general restorative massage, with the objectives of pain relief, enhancement of sleep, reduction of fascial shortening (especially lumbodorsal fascia), as well as offering attention to shortened latissimus dorsi, hamstrings, psoas, paraspinals and quadratus lumborum.

The general treatment plan for massage involves 60 minutes, twice a week, for 12 weeks. The massage follows a relatively classic style using gliding, kneading, compression, etc. in a relaxing and rhythmic manner.

Active and passive joint movement and palpation assess the current condition of tissue short-ening at each session. Specific connective tissue methods are used on shortened fascial areas, and MET is used to address muscles that have shortened due to increased motor tone.

The following describes a typical massage session as part of the prescribed treatment plan.

- Massage begins with the patient prone.

- When the tissues are warm and more pliable, deep slow gliding along the paraspinal muscles commences.

- When an area is identified by the client as contributing to the back pain, the glide stops, and ischaemic compression is used.

- As this is being done the client is asked to extend the spine and rotate towards the pain to create an isolated contraction at the point of the compressed tissue.

- The contraction is held for 7–10 seconds and then the client is asked to rotate away from the pain and to push down into the table with the anterior torso, and to draw the abdominals in, thereby contracting anterior torso muscles to create reciprocal inhibition of spinal muscles.

- At the same time the massage therapist slightly increases the compressive force and again begins to use gliding strokes through the tissues, which effectively produces isolated stretching of the shortened area that is creating symptoms.

- This process continues until about 50% of the muscle's increased motor tone is reduced. Since a possible reason for the muscle shortening is protection of the spine, the goal should be to manage the excessive muscle tension rather than trying to eliminate it.

- The massage then becomes more general to increase fluid movement in the area and to assist in integration of the changes.

- While the client remains prone the massage application addresses the gluteals, hamstrings, and calves.

- General massage application is used to assess and warm the area.

Since the hamstrings are one of the areas to be specifically addressed in the treatment plan, MET methods may well be useful.

- In the prone position it is difficult to lengthen the hamstrings but slow compressive gliding from distal attachments to proximal attachments, while the client slowly flexes and extends the knee in combination with compression and tension force with active movement, could be considered a form of manipulation of the proprioceptors. This type of application also addresses the connective tissue shortening.

- The massage then becomes general again.

- The client is placed in the side-lying position to more easily access latissimus dorsi and quadratus lumborum, and the general massage application resumes.

- Gliding over the latissimus dorsi begins at the hip and progresses to the shoulder.

- To lengthen the latissimus dorsi the client's arm is positioned with the arm placed over the client's head with the lateral aspect of the arm against the side of her face (Fig. 10.7).

- A resistance force is applied by the massage therapist at the medial arm near the elbow, and the client is asked to move the arm away from her face and back towards her side, resulting in an isometric contraction of the latissimus dorsi.

- The amount of effort asked for would be about 10% of maximal strength and duration for approximately 7–10 seconds.

- The massage therapist then reverses the focus of the resistance force and the client attempts to move the arm towards her head, resulting in an isometric contraction of the deltoid and inhibition of the latissimus dorsi.

- This alternating contraction application is repeated two or three times after which the client is asked to take the arm through the resistance barrier in order to stretch the shortened muscle while the massage therapist assists the lengthening process.

- When the new barrier is identified the client repeats the sequence of resisted contractions and assisted stretching. This is an example of a muscle energy procedure that can be summarised as contract–relax antagonist contract – lengthen and then stretch.

- The tissues would subsequently be gently returned to neutral position.

- The soft tissue is massaged again, both to palpate for changes and to support adaptation of the soft tissue to the new length.

- If additional areas of bind are identified then the massage therapist introduces bend and torsion forces (kneading) on the short binding tissue to directly stretch it (Fig. 10.8).

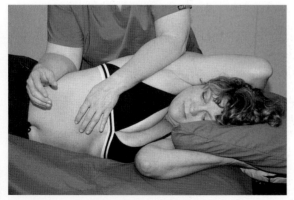

Figure 10.7 Position of arm, side-lying.

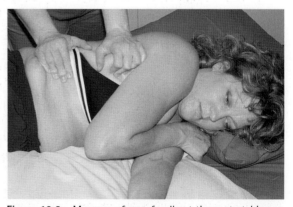

Figure 10.8 Massage of area for direct tissue stretching.

- When sufficient length has been achieved, the area is then generally massaged to help integrate the changes.

- While the client is in the side-lying position, quadratus lumborum and adjacent soft tissue can be lengthened by stabilising the iliac crest and having the client tilt (hike) the hip activating the muscle.

- Then the tissues are lengthened by having the client lower the leg behind the trunk, coupled with stretching by the massage therapist.

- MET can be used to address the psoas while the client is in the side-lying position. The client is positioned so that while lying on her side both hips are flexed to about 90° with one leg on top of the other. The knees are also flexed to about 90°.

- The massage therapist stands behind the client, grasps the upper leg, and extends the hip to 0°, while the knee remains flexed.

- The client maintains this position as the massage therapist applies a resistance force by placing a hand or forearm near the proximal attachment of the hamstring on the upper leg.

- The client attempts to move the hip into hyperextension against the resistance force, resulting in isometric contraction of the gluteus maximus and hamstrings, which would inhibit psoas through reciprocal inhibition. The contraction force only needs to be 15–20% of maximal strength and held for about 10 seconds.

- The client maintains the contraction and the position, as the massage therapist changes hand position to be able to stretch the psoas.

- The massage therapist grasps the client's anterior thigh, just above the knee (the knee remains flexed), stabilises the client in the lumbar area, and moves the leg back to stretch psoas while the client assists the movement by again attempting to hyperextend the hip. This procedure is repeated two or three times (Fig. 10.9).

- The massage application continues to generally address the rest of the body in the side-lying position.

- The client is positioned on the other side and the process is repeated.

- The client is positioned supine. Massage continues, beginning at the feet and progresses towards the hips.

- The leg is flexed at the hip and the knee is extended (straight leg raise) to assess for the shortening of the hamstrings.

- When the barrier is identified the client contracts against a resistance force applied by the massage therapist on the gastrocnemius, near the knee, by bringing the leg down towards the table using 10–20% contraction force, for about 7 seconds.

- The hamstrings are then stretched by raising the leg.

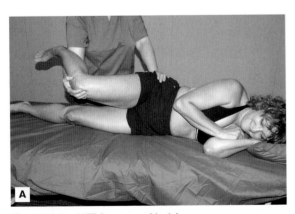
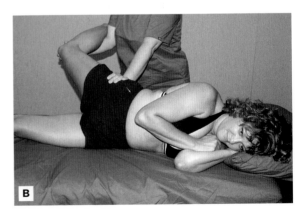

Figure 10.9   MET for psoas, side-lying.

- The knee remains extended while the massage therapist slowly flexes the hip until the barrier is again identified. The procedure is then repeated.

- The process is repeated on the other side.

At this point in the massage session all target areas have been addressed using MET and the therapist can generally massage the rest of the body in the supine position.

This case study example provides suggestions for integrating MET into massage to address a specific condition.

Summary

The flow of the massage session involves the skilled weaving of MET elements into a full body rhythmic, soothing, effective massage experience. Based on the examples provided, it is easy to see how muscle energy methods can be integrated into the massage session. It is difficult for this author to imagine performing a massage session without incorporating MET methods as an intervention tool.

MET methods are generally safe and well accepted by clients.

To effectively integrate MET methods into the massage the massage therapist needs to be knowledgeable about joint movement patterns and normal ranges of motion. With practice and a shift in perception, the massage professional should be able to introduce these methods, and the underlying concepts into the massage session, which results in greater benefits to the client.

References

Cassar M-P 1999 Handbook of massage therapy. A complete guide for the student and professional massage therapist. Butterworth-Heinemann, Oxford, pp 5–6

Chaitow L, DeLany J 2002 Clinical application of neuromuscular techniques, vol 2. The lower body. Churchill Livingstone, Edinburgh, pp 35–37

DeDominico G, Wood E C 1997 Beard's massage, 4th edn. W B Saunders, Philadelphia, pp 56–69, 75–76

Lederman E 1997 Fundamentals of manual therapy, physiology, neurology and psychology. Churchill Livingstone, Edinburgh, pp 7–8, 23–25, 39–40, 55–56, 66–67, 95–96, 126, 133–137, 213–221

Lewit K 1999 Manipulation in rehabilitation of the locomotor system, 3rd edn. Butterworths, London

Lowe W W 2003 Orthopedic massage theory and technique. Mosby, St Louis, MO, pp 49–58

Neumann D A 2002 Kinesiology of the musculoskeletal system foundations for physical rehabilitation. Mosby, St Louis, MO, pp 16, 18–9, 41, 308

Salvo S G, Anderson S K 2004 Mosby's pathology for massage therapists. Mosby, St Louis, MO, p 423

Simons D, Mense S 1998 Understanding and measurement of muscle tone as related to clinical muscle pain. Pain 75(1): 1–17

Tappan F M, Benjamin P J 1998 Tappan's handbook of healing massage techniques, holistic, classic, and emerging methods, 3rd edn. Appleton and Lange, Norwalk, CN, p 147

MET in treatment of athletic injuries

Ken Crenshaw, Nathan Shaw and
Ron Porterfield

CHAPTER CONTENTS

Adaptation of athletes	**312**
Dysfunction in sports	**314**
Screening for dysfunction	**315**
Pre-season screen	315
Spine measurements	315
Hip region measurements	317
Abdominal strength and coordination	321
Lower extremity measurements	321
Upper extremities	322
Manual assessment	323
Corrective/preventative strategies	**323**
Dynamic flexibility versus static stretching	323
Warm-up	325
Recovery techniques	327
Common injuries	329
Standard care of injuries	329
Acute injury care	329
Muscle energy techniques (MET) and integrated neuromuscular inhibition techniques (INIT) in sports injuries	**331**
Prevention of injury using MET, INIT and other techniques	331
Acute injury care with MET and other therapies	332
Chronic injury and long-term rehabilitation using MET	332
MET using isotonic, isometric and isokinetic contractions for strengthening weak postural muscles	**333**
Case A: Sub-acute low-back strain	333
Case B: Acute hamstring strain	334
Case C: Shoulder tendonitis (subacromial long head of biceps)	336
Summary	**337**
References	**337**
Further reading	**338**

It is the nature of competitive athletics to contain inherent risks of physical injury and dysfunction for those actively participating. Each sport creates the possibility of unique injuries and specific physical adaptations as a result of the particular physical demands of the sport and the position played within the sport. As competitive athletics (especially one-sport specialisation) continues to increase in popularity, so does the risk of injury and/or dysfunction. Specialised health care providers for athletes are essential for the prevention, recognition, assessment, management, and rehabilitation of sport injuries. The very special nature of returning athletes to sport after injury, or prevention of injury, is very complex. Understanding that injury and dysfunction go hand in hand, as one may be causative of the other, creates the need for in-depth knowledge of human tissue function. The elite competitive athlete is highly pressured by multiple social, physical, economic and emotional demands. These pressures, combined with increasing demands from team management and their own economic concerns, place an enormous responsibility on the sports medicine team to keep athletes participating.

This chapter will:

1. Examine the roles of the physician, athletic trainer, physical therapist, massage therapist, and strength and conditioning coordinator as parts of the primary sports medicine team.

2. Provide sound assessment techniques, classification systems, treatment and rehabilitation options for the most common musculoskeletal problems.

3. Explain how muscle energy techniques (MET) are used within the total health care package for the athletes.

4. Explain specific injury/dysfunction scenarios and give systematic therapy options utilising MET and other neuromuscular techniques (NMT).

It is not the intention of the authors, nor within the scope of this chapter, to provide gruelling details of every possible sport-related musculoskeletal problem, but rather to suggest ways in which MET, in combination with other therapies might be used in the treatment of the most common athletic injuries and/or dysfunctions. The authors concur that it is not currently mainstream practice for the majority of western sports medicine providers to use neuromuscular therapy that includes the use of MET, in the prevention, management and rehabilitation of athletic injuries. The principles and methods outlined in this chapter represent the combined experience of its authors, and are presented in the hope that they will stimulate interest in others whose work involves helping injured athletes and/or who aim to prevent athletic injuries.

Adaptation of athletes

Sport in general requires high levels of repetitive physical activity and training to achieve specific objectives. Exercise regimens to improve athletic qualities require physical adaptation. The combining of these two components requires tactful planning and constant assessment to avoid overload of the musculotendinous and neuromuscular systems. An athlete will inherently adapt to the imposed demands of his sport, the physical requirements of the position played within the sport, and his exercise regimens, or else he will become prone to injury or inadequate performance. This philosophy is based on the specific adaptation to imposed demands (SAID) principle discussed by Kraemer & Gomez (2001). Specific tissue (be it joint, muscular, tendinous, fascia, osseous, or ligamentous/capsular) will accommodate uniquely in each athlete. For example, generalised patterns of adaptation are recognised in the overhead throwing athlete (Box 11.1). However precisely a particular tissue or tissues have adapted in relation to such activities remains controversial. Various experts (Crockett et al 2002, Osbahr et al 2002, Reagan et al 2002, Wilk et al 2002, Borsa et al 2004) have described a variety of adaptation possibilities in the throwing shoulder. The common pattern of the throwing shoulder, to develop an increased range of external rotation and decreased internal rotation is one of many adap-

---

Box 11.1 **Personal view on adaptation in the athlete**

Age seems to be a key feature in the adaptation process. As discussed earlier, humeral retroversion occurs in overhead throwers, and the authors are currently researching the influence of age on this process. Presumably the process occurs between 12 and 13 years of age, prior to growth plate closure and dependent upon the amount of throwing involved (Meister 2005).

Any repetitive activity produces specific demands for adaptation. In sport trainers, coaches and therapist/practitioners are responsible for encouragement of healthy adaptation. It is essential for a certain level of adaptation to occur for athletes to compete at elite levels, for without specific adaptation to the imposed demands, the musculoskeletal system would almost certainly fail to function efficiently. In essence the adaptation helps to pre-position the body for the sport demands. There seems to be a fine line as to the degree of adaptation that is desirable, beyond which deleterious effects such as injury (shoulder laxity for example) become more likely (Pieper 1998).

Following injury the musculoskeletal system is required to adapt to the new situation and function of injured, or healing tissue. It is in this state that care is required to prevent re-injury and reduce dysfunctional patterns of use, so that appropriate and functional adaptation can occur. Following further injury, multiple injuries or extreme injury, functional adaptation may not be possible, so that decompensation and dysfunction become almost inevitable. In elite athletes a minute degree of dysfunction makes the difference between winning and losing, whereas in the non-athlete the same degree of dysfunction may create no more than minor annoyance.

Excluding injuries, the consequences of specialised adaptation, required to compete at elite levels of sport, do not seem to affect the athlete's lifestyle.

tations (Fig. 11.1A–C). The ability of the athlete to adapt adequately seems to be what allows him to compete at the top levels of his chosen sport. As adaptations from sport occur it is necessary to take into account an athlete's daily living habits. Any repetitive or prolonged activity will create adaptation and often it will negatively affect the athlete. Greenfield et al (1995), demonstrated that posture degradation such as forward head position, can effect the shoulder of the throwing athlete. The practitioner must constantly assess postural adaptations, and other specialised training adap-tations, in order to maintain optimal function of the athlete.

Not only are athletes challenged physically, they must adapt to many other stressors as well. Mental, social, environmental, nutritional stressors combined with ageing, competition requirements, travel, and sleep pattern disruption, all add to the athlete's adaptation burden. General health depends on more than the absence of disease. It is critical to keep stressors to a minimum and/or to use mech-anisms such as recovery and relaxation techniques to improve stress-coping potentials (Selye 1956).

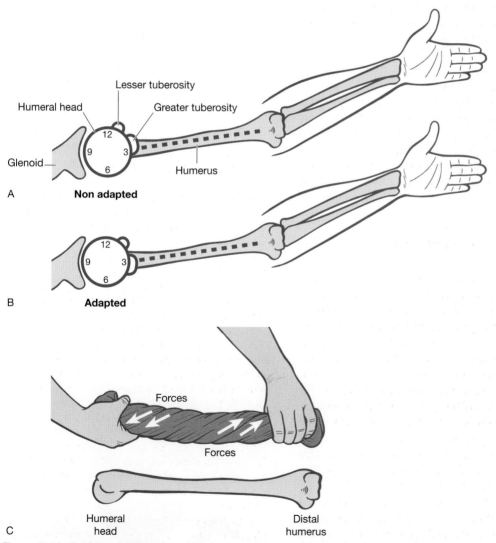

Figure 11.1A–C Osseous adaptation of the humerus from repetitive overhead throwing (humeral retroversion) is one of several adaptations in athletes.

Dysfunction in sports

Optimal physical function is critical for the success of the elite athlete. Strength, balance, power, speed, agility, coordination, endurance and mobility are important elements in most sports (Kraemer & Gomez 2001). These elements will almost certainly be hindered in the presence of musculoskeletal dysfunction. Whether postural imbalance, local tissue disturbance, psychosocial influences or some other factor is involved, the sports medicine team needs to be able to recognise and address the problem, in order to retain optimal performance.

As competitive seasons wear on, athletes may demonstrate the cumulative effects of the many stressors encountered. These effects range from spinal dysfunction, to digestive disturbances and specific inflexibility patterns that may lead to a decrease in performance and susceptibility to injury.

Training methods that focus on achieving strength and power that, according to Kramer & Gomez (2001), require using Type II fibres (fast twitch, fatigue-sensitive fibres) are widely used in many sports. Many of these training variations promote faulty movement patterns. Therefore, faulty training approaches may be as much to blame for injury as overtraining or overuse.

Furthermore, specific neuromuscular firing patterns described by Fritz & Grosenbach (2004) can be altered by daily living habits or adaptation to sport demands. Muscles that are required to undergo strength training to improve particular athletic qualities may become dysfunctional, and/or prone to inappropriate firing patterns. According to Chaitow & DeLany (2002) 'Excessive strength training frequently results in muscular imbalances between opposing muscle groups, as those which are being strengthened inhibit and overwhelm their antagonists ... This effect is not inevitable but reflects poorly designed training programs.' Norris (2004) mentions that 'to strengthen a muscle for a specific movement, an exercise must mimic the movement as closely as possible'.

Traditionally strength and power training has utilised bilateral extremity exercises, such as barbell squats or bench press exercises. Most training regimens were developed towards anterior musculature or accelerator dominant exercises (Fig. 11.2A, B). The posterior dominant chain decelerators and stabilisers were an afterthought. This method of training is another factor that may lead to increases in injury and dysfunction of the athlete as it may train muscles and not movement patterns required in a particular sport.

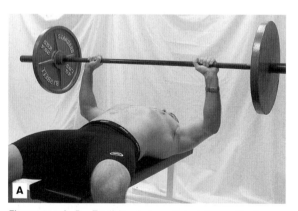

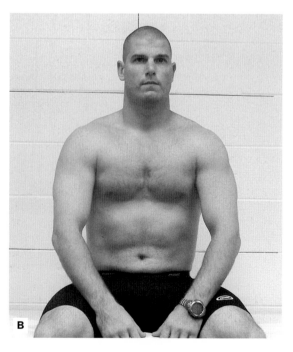

Figure 11.2A, B Traditional strength training methods may lead to faulty posture and neuromuscular firing patterns.

According to Myrland (2004) athletes must be able to produce and reduce force with balance and control on one leg. Proficiency in one-legged or one-armed exercises with a combination of core activation is paramount to athletic development (Fig. 11.3A, B).

Boyle (2004) states that conditioning programmes should include acceleration, deceleration and change of direction, as most injuries occur during these phases of movement.

It is also important to develop muscle specificity and movement specificity. Fritz & Grosenbach (2004) and Riley & Bommarito (2004) described the cross extensor and flexor reflexes that many athletes utilise in sport. Their views show the need to train in an ipsilateral manner for proper neural firing patterns. These concepts can be programmed into a corrective/preventative plan for each athlete (Figs 11.4A, B and 11.5 A–D).

It is the authors' experience that strategies to counteract postural misalignment, faulty training programmes, and other dysfunction promoters will minimise damage or potential damage to tissues. These strategies may include muscle energy techniques (MET), soft tissue work, corrective exercise programmes, biomechanical adjustments, and modification of training volume/recovery.

Screening for dysfunction

A meticulous and thorough screen for dysfunction is imperative as it may identify and help correct any problems before they cause irreparable tissue damage. The screening should look for overall gross movement dysfunction, postural abnormalities, flexibility, bilateral symmetry, muscle and joint function. It is the authors' view that, in the presence of altered muscular length–tension relationships, optimum movement may not be anatomically possible. There are many general and specific tests that can help in determining dysfunction. Since many have been explained in detail previously in Ch. 5, the authors have chosen to describe several specific tests that work well in the sport environment in addition to the previously mentioned tests. This should give the practitioner a reasonable picture of an athlete's current state of functionality.

Pre-season screen

An orthopaedic physician exam (of joint, ligamentous, cartilage and general neuromuscular function) should be coupled with a general well-being exam (internal organ, optical, dental, urinalysis, blood work) by a general medical physician.

A six-category screen should follow these exams:

1. Static posture
2. Dynamic posture
3. Spine angle symmetry assessment
4. Abdominal function
5. Overall flexibility
6. Manual assessment.

Static posture is the position from which all movement begins and ends. Therefore, the initial assessment of length–tension relationships begins here. Each athlete should have a static photograph taken from an anterior view, posterior view and lateral views, both right and left. The photographs can be taken in reference to a plumb line or grid chart, offering a reference point for future viewing. The static abnormalities are noted and compared with further screening data.

Assessment of dynamic posture should be done with the same four views, utilising digital video as the recording device. The initial dynamic test is the overhead squat test. The athlete should be instructed to keep a dowel or foam roll overhead with arms extended. Two complete full squats in each of the four directions should be completed (Fig. 11.6A–D). A single leg squat will increase load and decrease stability for a more specific test (Fig. 11.7A, B). Dynamic scapulothoracic motion is noted by the athlete abducting his/her arms into a palm-touching position overhead and/or horizontally abducting (rowing) the arms with elbows bent to 90° of flexion. These tests look for general kinetic chain movement patterns. They can help identify quality of movement and segmental stabilisation in the scapulospinal and scapulohumeral musculature (Fig. 11.8A–F).

Spine measurements

After all posture media and dynamic movement tests are compiled, a battery of goniometric/inclinometer measurements can be taken. This will

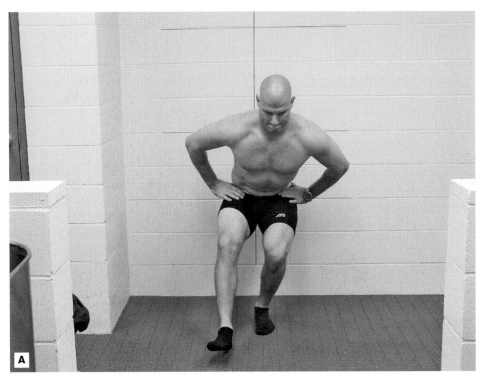

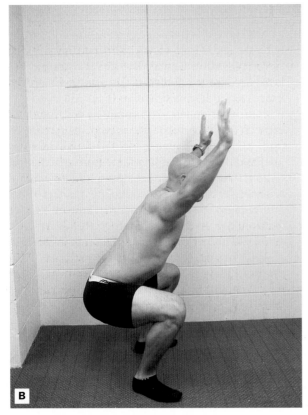

Figure 11.3A, B Exercises that utilise unilateral movements may be more advantageous than bilateral movements.

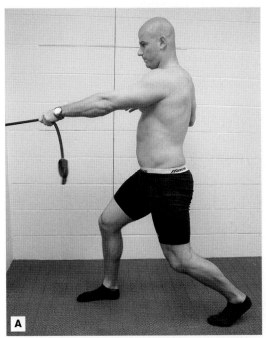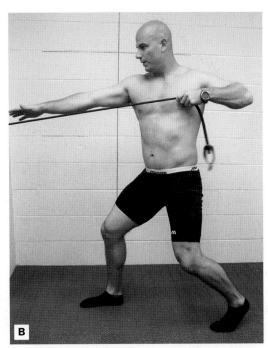

A **B**

Figure 11.4A, B Training in a contralateral manner may help to activate the cross-extensor or cross-flexor reflexes, therefore aiding motor control in sport-specific movements.

allow specific variances to be noted of particular joints and give detail for corrective strategies.

It is important to have a fundamental understanding of the spine and joint movements available prior to analysing the data. The spine has a total movement package available and each vertebral segment contributes to that total package. In all sports the spine plays a central role in accomplishing the objective of the sport (Farfan 1996). Therefore, proximal stability will help promote distal mobility.

According to Chek (2003) the standing curvature of the lumbar spine and the thoracic spine can be assessed via dual inclinometer in the following manner. To assess static thoracic curvature and thoracic extension, the practitioner should place the superior inclinometer on a central point between the C7–T1 spine junction, and place the inferior inclinometer on a central point between the T12–L1 junction and obtain readings in neutral and extended positions. Another measurement of thoracic extension can be done with the shoulders fully flexed overhead,

elbows extended and palms in neutral position. This measurement allows the practitioner to see how the upper extremities and thoracic extension function together (Fig. 11.9A–D).

Lumbar curvature can be measured in neutral, extended and flexed positions by placing the superior inclinometer between the T12–L1 junction and inferior inclinometer between the L5 (or L6)–S1 junction and obtaining angles in the three different positions (Fig. 11.10A–D).

The normal range for static thoracic and lumbar curvature is 30–35° according to Chek (2003). The available thoracic extension motion should be to the same degree as its measurement (e.g. a 30° thoracic curve should have 30° of extension). With the arms overhead, the thoracic extension in the spine should allow for at least 14° of movement (Chek 2003).

Hip region measurements

General assessment of the medial hamstring/hip adductors, rectus femoris/iliopsoas, hamstring,

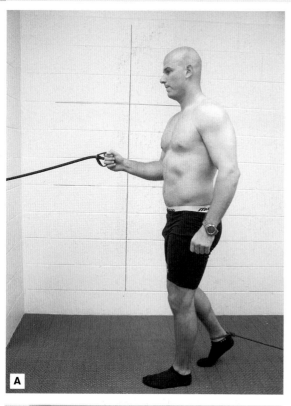
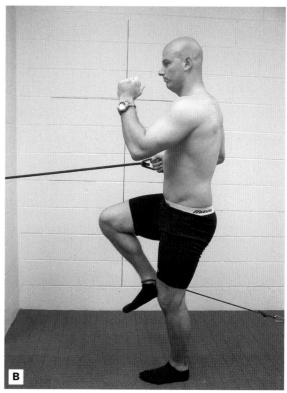
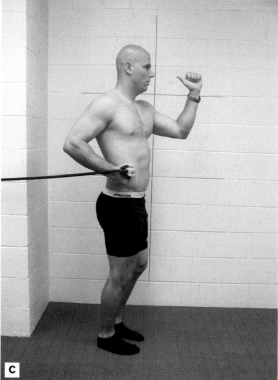
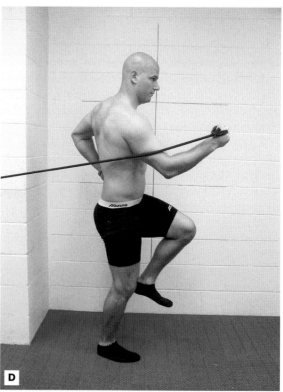

Figure 11.5A–D   Contralateral training exercises, which utilise specific firing patterns, may help performance and injury prevention.

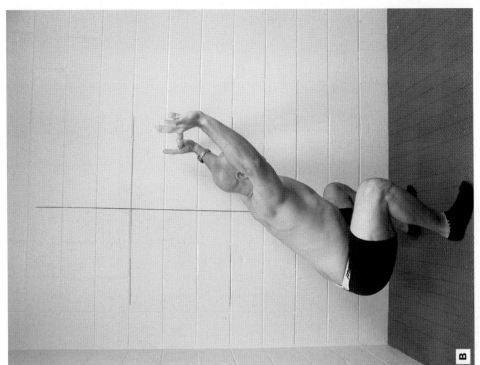

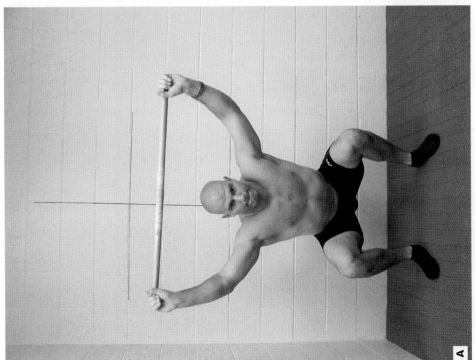

continued

Figure 11.6A–D Screening for dynamic dysfunction should include the overhead squat assessment in all directions.

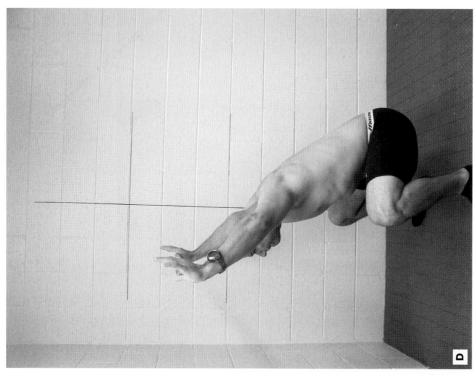

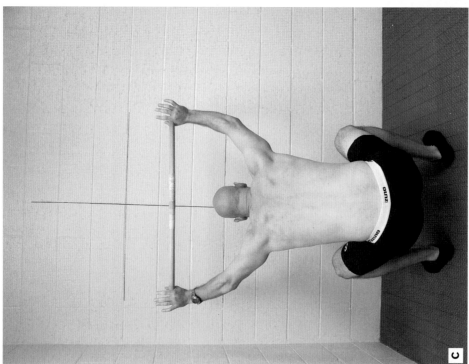

Figure 11.6A–D *continued*

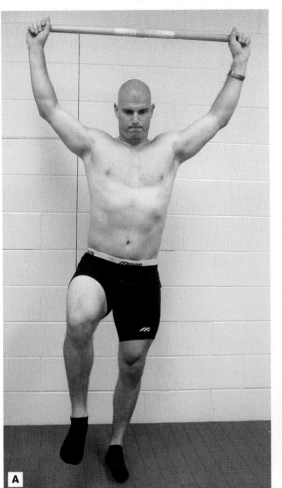 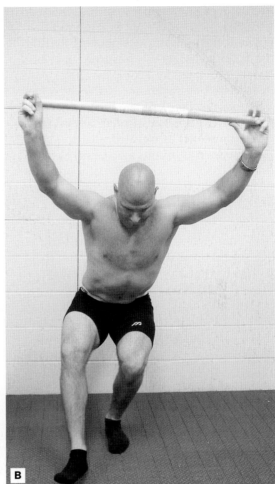

Figure 11.7A, B A single-leg squat will increase load, decrease stability and show faulty movement patterns more specifically than the overhead squat.

tensor fascia lata and quadratus lumborum were explained in Ch. 5. In addition, goniometric measurements of hip flexion/extension/internal rotation/external rotation, and pelvic tilt should be performed.

Abdominal strength and coordination

Abdominal coordination and strength may be tested by having the athlete (lying supine) lower their straightened legs, from a hips flexed position, towards the floor. Special attention should be given to movement of the spinous processes of L3–L5 when lowering the legs. When the processes migrate away from the examiner's hand the lower abdominal strength threshold has been met (Fig. 11.11A–C).

Lower extremity measurements

Knee and ankle movements can be assessed via goniometric measurements. A navicular drop test of the foot can be done to assess pronation and its possible effects up the kinetic chain (DeLany, personal communication, 2004). Finding the neutral position for the subtalar joint is done as follows. The medial prominence of the navicular bone is noted in a non-weight-bearing position. The athlete is then asked to weight bear and the drop in navicular height is measured, described as a navicular drop test by Thompson (2005). Also to be considered as significant is the degree of elevation (off the floor) of the first metatarsal when the foot is placed in subtalar neutral position. When presented as elevated, this condition has been described as primus metatarsus elevatus by Rothbart (2002), which he hypothesises has significant whole body postural implications (Fig. 11.12A, B).

Upper extremities

In the throwing athlete special attention should be given to the shoulder and elbow. All joint movements should be assessed and compared bilaterally. Values will frequently differ between dominant and non-dominant sides; however, these measurements may still be within the normal range, comparatively speaking. Wilk (2004) presented an example in professional baseball pitchers of the norm (external rotation at 90° abduction: dominant side 129° ± 9°, non-dominant side 122° ± 10°; internal rotation at 90° abduction: dominant side 62° ± 9°, non-dominant side 70° ± 10°) (Fig. 11.13).

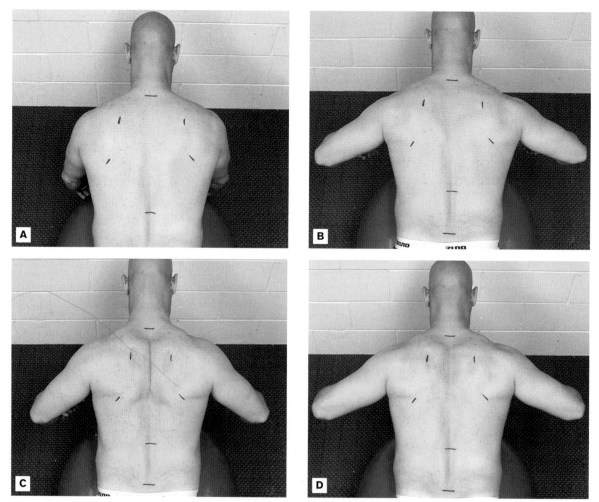

Figure 11.8 The practitioner should assess movement in both scapulospinal and scapulohumeral musculature for proper firing sequences and quality of motion. **A** Beginning position for assessing scapulohumeral and scapulospinal. **B** Excessive scapulohumeral motion. **C** Excessive scapulospinal motion. **D** Normal motion.

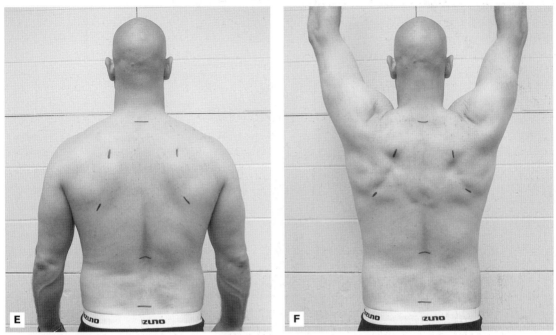

Figure 11.8 E Beginning position for scapular overhead motion. F Normal scapular overhead motion.

Manual assessment

The last screening component is a thorough manual assessment of the skin, fascia and muscular status to confirm identified dysfunctions from previous assessment.

Corrective/preventative strategies

After a meticulous screening for dysfunction, an individualised corrective/preventative programme should be developed from the data collected. The programme may include stretching, strengthening, inhibition or some other form of correcting identified musculoskeletal imbalances and dysfunction.

Dynamic flexibility versus static stretching

Flexibility, or better stated, mobility, in the athlete is important for athletic performance if the motions can be dynamically controlled. Any athlete or human in general will compensate for the lack of flexibility by using alternate movement patterns. It is possible for an athlete to perform well even when poor biomechanical motions are used, but eventually a decrease in optimal tissue function will be experienced. It is important to discuss what type of stretching programme to use and when to use it.

There are many variations of stretching including proprioceptive neuromuscular facilitation (PNF), static stretching, MET and dynamic methods. These methods have been discussed by McAtee (1993), Kurz (1994) and Chaitow (2001). Although the optimum method for improving athletic performance and decreasing injury may be debatable, the authors of this chapter prefer a systematic choice based on research evidence, clinical experience and athlete needs. Gleim & McHugh (1997) and Thacker et al (2004) have shown evidence that stretching does not prevent sports injury. The more critical component to injury prevention appears to be active warm-up. Young & Behm (2002) indicated that static stretching may inhibit maximal force production if done within 1 hour prior to competition. This may

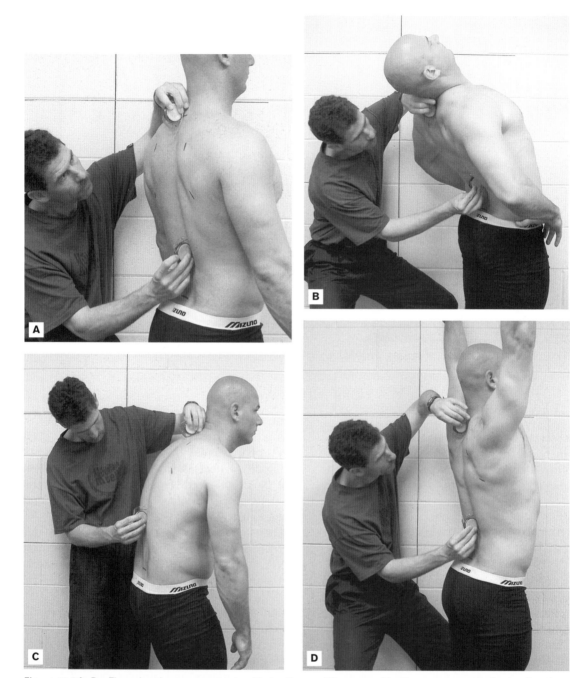

Figure 11.9A–D Thoracic spine measurements will give the practitioner an objective measurement of spine function (Chek 2003).

reduce an athlete's ability to succeed in his/her competition. These findings support a more dynamic or active form of stretching/warm-up prior to competition (Fig. 11.14A–F). Static stretch-ing, PNF, MET and other methods appear to be more beneficial post-competition, or at least 3–4 hours pre-competition, and/or in the rehabili-tation process.

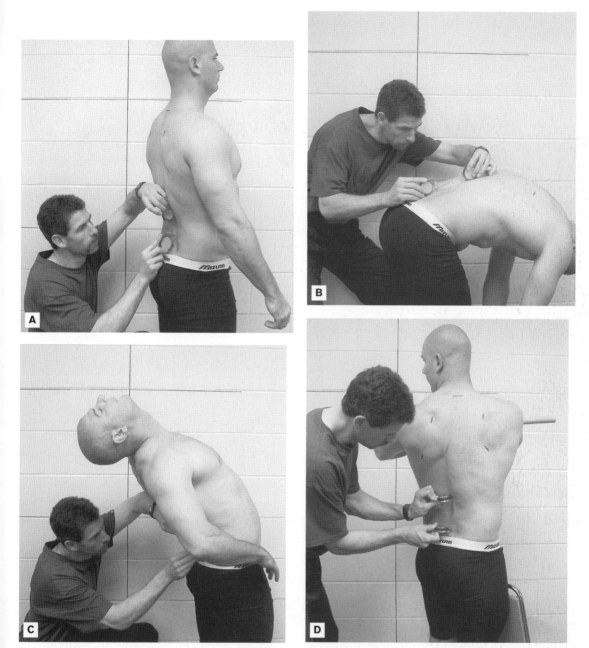

Figure 11.10A–D Lumbar spine measurements to assess curvature and movement will help the practitioner with screening (Chek 2003).

Warm-up

As Gleim & McHugh (1997) and Thacker et al (2004) have demonstrated, warm-up is critical to injury prevention. A general increase in blood flow will aid in any flexibility programme. An ade-quate warm-up may consist of 5–10 minutes of cardiovascular activity at 40–50% maximum heart rate. It is the authors' preference to have all athletes do a general warm-up prior to any flexibility/corrective exercise session.

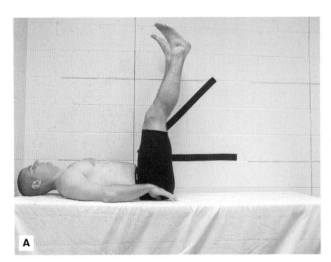

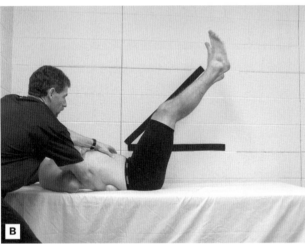

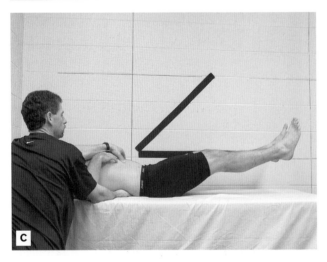

Figure 11.11A–C Abdominal function is critical to athletic movement and can be assessed with the leg-lowering test.

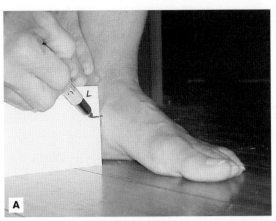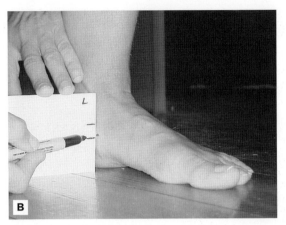

Figure 11.12A, B The navicular drop test can help determine dysfunction beginning in the foot and being transferred up the kinetic chain. (Reprinted with permission from Thompson 2005.)

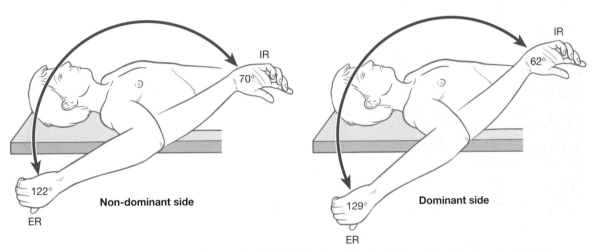

Figure 11.13 The total motion concept discussed by Wilk (2004) shows the adaptation of the throwing shoulder in the professional baseball pitcher. (Reprinted with permission from Wilk 2004.)

Recovery techniques

As in any sport it is not the amount of work the athlete does that determines good health, instead it is the recovery that takes place between exercise and/or athletic competition. Stress is simply a stimulus that interacts with the physiology of the body. Depending on the intensity of the stress, it can either injure or improve the athlete. In order to improve there must be a balance between stress and recovery. According to Calder (1990) the following techniques can help athletes with their recovery from exercise or competition:

1. Proper nutrition and hydration
2. Hot/cold hydrotherapy techniques
3. General sports massage
4. Relaxation techniques (breathing, meditation, visualisation, music, etc.)
5. Rest or sleep.

In the presence of good general body conditioning and adequate recovery techniques, injury recovery will be optimal.

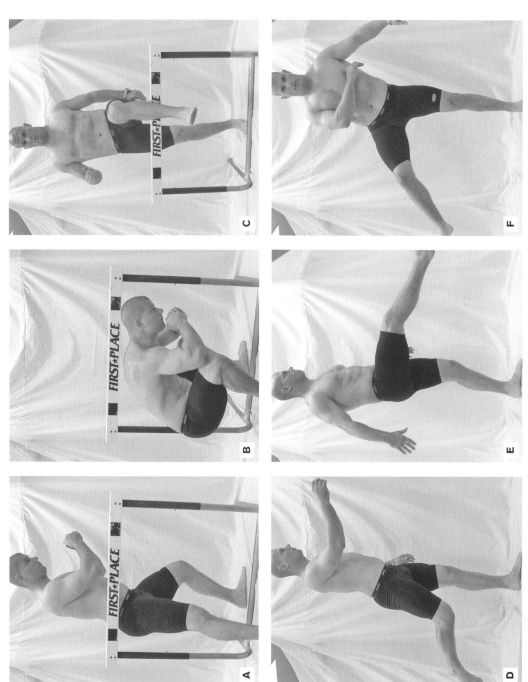

Figure 11.14A–F Dynamic warm-up exercises may be more beneficial than static stretching prior to competition.

Common injuries

Human movement during sport and exercise is typically faster and produces greater force than activities of daily living. As a result, the potential for injury is increased. Injury trends in athletes vary from sport to sport. It is not uncommon to have soft tissue and joint injury in any sport. Injuries can be classified as: strain, sprain, contusion, fracture and inflammation (tendonitis, tenosynovitis, bursitis, neuritis, etc.). Most inflammation-type injuries are commonly caused by overuse. To further describe an injury one can use a sub-classification system of acute, sub-acute or chronic, which will aid the practitioner in assessment and treatment.

Data collected by the National Collegiate Athletic Association's Injury Surveillance System (NCAA 2004) showed that American football had the highest occurrence of injuries (33) per 1000 exposures followed by wrestling (25.7) and men's soccer (18.8). When looking at a 15-year average of which body parts were most involved in injury the system showed knee, ankle and upper leg as the most commonly injured. The most prevalent types of injuries were sprain, contusion and strain in descending order.

Other data from the NCAA's Injury Surveillance System showed common types of injuries in baseball from 1997 to 2004. They were classified from the most common to least common, as follows: strain, sprain, tendonitis, and contusion. The body parts involved, listed from most common to least common, were as follows: shoulder, elbow and upper leg.

Data from the 2003 Redbook (American Specialty Companies 2003), which is a disability analysis of major league baseball in the United States, showed that from the years 1999 to 2003 the most common injuries were shoulder, elbow, knee and back. The type of injury was listed from most prominent to least as follows: strain, sprain and inflammation.

Although this data shows only a small spectrum of injury in competitive sports, it gives the practitioner a good sense of what preventative and standard care measures are required to help the athlete. For the purpose of this chapter, soft tissue and joint dysfunction will be the primary focus.

Standard care of injuries

Any practitioner should be able to recognise that a quick and accurate evaluation will lead to a rapid initiation of acute care, which, in turn, leads to a more rapid return to function. The goal should be to safely return the athlete to competition in the shortest time possible. Appropriate pre-injury screening data can be consulted to help in this process. The severity of the injury and what medical intervention is required (surgery, immobilisation, etc.) will determine when and how each member of the sports medicine team will intervene.

Because the normal healing process takes place in a regular and predictable fashion the health care provider can follow the various signs and symptoms exhibited to monitor the healing process. Knowing when it is appropriate to begin new interventions is paramount to the recovery process. The natural healing process usually cannot be accelerated, but several things can inhibit or slow recovery. Medicine, modalities, manual therapies, psychological ease, nutrition and exercise are factors that can assist the body in obtaining the optimal healing environment. Utilising the many tools available will give the practitioner the best results. Therapeutic modalities such as hydrotherapy, cryotherapy, moist heat, ultrasound, microcurrent, soft tissue oscillation units and others can be used in combination with exercise and manual techniques for injury recovery. All modalities and manual techniques should have a specific physiological purpose. Examples of specific objectives could include lymphatic drainage, vasoconstriction, vasodilation, neural inhibition, etc.

As athletes may present with a similar injury but have a different set of problems, different treatment options will provide the best results. Each athlete requires an in-depth and individualised assessment/management plan to optimise recovery.

Acute injury care

Understanding the stages of healing and repair are important in acute care of injuries. It is not the scope of this text to belabour the details of tissue healing but a general overview may be helpful.

After any trauma the body has an acute response or reaction (inflammation), which lasts 24–48 hours. A repair and regeneration phase begins, which overlaps the acute response and lasts from 2 days to 6–8 weeks. The final healing phase is remodelling. The remodelling phase begins at about 3 weeks and continues for a year or more it also has some overlap of the repair and response phase (Fig. 11.15).

According to Mangine et al (2004) the primary role of the practitioner is to decrease inflammation and prevent damaging secondary effects such as decreased range of motion, decreased muscle strength, and prolonged edema. Inflammation control can be best achieved by rest, cryotherapy, compression, elevation, massage techniques, lymphatic drainage via tissue oscillation units, and various other modalities (microcurrent, etc.) (Merrick 2004).

Secondary effects can be prevented with range of motion exercises, isometrics, proprioceptive exercises and manual therapies, all of which depend on tissue or type of joint injured. If immobilisation or surgery is required the practitioner must consider the influence of reflex inhibition caused by the muscle spindle. When a muscle is immobilised in a shortened or lengthened position the spindle will assume a new resting length (Mangine et al 2004). Therefore while waiting for protected tissues to heal, attention can be focused to the rest of the kinetic chain and any other dysfunctions. Once injured tissues have adequately healed, specific deficiencies can then be addressed (Fig. 11.16A, B).

Injury in the sub-acute and chronic phases can be treated by, evaluating the symptoms and probable causes. A systematic rehabilitation plan can then be formed using many of the previously mentioned therapies. Sub-acute and chronic

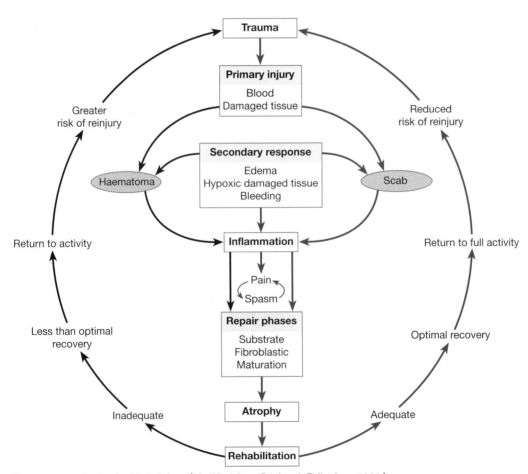

Figure 11.15 Cycle of athletic injury. (Modified from Booher & Thibodeau 1989.)

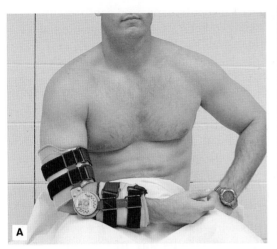 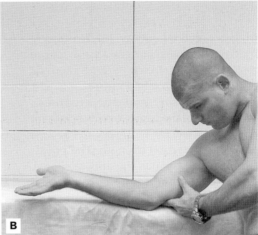

Figure 11.16A, B   After periods of immobilisation, musculature may shorten and therefore need to be assessed and treated by the practitioner.

injuries are commonly more problematic and require advanced manual therapies such as MET and NMT.

Muscle energy techniques (MET) and integrated neuromuscular inhibition techniques (INIT) in sports injuries

As has been discussed, athletes may be injured or develop a variety of dysfunctional biomechanics. The prevention, treatment, rehabilitation and return to activity are critical components to an athlete's and a team's success. MET can be very useful and easily integrated into the total care package for each athlete. It is important to understand that MET is only one element of the many possible therapies. MET and its use will be described in combination with other therapies. Emphasis on managing each individual and his symptoms is paramount to success.

Prevention of injury using MET, INIT and other techniques

The authors feel that the many acute dysfunctions that are described daily by athletes as 'general stiffness' or 'general soreness' can be managed by the following sequence:

1. Assessment of movement limitations
2. Assessment of skin mobility for underlying pathology
3. Trigger point assessment
4. General body warm-up or localised warm-up using moist heat or hydrotherapy
5. General massage (gliding primary application)
6. Modified version of INIT
7. MET for shortened structures
8. Isotonic/isometric/isokinetic corrective exercise programme
9. Post-exercise or post-competition recovery techniques
10. Appropriate nutrition and hydration.

The INIT used in this sequence was first described by Chaitow (1994) although the method used is a slightly different version. Palpate the trigger point 'by direct finger or thumb pressure, and when the very tissues in which the trigger point lies are positioned in such a way as to take away the pain (entirely or at least to a great extent), that the most (dis) stressed fibres in which the trigger point is housed are in a position of relative ease. The trigger point would then be receiving direct inhibitory pressure (mild or perhaps intermittent) and (using strain/counterstrain methods) would have been positioned so that tissues housing it are relaxed (relatively or completely).' It is the view of the authors of this chapter to hold this position intermittently for 20–40 seconds or until muscle release occurs.

After trigger point inhibition, MET, utilising an isometric contraction of shortened musculature with a postfacilitation stretch would then be initiated.

Contraction starting point should be at the resistance barrier. The shortened muscles (agonist) are isometrically contracted for 5–10 seconds at 20% of their maximal contraction strength. The practitioner should meet and match the athlete's force. The athlete is asked to inhale prior to contraction using an outward abdominal movement. After isometric contraction the athlete is asked to exhale, relax and breathe normally. Within a 5-second period, a stretch of the shortened muscle is commenced. The muscle is taken to its new barrier and slightly beyond, and held for at least 10 seconds and up to 60 seconds. This process is repeated three to four times with a 5-second break between repetitions. Each isometric contraction begins from the new barrier position.

Indications

- Stretching contracted soft tissue (fascia, muscle) or tissues housing active trigger points
- To optimise length tension relationships
- To maximise neuromuscular function thus increasing biomechanical efficiency.

Acute injury care with MET and other therapies

From a practitioner's perspective, the acute injury is the most fragile of all cases. Care to prevent further damage while helping set up the optimal healing environment is important and requires precise protocols.

The authors prefer the following treatment sequence in most acute muscle injuries. Joint, ligament, cartilage or bone damage may alter the sequence. The practitioner can use these guidelines in applying treatment to the previously mentioned conditions when their healing parameters allow.

1. Immediate cryotherapy, compression, and elevation to moderate inflammation
2. Within 24 hours of injury, tissue oscillation therapy for lymphatic drainage and/or

microcurrent therapy used concurrently with cryotherapy for pain and control of inflammation
3. Deactivation of surrounding kinetic chain trigger points
4. Skin release or gliding technique of underlying fascia
5. Neural stretching in specific cases
6. 24–48 hours post injury, INIT/MET in injured tissue and/or surrounding tissues
7. Proprioception exercises as tolerated
8. Any other acute therapies and progression to rehabilitation.

The following INIT/MET sequence is used in the acute injury: identify any trigger points in the injured muscle or surrounding muscles with direct finger or thumb pressure. Gently compress, either intermittently or persistently, the trigger point. Take the muscle into a position of ease that does not violate injured tissue, and hold for 20–40 seconds, after which a contraction in the antagonist muscle is initiated. The contraction should be 20% or less of maximum contraction and held for 5–10 seconds. The practitioner's force should meet and match athlete's force. This is thought to create reciprocal inhibition in the injured muscle (Lewit 1999). The athlete should inhale prior to contraction, exhale and relax after contraction. Within 5 seconds of relaxation a very gentle movement of the injured muscle to its barrier may be initiated provided there is no pain. This may be repeated two or three times.

This technique may be modified for the sub-acute injury by adding an isometric contraction of injured tissue followed by postisometric relaxation and mild stretch.

Indications

- Relaxation of acute muscle spasm or trigger points
- Stimulation of neuromuscular firing to prevent muscle shutdown.

Chronic injury and long-term rehabilitation using MET

Although chronic injuries are not particularly delicate they are often the most difficult to treat because they may be perpetuated by deep-seated dysfunction. Adequate time and therapy are required to correct this type of injury. Rehabilitation from injury that may have required surgery or immobilisation can be managed in a similar fashion to the chronic injury. Both cases require thorough assessment of the entire kinetic chain for possible contributors to the injury. Once dysfunctions are identified, specific manual therapies, modalities and other techniques can be applied.

MET, INIT and a corrective isometric/isotonic/isokinetic exercise programme can be implemented in the following sequence:

1. General body warm-up
2. Specific modality treatment to increase blood flow
3. Specific modality treatment to promote lymphatic drainage, decrease pain/spasm if indicated
4. General massage to loosen overlying and surrounding tissues
5. INIT and MET
6. Corrective exercise programme
7. Recovery techniques.

The specifics of INIT and MET as they are used in the above sequence are as follows: tissues containing trigger points and shortened tissues are identified. Trigger points are treated first by applying a direct ischaemic pressure with the fingers or thumb, either intermittently or constantly. The tissues containing the trigger points/pain/tenderness are taken to a position of relative ease of the pain. This position is held for 30–60 seconds or until the trigger point releases. The athlete is instructed to maintain a consistent respiratory rhythm throughout. After trigger points are assessed and treated, MET utilising one of the two following methods should be applied to shortened muscles.

- *Method 1:* Utilise an isometric contraction of the agonist muscle followed by a postfacilitation stretch. Contraction should be painless and should involve 20–40% of maximum available strength for 5–10 seconds against the practitioner's matching force, commencing from just short of the muscle's restriction barrier. The athlete should inhale prior to

contraction, exhale and relax thereafter. Within 5 seconds after contraction and with total relaxation, the muscle should be stretched to the new barrier and slightly beyond and held for 10–30 seconds. This process may be repeated three to five times.

- *Method 2:* Utilise an isometric contraction of the antagonist muscle, which will create reciprocal inhibition in the shortened muscle and allow for stretch (Lewit 1999). All other criteria are the same as method 1.

Indications

- Stretching of chronic shortened tissues (myofascial, muscle, fibrotic)
- Stretching tissues with active trigger points.

MET using isotonic, isometric and isokinetic contractions for strengthening weak postural muscles

As explained in Ch. 5, these MET procedures are used in various aspects of injury rehabilitation, preventative and corrective programmes. Their use is dependent on athlete and injury assessment.

All athletes are treated on a daily basis, therefore anything other than posture awareness exercises and breathing techniques is not prescribed to athletes for self or home care. If athletes are not available for treatment on a daily basis then a home programme should be implemented. In the cases of rehabilitation and immobilisation, specific self-stretching, mobilisation and strengthening exercises may be necessary for home care.

The following are some specific athletic injuries and useful management options using MET or INIT.

Case A: Sub-acute low-back strain

An athlete reports with low-back pain. His subjective pain is a 6/10, 10 being the most intense. His activity level is compromised. He states that he first felt the pain following a series of flexion movements during skills practice 7 days prior. His chief complaint is generalised low-back pain that is located in the L4/L5/S1 area, and as the pain increases with an activity it migrates laterally to both PSIS regions. Orthopaedic physician exam shows no remarkable findings, x-rays are negative for spondylolysis/spondylolisthesis, neurologic exam is normal. Athlete has no previous history of back injury.

The diagnosis is low-back strain. Objective evaluation information was as follows:

Test/measurement	Finding	Norms (Chek 2003)
Forward head posture (cm)	5	0–3
1st rib angle (deg.)	31	25
SCM (deg.)	75	45–60
Thoracic curve (deg.)	57	30–35
Thoracic extension (deg.)	20	57 (reverse of T-curve)
Thoracic ext. arms overhead (deg.)	7	<14
Lumbar curve (deg.)	15	30–35
Lumbar extension (deg.)	15	20–35
Lumbar flexion (deg.)	24	40–60
Pelvic tilt: ASIS to PSIS (deg.)	12R, 13L	4–7
Abdominal function	poor/ weak	

General testing shows bilateral rectus femoris, psoas and spinal erector tightness. The athlete shows bilateral foot pronation, and general internal rotation of femurs, as well as genu recurvatum.

Manual assessment indicates skin restrictions over bilateral spinal erector region. Several trigger points were found in the quadratus lumborum and spinal erector musculature. The athlete has bilateral psoas hypertonicity and tender points that are localised in iliacus. He also has bilateral adductor mass and piriformis hypertonicity.

Treatment

Treatment was initiated with a 5-minute stationary bike ride, followed by tissue oscillation modalities and general massage from gluteal to mid-thoracic region. Trigger point areas previously identified were addressed with INIT, described earlier in this chapter. MET using isometric contraction of agonist/post facilitation stretch, as described earlier in the chapter, was applied bilaterally to ilopsoas, rectus femoris, and hip adductors. Self-mobilisation of thoracic spine was performed with use of a foam roll. Corrective exercises were implemented as follows:

1. Abdominal muscle toning manoeuvre with associated stabilisation exercises and progressions are initiated with primary focus on lower abdominal endurance and control.

2. Posterior kinetic chain exercises to promote strength and endurance in the gluteals and thoracic extensor musculature. Time under tension is a key variable to promote endurance. Extension exercises to correct lumbar spine deficit would be initiated if there were no associated pain or discomfort.

3. Exercises to strengthen the deep neck flexors.

Following the corrective programme, the athlete tolerated light skills activity well. After skills practice a second session of treatment, as described above, excluding trigger point deactivation, was conducted. The second session ended with recovery hydrotherapy techniques and cryotherapy. Return to full activity was based on symptoms and tolerance.

Case B: Acute hamstring strain

An athlete is running a maximum speed sprint and experiences a sharp pain in middle portion of right hamstring (semi-tendinosis). His subjective pain scale is 7/10 with 10 being the most intense. He is unable to ambulate normally and indicates that his chief complaint is pain with full extension in posterior thigh. He has no previous history of hamstring injury.

Objective evaluation prior to injury is as follows:

Test/measurement	Finding	Norms (Chek 2003)
Forward head posture (cm)	5	0–3
1st rib angle (deg.)	31	25
SCM (deg.)	80	45–60
Thoracic curve (deg.)	37	30–35

Thoracic extension (deg.)	22	37 (reverse of T-curve)
Thoracic ext. arms overhead (deg.)	8	<14
Lumbar curve (deg.)	20	30–35
Lumbar extension (deg.)	20	20–35
Lumbar flexion (deg.)	22	40–60
Pelvic tilt: ASIS to PSIS (deg.)	14R, 9L	4–7
Abdominal function	poor/ weak	

General testing shows a lack of full knee extension and hip flexion compared with opposite extremity. He has no discoloration or obvious deformity. Manual muscle testing shows a deficit (3/5) in knee flexion in injured extremity. Manual muscle testing scale is 5/5 normal contraction (1/5 is no muscle contraction). Hip extension and hip adduction are 4/5 on muscle testing and both tests produce mild discomfort. All other manual muscle tests are normal.

General observation in standing position shows that his feet supinate bilaterally and he presents with external rotation in both legs but slightly more in right leg.

Manual assessment indicates skin restrictions with skin rolling technique in bilateral spinal erector region and right posterior hamstring region, which suggests underlying problems (Fritz 2000).

Bilateral iliopsoas, rectus femoris, and hip adductors all display hypertonicity. Iliotibial band presents with tightness bilaterally. In addition the athlete presents with some left latissimus dorsi tightness.

Treatment

Initial treatment (first 24 hours) was to control any possible inflammation in injured tissues. A combination of cryotherapy, tissue oscillation for lymphatic drainage, microcurrent and compression were applied. These treatments were performed multiple times. During the following 24 hours, symptoms were minimal, continued inflammation control and manual therapy to hypertonic musculature was addressed. Care was taken to not disrupt healing tissue. A skin/fascia release of hamstring, utilising a gliding technique was initiated. Utilising the acute injury version of INIT/MET the hamstring was treated. Neural stretching technique of the lower extremities was performed (Fig. 11.17A–C). Standing proprioception exercises were performed with no discomfort to injured tissue. Utilising INIT and MET, as previously explained, the hypertonic iliopsoas, rectus femoris, hip adductors, iliotibial band and lower spinal erectors were treated, along with a general effleurage of the same musculature. In addition, self-mobilisation of the iliotibial band, thoracic spine, and left latissimus dorsi was performed via foam roll.

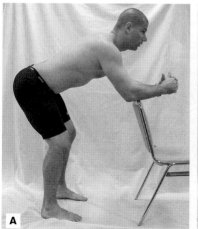 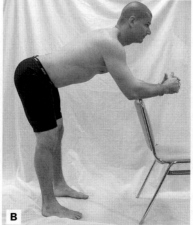 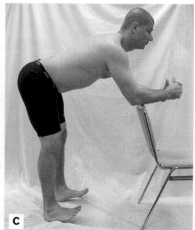

Figure 11.17A–C Neural stretching technique after an acute hamstring injury.

Corrective exercises were implemented as follows:

1. Abdominal muscle toning manoeuvre with associated stabilisation exercises and progressions were initiated with primary focus on lower abdominal endurance and control.

2. Posterior kinetic chain exercises to promote strength and endurance in the gluteals and thoracic extensor musculature. Time under tension is a key variable to promote endurance. Neurological firing sequence is also a vital component, as the athlete should learn to fire gluteals before hamstring. Lumbar extension exercises to correct spine deficits were also addressed.

3. Psoas exercises aimed at restoring normal length–tension relationships.

4. Exercises to strengthen deep neck flexors.

Following the corrective exercise programme a second session of treatment, as included above, without trigger point treatment was started. The second session ended with recovery hydrotherapy techniques and cryotherapy.

As soon as functional strengthening of hamstring as a hip extensor and a knee flexor could be tolerated, skills practice was slowly initiated. An in-depth look at running mechanics and biomechanical changes was necessary to prevent further strain. Return to full activity was based on symptoms, tolerance and functional capability.

Case C: Shoulder tendonitis (subacromial long head of biceps)

An overhead-throwing athlete reports post-game-presenting right anterior shoulder soreness. He has been experiencing periodic soreness in anterior shoulder in subacromial region. The athlete states that his initial soreness started after a biomechanical change in throwing 2 weeks prior. He states that soreness is tolerable when he gets warmed up. He has no previous history of shoulder injury/pain. Subsequent exam by orthopaedic physician and MRI reveals subacromial inflammation in long head of the biceps.

The diagnosis is subacromial impingement/tendonitis. Objective evaluation prior to injury was as follows:

Test/measurement	Finding	Norms (Chek 2003)
Forward head posture (cm)	6	0–3
1st rib angle (deg.)	35	25
SCM (deg.)	82	45–60
Thoracic curve (deg.)	47	30–35
Thoracic extension (deg.)	20	47 (reverse of T-curve)
Thoracic ext. arms overhead (deg.)	6	<14
Lumbar curve (deg.)	38	30–35
Lumbar extension (deg.)	20	20–35
Lumbar flexion (deg.)	15	40–60
Pelvic tilt: ASIS to PSIS (deg.)	12R, 13L	4–7
Abdominal function	poor/weak	

General evaluation shows that the athlete has pronounced bilateral protraction of shoulders and internal rotation of arms in general. He has a decrease of internal rotation and increase of external rotation in the right shoulder when compared with the left. Tests show tightness of pectorals and latissimus dorsi. Manual muscle testing shows weakness (of injured arm) in flexion of shoulder (4/5), prone horizontal abduction with thumb pointing upward (3/5), and external rotation at 0° abduction.

Manual assessment indicates bilateral pectoral tightness. The athlete has hypertonic levator scapula, upper trapezius, subcapularis and infraspinatus.

Treatment

Initial treatment included deep tissue oscillation modality, moist heat, general body warm-up in conjunction with anti-inflammatory medications prescribed by physician, and general massage of pectoral and latissimus dorsi muscles. Hypertonic or trigger point tissues, previously identified were treated with chronic injury version of INIT technique. MET using isometric contraction of antagonist (method 2), as explained previously, were applied to hypertonic musculature. Corrective exercises were implemented as follows:

1. Abdominal muscle toning manoeuvre with associated stabilisation exercises and progressions were initiated with primary focus on lower abdominal endurance and control.

2. Posterior kinetic chain exercises to promote strength and endurance in the gluteals and thoracic extensor musculature. Time under tension is a key variable to promote endurance.

3. Exercises to strengthen deep neck flexors.

4. Thoracic mobilisation via foam rolls.

5. Specific isotonic/isokinetic/reactive stabilisation exercises for the rotator cuff and scapular muscles.

Following the corrective exercise programme, the athlete was allowed to participate in any skills activity that did not produce pain. After skills practice, recovery hydrotherapy techniques, cryotherapy and microcurrent treatment concluded the session. Return to full activity was based on symptoms and tolerance of functional activities.

Summary

Athletic injuries present the practitioner with many different scenarios. As each athlete responds in a unique way, the practitioner must adapt his skills through knowledge and experience to the athlete, specific injury and surrounding variables that may inhibit adequate recovery.

MET, if utilised properly, can play a very important role in the overall health care of athletes. Further understanding of MET and the many other manual therapies is an ever-evolving process for the sports practitioner.

References

American Specialty Companies 2003 Redbook: Major league baseball disability analysis, 2003 edn. American Specialty Companies, Roanoke

Booher J M, Thibodeau G A 1989 Athletic injury assessment, 2nd edn. Times Mirror/Mosby, St Louis

Borsa P A, Wilk K E, Jacobson J A et al 2004 Instrumented measurement of gleno-humeral translation in professional baseball pitchers. Medicine and Science in Sports and Exercise 36: S200

Boyle M 2004 Functional training for sports. Human Kinetics, Champaign

Calder A 1990 Recovery: Restoration and regeneration as essential components within training programs. Excel 6(3): 15–19

Chaitow L 1994 Integrated neuromuscular inhibition technique. British Journal of Osteopathy 13: 17–20

Chaitow L 2001 Muscle energy techniques, 2nd edn. Churchill Livingstone, Edinburgh

Chaitow L, DeLany J W 2002 Clinical application of neuromuscular techniques, vol 2: The lower body. Churchill Livingstone, Edinburgh

Chek P 2003 Certified high-performance exercise kinesiology practitioner certification level 1. Peak Performance, Manhattan, 10–19 November 2003

Crockett H C, Gross L B, Wilk K E et al 2002 Osseous adaptation and range of motion at the gleno-humeral joint in professional baseball pitchers. American Journal of Sports Medicine 30(1): 20–26

Farfan H F 1996 Biomechanics of the spine in sports. In: Watkins R G (ed) The spine in sports. Mosby, St Louis, pp 13–20

Fritz S 2000 Mosby's fundamentals of therapeutic massage, 2nd edn. Mosby, St Louis

Fritz S, Grosenbach J M 2004 Mosby's essential sciences for therapeutic massage, 2nd edn. Mosby, St Louis

Gleim G W, McHugh M P 1997 Flexibility and its effects on sports injury and performance. Sports Medicine, New Zealand 24(5): 289–299

Greenfield B, Catlin P A, Coats P W et al 1995 Posture in patients with shoulder overuse injuries and healthy individuals. Journal of Orthopaedic and Sports Physical Therapy 21(5): 287–295

Kraemer W J, Gomez A L 2001 Establishing a solid fitness base. In: Foran B (ed) High performance sports conditioning. Human Kinetics, Champaign, pp 3–17

Kurz T 1994 Stretching scientifically: A guide to flexibility training. Stadion, Island Pond

Lewit K 1999 Manipulative therapy in rehabilitation of the motor system, 3rd edn, Butterworths, London

Mangine B, Nuzzo G, Harrelson G L 2004 Physiologic factors of rehabilitation. In: Andrews J R, Harrelson G L, Wilk K E (eds) Physical rehabilitation of the injured athlete, 3rd edn. Saunders, Philadelphia, pp 13–33

McAtee R E 1993 Facilitated stretching. Human Kinetics, Champaign

Meister K 2005 Throwing adaptations in youth and adolescents in baseball. Presentation, American Sports Medicine Institute Injuries in Baseball Course, 15 January 2005

Merrick M A 2004 Therapeutic modalities as an adjunct to rehabilitation. In: Andrews J R, Harrelson G L, Wilk K E (eds) Physical rehabilitation of the injured athlete, 3rd edn. Saunders, Philadelphia, pp 51–98

Myrland S 2004 No ice? No problem! Training and Conditioning 24(7): 43–47

NCAA 2004 Injury surveillance system. National Collegiate Athletic Association, Indianapolis

Norris C M 2004 Sports injuries, diagnosis and management, 3rd edn. Butterworth-Heinemann, London

Osbahr D C, Cannon D L, Speer K P 2002 Retroversion of the humerus in the throwing shoulder of college baseball pitchers. The American Journal of Sports Medicine 30: 347–353

Pieper H G 1998 Humeral torsion in the throwing arm of handball players. The American Journal of Sports Medicine 26: 247–253

Reagan K M, Meister K, Horodyski M B et al 2002 Humeral retroversion and its relationship to gleno-humeral rotation in the shoulder of college baseball players. The American Journal of Sports Medicine 30(3): 354–360

Riley J, Bommarito P 2004 Position specific training for football: An application to the high school, college, and professional levels. Presentation, National Strength and Conditioning Association Sports Specific Conference, Orlando, 10 January 2004

Rothbart B A 2002 Medial column foot systems: an innovative tool for improving posture. Journal of Bodywork and Movement Therapies 6(1): 37–46

Selye H 1956 The stress of life. McGraw Hill, New York

Thacker S B, Gilchrist J, Stroup D F et al 2004 The impact of stretching on sports injury risk: A systematic review of the literature. Medicine and Science in Sports and Exercise 36(3): 371–378

Thompson B 2005 Ankle pain (chronic) with associated low back pain. In: Chaitow L, DeLany J (eds) Clinical application of neuromuscular techniques – practical case study exercises. Churchill Livingstone, Edinburgh

Wilk K E 2004 Rehabilitation guidelines for the thrower with internal impingement. Presentation, American Sports Medicine Institute Injuries in Baseball Course, 23 January 2004

Wilk K E, Meister K, Andrews J R 2002 Current concepts in the rehabilitation of the overhead athlete. American Journal of Sports Medicine 30(1): 136–151

Young W B, Behm D G 2002 Should static stretching be used during a warm up for strength and power activities? Strength and Conditioning Journal 24(6): 33–37

Further reading

Anderson J E 1983 Grant's atlas of anatomy, 8th edn. Williams and Wilkins, Baltimore

Anderson M K, Hall S J 1995 Sports injury management. Williams and Wilkins, Baltimore

Andrews J R, Harrelson G L, Wilk K E 2004 Physical rehabilitation of the injured athlete, 3rd edn. Saunders, Philadelphia

Apostolopoulos N 2001 Performance flexibility. In: Foran B (ed) High performance sports conditioning. Human Kinetics, Champaign, pp 49–61

Bandy W D, Irion J M, Briggler M 1998 The effect of static stretch and dynamic range of motion training on the flexibility of hamstring muscles. Journal of Orthopaedic and Sports Physical Therapy 27(4): 295–300

Basmajian J V, DeLuca C J 1985 Muscles alive, 5th edn. Williams and Wilkins, Baltimore

Bompa T O 1999 Periodization training for sports. Human Kinetics, Champaign

Brotzman S B, Wilk K E 2003 Clinical orthopaedic rehabilitation. Mosby, Philadelphia

Burkhart S S, Morgan C D, Kibler W B 2000 Shoulder injuries in overhead athletes. The 'dead arm' revisit. Clinical Sports Medicine 19(1): 125–158

Burkhart S S, Morgan C D, Kibler W B 2003 The disabled throwing shoulder: spectrum of pathology. Part I: Pathoanatomy and biomechanics. Arthroscopy 19(4): 404–420

Burkhart S S, Morgan C D, Kibler W B 2003 The disabled throwing shoulder: spectrum of pathology. Part III: The SICK scapula, scapular dyskinesis, the kinetic chain and rehabilitation. Arthroscopy 19(6): 641–661

Chaitow L 2002 Positional release techniques, 2nd edn. Churchill Livingstone, Edinburgh

Chaitow L 2003 Palpation and assessment skills, 2nd edn. Churchill Livingstone, Edinburgh

Chaitow L, DeLany J W 2001 Clinical application of neuromuscular techniques, vol 1: The upper body, 2nd edn. Churchill Livingstone, Edinburgh

Church J B, Wiggins M S, Moode F M et al 2001 Effect of warm-up and flexibility treatments on vertical jump performance. Journal of Strength and Conditioning Research 15(3): 332–336

Colgan M 1993 Optimum sports nutrition. Advanced Research Press, New York

Colgan M 2002 Sports nutrition guide. Apple Publishing Company, Vancouver

Cook G 2001 Baseline sports-fitness testing. In: Foran B (ed) High performance sports conditioning. Human Kinetics, Champaign, pp 19–48

Cramer J T, Housh T J, Johnson G O et al 2004 Acute effects of static stretching on peak torque in women. Journal of Strength and Conditioning Research 18(2): 236–241

Derosa C, Porterfeild J A 1998 Mechanical low back pain: Perspectives in functional anatomy, 2nd edn. Saunders, Philadelphia

Ellenbecker T S 2001 Restoring performance after injury. In: Foran B (ed) High performance sports conditioning. Human Kinetics, Champaign, pp 327–344

Frederick G A, Syzmanski D J 2001 Baseball (part I): Dynamic flexibility. Strength and Conditioning Journal 23(1): 21–30

Goering E, Jones L H, Kusunose R 1995 Jones strain-counterstrain. Jones Strain-Counterstrain, Boise

Janda V 1978 Muscles central nervous regulation and back problems In: Korr I (ed) Neurobiological mechanisms in manipulative therapy. Plenum Press, New York

Kain K, Berns J 1997 Ortho-bionomy: A practical manual. North Atlantic Books, Berkeley

Kendall F P, McCreary E K 1983 Muscle testing and function, 3rd edn. Williams and Wilkins, Baltimore

Knudson D V, Noffal G J, Bahamonde R E et al 2004 Stretching has no effect on tennis serve performance. Journal of Strength and Conditioning Research 18(3): 654–656

Korr I 1980 Neurobiological mechanisms in manipulation. Plenum Press, New York

Leahy P M, Mock L E 1991 Altered biomechanics of the shoulder and subscapularis. Chiropractic Sports Medicine 5(3): 62–66

Liebenson C 1990a Muscular relaxation techniques. Journal of Manipulative and Physiological Therapeutics 12(6): 446–454

Liebenson C 1990b Active muscular relaxation techniques (Part 2). Journal of Manipulative and Physiological Therapeutics 13(1): 2–6

Liebenson C (ed) 1996 Rehabilitation of the spine. Williams and Wilkins, Baltimore

Liebenson C 2001 Sensory motor training. Journal of Bodywork and Movement Therapies 5(1): 21–27

Lukasiewiscz A C, McClure P, Michener L et al 1999 Comparison of 3-dimensional scapular position and orientation between subjects with and without shoulder impingement. Journal of Orthopaedic and Sports Physical Therapy 29(10): 574–586

Lum L C 1987 Hyperventilation syndromes in medicine and psychiatry: a review. Journal of the Royal Society of Medicine 80(4): 229–231

Magee D 1997 Orthopedic physical assessment, 3rd edn. Saunders, Philadelphia

McGill S 2004 Ultimate back fitness and performance. Wabuno, Waterloo

Myers T 2002 Anatomy trains myofascial meridians for manual and movement therapists. Churchill Livingstone, Edinburgh

Norris C 2000 Back stability. Human Kinetics, Champaign

Peri M A, Halford E 2004 Pain and faulty breathing: A pilot study. Journal of Bodywork and Movement Therapies 8(4): 297–306

Sahrmann S A 2002 Diagnosis and treatment of movement impairment syndromes. Williams and Wilkins, Baltimore

Shrier I 1999 Stretching before exercises does not reduce the risk of local muscle injury; a critical review of the clinical and basic science literature. Clinical Journal of Sports Medicine 9(4): 221–227

Simons D, Travell J, Simons L 1999 Myofascial pain and dysfunction: the trigger point manual, vol 1: Upper half of body, 2nd edn. Williams and Wilkins, Baltimore

Travell J, Simons D 1993 Myofascial pain and dysfunction; the trigger point manual, vol 2: The lower extremities. Williams and Wilkins, Baltimore

Solem-Bertott E, Thuomas K A, Westerberg C E 1993 The influence of scapular retraction and protraction on the width of the subacromial space: An MRI study. Clinical Orthopedics 296(Nov): 99–103

Warner J P, Micheli L J, Arslanian L E et al 1992 Scapulothoracic motion in normal shoulders and shoulders with glenohumeral instability and impingement: A study using Moire topographic anaylsis. Clinical Orthopedics 285(Dec): 191–199

Wenos D L, Konin J G 2004 Controlled warm up intensity enhances hip range of motion. Journal of Strength and Conditioning Research 18(3): 529–533

Index

Page numbers in bold indicate pictures.

A

Abdominal muscles, **103**
  strength and coordination, 321, **326**
  see also specific muscle
Acromioclavicular dysfunction, 223–4, **224**
Active isolated stretching (AIS), 4–5
Acute, definition of, 138
Adaptation
  of athletes, 312–13, **313**
  cellular, 25, **25**
  functional and structural, 24
Adductors, thigh, 79–81, **80**, 143–5, **145**
Adenosine triphosphate (ATP), 12
Adhesions, 92
Agency for Healthcare Research and Quality (AHCPR) guidelines, 275–7
Agonists, 11–12
  agonist contract-relax (ACR), 3, 110, 111
  versus contract-relax, 114–15
  contract-relax agonist contract (CRAC), 3, 4, 110, 111, 114–15
Algometrics, 252
Altered movement patterns, 49–50
Analgesia, 14
Ankle
  movement assessment in athletes, 321–2, **327**
  sprains, 281, 282
Antagonists, 3, 4, 11–12
  coactivation of and upright posture, 263–4
  reciprocal inhibition (RI) of, 9
Anterior superior iliac spine (ASIS), **239**, 239–40, **240**

B

Back muscles, **100, 101**
Back of the arm lines, 29, **29**
Ballistic stretching, 5
Banana position, 168, **168**
Barriers, 137
  identifying, 258, **258**
  resistance, 79, **80**
Beal's springing assessment, 66–7, **67**

Arm
  flexors, 191–3, **192**
  movement assessment in athletes, 322, **327**
Assessment, 95
  of ankle movement in athletes, 321–2, **327**
  of arm movement in athletes, 322, **327**
  Beal's springing, 66–7, **67**
  of bind, **80**
  of elbow movement in athletes, 322, **327**
  form/force closure, 233–6, **235, 236**
  of joints, 300
  of knee movement in athletes, 321–2, **327**
  massage methods for, 299–300
  mobility, 11
  muscle shortness, 136–7
  of postural muscles, 140–97
  of shoulder movement in athletes, 322, **327**
  of soft tissues, 43–6, 300
  and use of MET, important notes, 137–40
Athletic injuries, MET treatment of, 311–37
  see also specific problem
Atrophy, muscle, 51

Biceps
  brachii, 193
  tendon, 191–2, **192**
Bind
  assessment of, **80**
  increased, 49–50
  see also Ease and bind
Biomechanical stress, 2
Breathing
  inappropriate, patterns of change with, 61–3, **62**
  instructions to patients, 138–9
  and MET, 86
  paravertebral muscle shortness test, 194, **194**
  scalene observation, 180–1, **181**
Brügger
  facilitation method, 267–8, **268–70**
  relief position, **261**, 261–2, **262**

C

Carpal tunnel syndrome (CTS), 48
Cellular adaptation, 25, **25**
Cervical application of MET, 212–16, **216**
Cervicothoracic (CT) area, 43–4
Chain reactions, dysfunction, 59
Chronic, definition of, 138
Classification models, low-back pain, 274–7
Clenched fists analogy, 33, **33**
Clinical prediction rule (CPR), 276–7
Coactivation of antagonists and upright posture, 263–4
Co-contraction MET method, hamstring treatment, 157
Cold, application of, 117
Collagen, 16–17, 41
Colloids, 41–2
Common compensatory patterns (CCP), 42–6

Compensation, 42–6
Compression, 303, **304**
Concentric contractions, 88, 288
Connective tissue changes, 16–17
Contractions, 51
    concentric, 89, 288
    duration of, 115–16
    force of, 116
    number of, 116
    see also specific type of contraction
    e.g. Isometric contraction
Contract-relax agonist contract
    (CRAC), 3, 4, 110, 111, 114–15
Contract-relax (CR), 3, 4, 8, 110, 111
    versus agonist contract-relax,
      114–15
    immediate effects of, 111–13
    long-term effects of, 113–14
Contraindications of MET, 85–6
Corrective strategies for athletes, 323–31
Coupling, spinal, 214
Creep, 24, 36, 42, 122
Cryotherapy, 117

D

Decompensation, 23–4, 42
Developmental influences on
    hypertonicity, 262–3
Direct action, 11–12
Discomfort, post-treatment, 140
    see also Pain
Drag palpation, 249
Dysfunction
    evolution of musculoskeletal, 46–50
    foot, 38
    nociceptively modulated, 37
    proprioceptive model of, 34, **35**
    route to, 1–2
    spinal, 126–8, 128–9
    in sports, 314–31

E

Ease and bind, 45–6, 78–81
Eccentric isotonic contraction *see*
    Isolytic contraction
Efficacy of MET, 110–20
Effleurage, 303, **304**
Elbow movement assessment in
    athletes, 322, **327**
Electromyographic (EMG) muscle
    activity, 51, 65
Emotions, role of in musculoskeletal
    dysfunction, 32
End-feel, 11, 45, 200

Endurance
    phase, segmental strengthening
      programme, 288
    tests, 57–8, **59**
Erector spinae muscle group, 39, **193**,
    194–5, 195–6
Errors during MET, 84–6
Evaluation *see* Assessment
Evolution of musculoskeletal
    dysfunction, 46–50
Exercises
    ease-bind palpation exercise, 79–81
    home exercise programme (HEP),
      281
    isolytic contraction, 90–1
    in MET, 81–4
    postisometric relaxation (PIR), 82–3
    psoas toning, 149
    reciprocal inhibition (RI), 83–4
    resistance, 283
    William's flexion, 149
Exhalation, 86
    see also Breathing
Eye
    movements, 9, 14, 139
    muscles, pulsed MET for, 187–8

F

Facet joint, 282–3
Facial pain, 60–1
Facilitated stretching, 4
Facilitation, **66**, 257
    and the central nervous system, 68
    local, 67, **67**, 248
    recognising a facilitated area, 66–7
    reflex patterns and, 65
    segmental, 65–6
    of tone in lower shoulder fixators,
      187
Fascia, 39–40, **40**, 63
    fascial trains, Myers', 27–30, **27–30**
    patterns, 42–6
    and posture, 41
    properties of, 40–1
    stiffness in, 17
    tension, 41
Fast muscle fibres, 52
Fatigue, 31
Fear Avoidance Brief Questionnaire
    (FABQ), 274–5
Fibromyalgia, 68–9, 134–5
Fibrosis, 16–17, 92
Firing patterns, 314
Fitness influences on dysfunction, 48–9
Flares, iliosacral, 239–40
Flexibility of athletes, 323–4

Foot dysfunction example, Prior's, 38
Force, patient/therapist, 9, 11–12, 207–8
Form/force closure assessment, 233–6,
    235, 236
Friction, skin, 249
Front of the arm lines, 29–30, **30**
Fryer, Gary, 3
Functional
    adaptation, 24
    problems, 18
    SCM test, 183
    screening tests, 264–5, **264–7**
    unit, Isaacson's, 38–9

G

Gastrocnemius, 141–3, **142, 143, 193**
Gene expression, 25
Gliding, 303, **304**
Global muscles, 55–9
Gluteus
    maximus, **40**, 58
    medius, **40**, 58
Goldthwaite's postural overview, 63–4
Golgi tendon organs, 8, **8**, 9, 19
Goodridge, J., 7
    ease-bind palpation exercise, 79–81
Gothic shoulders, 176
Gracilis, 143–5
Gravity-induced MET, 169–70
Greenman, Philip, 3, 6
    cervical palpation, 214–15, **216**
    TFL treatment, 160–1, **161**
Grids, creating, 26
Grieve's low-back approach, 209–10,
    210

H

Haemophilia, joints damaged by, 202–3
Hamstrings, 154–7, **155**
    acute strain, 334–6, **335**
    assessing for shortness, 143–5, **144**
    contract-relax techniques, 111–13,
      113–14, 114–15
    efficacy of MET, 110
    excessive substitution of, **264**
    massage including MET, 302–3, **303**
    slow eccentric isotonic stretching,
      150
    tight, **193**
Harakal's cooperative isometric
    technique, 208, **208**
Head and neck muscles, **98**
High-velocity/low-amplitude (HVLA)
    thrust, 3, 201, 281

Hip
  abduction test, 159, **159**
  flexors, 145–54, **147, 150–4**
  region measurements, 317–21
History of MET, 3–9
Hold-relax (HR), 4, 8, 257
Home exercise programme (HEP), 282
Hooke's law, 24
Hyperirritable neural feedback, 65, **66**
Hypermobility influences on
    dysfunction, 48–9
Hypertonicity, 47, 49–50, 262–3, 284
Hypertrophy, segmental
    strengthening programme, 288
Hyperventilation, 61–3
Hypotheses, 250
Hypotonia, 48–9

I

Ice massage, 282
Iliac rotation, 241–3
Iliopsoas, 58, 145–6
Iliosacral (IS) joint, 232–43, **238, 239,
    240, 242**
Impairments, addressing, 282–90
Indirect action, 11–12
Ineffective MET, 18
Inflare, iliosacral, 239–40, **240**
Infraspinatus, 187–9, **188, 189**
Inhalation, 86
    see also Breathing
Inhibited muscle chains, 265–8
INIT, 10, 72, 247–54, **253, 254,** 331–3
Injuries, sporting, **330, 331**
  acute injury care, 329–31, 332
  chronic and long-term
    rehabilitation, 332–3
  common, 329
  MET and INIT in, 331–3
  standard care of, 329
Inner range holding tests, 57–8, **59**
Integrated neuromuscular inhibition
    technique (INIT), 10, 72, 247–54,
    253, 254, 331–3
Integrins, 25
Intersegmental muscles, 282
Isaacson' functional unit, 38–9
Ischaemic compression
  piriformis, 163, **165**
  trigger point deactivation, 251–2
  validation, 250–1
Isokinetic contraction, 15, 106–7
  strengthening joint complexes,
    91–2
  strengthening weak postural
    muscles, 333–7

Isolytic contraction, 15–16, **16**
  definition of, 7
  exercises, 90–1
  reduction of fibrotic changes, 92, 102
  segmental strengthening
    programme, 287
  strengthening weak postural
    muscles, 104–6
  tensor fascia lata, 161
Isometric contraction
  definition of, 7
  degree of effort with, 86–7
  effect on skeletal muscle, 8, **8, 9**
  Harakal's approach, 208, **208**
  latency period after, 12
  strengthening weak postural
    muscles, 333–7
  using postisometric relaxation, 96–7
  using reciprocal inhibition, 96,
    97–100
Isotonic
  concentric contraction, 90, 100–2
  contraction, 7, 333–7
  eccentric contraction see Isolytic
    contraction

J

Janda, Vladimir
  hypertonicity, 49–50
  model of muscle imbalance, 260
  postfacilitation stretch method, 14,
    83
  primary and secondary response, 38
  view on strength testing, 87–8
Jaw pain, 60–1
Joints, 140, 197, 216–45
  assessment of, 300
  cervical application of MET, 212–16
  direction of movement, 13, **13**
  dysfunction, 57–9
  MET for, 20–1, 93–4, 199–203
  mobilisation using MET, 204–5
  posterior-anterior (PA) joint
    mobilisations, 281
  preparing for MET, 203–4
  questions and answers, 212
  restriction, basic criteria for
    treating, **205–6,** 205–9, **208–9**
  see also specific joint

K

Kinematic imbalances due to
    suboccipital strain (KISS), 42
Kneading, 303, **304**

Knee movement assessment in
    athletes, 321–2, **327**
Korr, Irwin, 2
  orchestrated movement concept, 33
  trophic influence research, 64
Kuchera, W., 7

L

Lateral line, 28, **28**
Latey, Philip, perspective, 33, **33**
Latissimus dorsi, **40,** 170, **170,** 174–6,
    176
Laxity of soft tissues, 300
Leg muscles, **103, 105, 106**
    see also specific muscle
Levator scapulae, 185–7, **186**
Lewit, Karel, 2, 3–5, 13–14
  TFL palpation, 158–9
  tight-loose thinking, 45–6
  use of postisometric relaxation
    (PIR), 83
Liebenson, Craig, 2, 3
Local muscles, 55–9
Locomotor system, 2
Loose-tight concept, 45–6, 78–81
Low-back
  low-back pain (LBP), 201–2, 273–80
    massage with MET, 306–9
    staging, 281–91
  MET and the, 209–12
  strain, 333–4
Lower crossed syndrome, 59–60, **60,** 263
Lumbar
  dysfunction, 207
  spine, **205**
  see also Low-back
Lumbosacral (LS) area, 44

M

Manual resistance techniques (MRT),
    257–71
    see also MET
Maps, creating, 26
Massage therapy setting, MET in,
    299–309
McAtee, Robert, 4
Mechanical stress, 2
MET
  basic exercises in, 82–4
  contraindications of, 84–5
  efficacy of, 110–20
  errors during, 84–6
  history of, 3–9
  important notes on, 137–40

MET—cont'd
  in massage therapy setting, 299–309
  in physical therapy setting, 273–95
  research, 109–10, 120–9, 133–5,
    200–3, 274–80
  terminology, 7
  in treatment of athletic injuries,
    311–37
Metatarsophalangeal joints (MTPJ), 38
Mitchell, Fred Snr, 3, 6
  strength test, 87–8, 146
Mobilisation with impulse, 3
Mobilisers, 54–5, 88
Mobility assessments, 11
Modes of massage, 301–2
Multifidus group, 39, 283
Muscle
  atrophy, 51
  chains, inhibited, 265–8
  different stress response of, 50–9
  direction of movement, 13, **13**
  effect of isometric contraction on,
    8, **8**, **9**
  energy sources, 12
  imbalance, 54, 57, 260–8
  intersegmental, 282
  maps, 107
  property change, 122–5
  resting, 165
  shortness, 57, 136–7
  stress response of, 50–9
  tone and contraction, 19
  working and resting, 165
  see also specific muscle/muscle group
Muscle energy techniques *see* MET
Musculoskeletal system, 2
Myers' fascial trains, 27–30, **27–30**
Myofascial
  extensibility, 110–18, 120–6, 128
  myofascial pain syndrome (MPS),
    68–9
  pain, 9, 134, **135**
  release, 12
  see also Fascia

N

Navicular drop test, 321–2, **327**
Neck muscles, **98**, **101**
  extensors, 196
  flexors, 196
Neuromuscular re-education,
  segmental strengthening
  programme, 288
Neuromuscular technique (NMT), 10, 16
Newton's third law, 24
Nociceptors, 34–8

Nottingham Health Profile
  Questionnaire, 278

O

Ober's test, 158, **158**
Objectives of manual treatment, 135–6
Observation, 57–8, 159, **159**
  levator scapulae, 185–6
  scalenes, 180–1
Occipitoatlantal (OA) area, 43
Oculopelvic reflexes, 38
Orchestrated movement concept,
  Korr's, 33
Oscillation, 303, **304**
Oswestry Disability Index (ODI), 274–5
Outflare, iliosacral, 239, 240–1, **241**

P

Pain, 14, 31
  during application of MET, 138
  facial and jaw, 60–1
  low-back *see* Low-back pain
  modulation, 281–4
  myofascial, 9, 68–9, 134, **135**
  pain/spasm cycle, 281
  spinal, 119–20, 126–7
  and the tight-loose concept, 46
Palpation, 11
  cervical, 214–15, **216**
  locating trigger points, 248–9
  piriformis, 162–3
  rib, **227**, 227–8, **228**
  skills, 78–84
  tensor fascia lata, 158–9
  three finger 'stacked,' 284–6, **286**
Paravertebral muscles, **193**, 193–7
Patient errors during MET, 84
Patterns
  of dysfunction, 59–64, 64–72
  of muscular imbalance, 57
  uncompensated, 43
Pectineus, 143–5
Pectoralis major, **170**, 170–5, **171**, **172**,
  174
Pelvic joint, 236–7
Pelviocular reflexes, 38
Percussion, 303, **304**
Petrissage, 303, **304**
Phasic muscles, 50–5
Physical therapy setting, MET in,
  273–95
Piriformis, **162**, 162–6, **163**, **165**
PNF *see* Proprioceptive
  neuromuscular facilitation

Post-contraction inhibition *see*
  Postisometric relaxation (PIR)
Post-contraction stretch, 116–17
Posterior-anterior (PA) joint
  mobilisations, 281
Postfacilitation stretch, 14, 97
Postisometric relaxation (PIR), **8**, 8–9,
  258–9
  basic exercise in MET, 82–3
  comparison to AIS, 4
  hypertonic muscles, 12
  Lewit's PIR method, 13–14
Post-treatment
  discomfort, 140
  interventions, 282
Postural
  changes, 32
  correction, **261**, 261–2, **262**
  imbalances, 46, **47**
  muscles, 50–5, **53**, 88, **193**
    sequential assessment and MET
      treatment, 140–97
    strengthening weak, 333–7
  patterns, 42–6
  problems, 18, **18**
Posture, 41
Practitioner errors in application of
  MET, 84
Prayer test, 225, **226**
Pre-season screen for athletes, 315
Preventative strategies for athletes,
  323–31, 331–2
Primary responses, Janda's, 38
Prior's foot dysfunction example, 38
Progressive resisted exercise *see*
  Isokinetic contraction
Proprioceptive neuromuscular
  facilitation (PNF), 3
  in athletes, 323
  facilitated stretching, 4
  rehabilitation, 257, **259**, 259–60
  spiral stretch, 221–2
Proprioceptor responses, 34, **35**
Psoas
  self-treatment, 153–4, **154**
  strength testing and toning
    exercise, 146–9, **147**, **149**
  treatment of, 150–3, **151**, **152**, **153**, **264**
Pulsed muscle energy technique, 10,
  89–90, 187–8

Q

Quadrant method, segmental
  strengthening, **283**, 283–4
Quadratus lumborum, 166–70, **167**,
  169, **264**

Quadriceps, massage including MET, 302, **302, 303**

R

Range of motion, 200–1
Rapid rhythmic resistive deduction, 10, 89–90, 187–8
Reciprocal inhibition (RI), 4, 8–9, **9**
    basic exercise in MET, 83–4
    variation, 15
Reciprocal innervation, 283
Recovery techniques for athletes, 327
Rectus femoris, 145–6, **147**, 149–50, **150**
Reflex, 19–20
    muscle relaxation, 120–2
    patterns, 65
    pelviocular and oculopelvic, 38
Rehabilitation, 65
    manual resistance techniques in, 257–71
    postural and phasic muscles, 53–4
    sporting injuries, 332–3
Relaxation, 13–14
    of soft tissues, 12
Release of soft tissues shortening, 12
Release techniques, 12
Research, MET, 109–10
    evidence, 133–5, 200–3
    low-back pain, 274–80
    into mechanisms of therapeutic effect, 120–9
Resistance, 10, 13–14
    exercise, 283
Respiratory synkinesis, 139
    see also Breathing
Resting muscles, 165
Restriction barrier *see* Barriers
Rhomboids, **40**
Rib dysfunction, 226–32, **227, 228**
    depressed ribs, 230–1, **231**
    elevated ribs, 229–30, **230**, 231–2, **232**
    restricted ribs, 229, **229**, 229–31
Rocking, 303, **304**
Ruddy, T. J., 3, 5–6
    pulsed MET, 10, 89–90, 187–8

S

Sacroiliac (SI) joint, 232–43, **234, 235, 236, 238**
Sacrotuberous, **40**
Sarcomeres, 2
Scalenes, 180–3, **181, 182**
Screening tests, 264–5, **264–7**
    in athletes, 315–23, **319–23**

Secondary responses, Janda's, 38
Segmental-specific strengthening, 283–90, **284, 287, 289–90, 291–5**
Self-treatment, **94**, 94–5
    psoas, 153–4, **154**
    quadratus lumborum, 169–70
    temporomandibular joint, 244–5
    tensor fascia lata, 162
Selye's concepts, 250
Semi-membranosus, 143–5
Semi-tendinosus, 143–5
Serratus posterior inferior, **40**
Shaking, 303, **304**
Shifting, 46
Shortened muscle, 57, 136–7
Shoulder
    abduction, 220
    adduction, **218**, 220
    circumduction with compression, **218**, 219
    circumduction with traction, **218**, 219–20
    extension, **217**, 218–19
    flexion, **217**, 219
    gothic, 176
    internal rotation, **218**, 220–1
    movement assessment in athletes, 322, **327**
    Spencer shoulder sequence, 3, **217–18**, 217–21
    spiral stretch, 221–2, **222**
    tendonitis, 336–7
Shrug test, 224, **225**
Side-effects of MET, 85–6
Skiers, muscular imbalances in, 54
Skin friction, 249
Slow eccentric isotonic stretching (SEIS), 16
    example of, 91
    of the hamstrings, 150, 157
    neck flexors, 196
    pectoralis major, 174
    for strengthening weak postural muscles, 104–6
    see also Isolytic contraction
Slow muscle fibres, 52
Slow stretching, 41–2
Soft tissues, assessment of, 300
Soleus, 141–3, **142, 193**
Somatic dysfunction, 34
Spasm, 49–50, 51
    pain/spasm cycle, 281
    psoas, 148
Specific adaptation to imposed demands (SAID), 25, 312
Spencer shoulder sequence, 3, **217–18**, 217–21

Spine
    coupling concepts, 214
    dysfunction, 126–8, 128–9 *see also* Low-back pain
    measurements, 315–17, **324–5**
    MET applied to the, 118–20
    motion, 38–9
Spiral
    lines, 28, **28**
    stretch, 221–2, **222**
Splenius
    capitis, **40**
    cervicis, **40**
Sport-induced compensation, 44–5
Sporting injuries *see* Injuries, sporting
Spring test for levator scapulae, 185
Squat test, 142
Stabilisers, 54–5
Staging, 274, 281–91
STAR palpation, 248–9
Static stretching, 5, 323–4
Sternoclavicular dysfunction, 224–6, **225, 226**
Sternocleidomastoid (SCM), 183–5, **185**
Sternosymphyseal syndrome, 261, **261**
Stiles, Edward, 6–7
    whiplash and MET, 213–14
Strain
    acute hamstring, 334–6, **335**
    low-back, 333–4
    suboccipital, 42
    on tissues, 24
Strain/counterstrain (SCS), 252–3
Strength
    influences on dysfunction, 48–9
    testing, 87–8
        Mitchell's strength test, 146
        piriformis, 163
        psoas strength test, 146–9, **147, 148**
    training, excessive, 314–15
Strengthening, 18
    segmental-specific, 283–90, **284, 289–95**
    variation, 15
Stress, 32
    factors leading to musculoskeletal dysfunction, 46–8, **47**
    fascial, 41
    response of muscles, 50–9
    on tissues, 24
Stressors, 247–8
Stretch, 13
    sensitivity, increased, 51
    tolerance, 125–6
Stretching, 18, 139–40
    slow, 41–2
    static, 323–4
    variations, 4

Structural adaptation, 24
Studies, review of, 278–80
Subscapularis, 189–90, **191**
Superficial back line (SBL), 27, **27**
Superficial front line (SFL), 27, **27**
Supraspinatus, 191, **191**
Symptoms, viewing in context, 31–42

T

TART palpation, 249
Temporomandibular joint (TMJ), 60–1,
 61, 243–5, **244**
Tendonitis, shoulder, 336–7
Tendons, 18–20
Tension
 fascial, 41
 muscle, 51
Tensor fascia lata (TFL), **147, 158,**
 158–62, **160, 264**
Terms used in MET, 7
Thigh muscles, **103**
Thoracic
 area, 63, **206**
 cage release, 232, **232**
 spine, **205**
 thoracic outlet syndrome (TOS),
 48

Thoracolumbar (TL) area, 44, 195
Three-dimensional patterns, 46
Three finger 'stacked' palpation, 284–6,
 286
Tight-loose concept, 45–6
Tissue preference assessment, 43–6
Tone, 92
 increased, 49–50
 toning exercise, psoas, 149
Transcutaneous electrical nerve
 stimulation (TENS), 282
Trapezius, upper, 176–80, **177, 178, 179**
Trigger points, 14, 40, **67**
 characteristics of, 69–72
 fibromyalgia and, 68–9
 locating and treating, 248–54, **253,**
 254
 myofascial, 46, 62, **62,** 65–8, 247–8
 target areas, **70–1**
 treatment of, 9
Trunk muscles, **101, 104**

U

Uncompensated patterns, 43
Upper chest breathing, 61–3
Upper crossed syndrome, 59–60, **60,**
 263, **263**

V

Van Buskirk's nociceptive model, 34–8
Vertebral column, movement of, 39
Viscoelasticity, 122–5, 139
Visual synkinesis, 14, 180
 see also Eye movements

W

Warm-up for athletes, 325
Water and fascial stiffness, 17
Weakening, muscle, 57
Weakness
 factor, 88
 influences on dysfunction, 48–9
Whiplash injury, 213–14
Williams' flexion exercises, 278–80
Wolff's law, 24
Working muscles, 165

Y

Yale, Sandra, 6
Yoga stretching, 5

Minimum system requirements

Windows®
Windows 98 or higher
Pentium® processor-based PC
16 MB RAM (32 MB recommended)
10 MB of available hard-disk space
2 X or faster DVD-ROM drive
VGA monitor supporting thousands of colours (16-bit)

Macintosh®
Apple Power Macintosh
Mac OS version 9 or later
64 MB of available RAM
10 MB of available hard-disk space
2 X or faster DVD-ROM drive

NB: No data is transferred to the hard disk.
The DVD-ROM is self-contained and the application runs directly from the DVD-ROM.

Installation instructions

Windows®
If you have enabled DVD-ROM autoplay on your system then the DVD-ROM will run automatically when inserted into your DVD-ROM drive. If you have not enabled autoplay, click on My Computer and double-click on your DVD-Rom drive. Your DVD-ROM drive should be represented by an icon labeled 'MET'.

Macintosh®
If you have enabled DVD-ROM autoplay on your system then the DVD-ROM will run automatically when inserted into your DVD-ROM drive. If you have not enabled Autoplay, click on the DVD-ROM icon that appears on your desktop, then click on 'MET' to open the application.

To enable the DVD-ROM to autorun, select the Control Panels from the Apple menu on your desktop. Select QuickTime settings, then select Autoplay. Click the Enable DVD-ROM Autoplay checkbox, and then save the settings.

Using this Product

Software Requirements
This product is designed to run with Internet Explorer 5.0 or later (PC) and Netscape 4.5 or later (Mac). Please refer to the help files on those programs for problems specific to the browser.

To use some of the functions on the DVD, the user must have the following:

a. DVD requires "Java Runtime Environment" to be installed in your system to use "Export" and "Slide Show" features. DVD automatically checks for "Java Runtime Environment" version 1.4.1 or later (PC) and MRJ 2.2.5 (Mac) if not available, it starts installing from the DVD. Please complete the installation process. Then click on the license agreement to proceed. "Java Runtime Environment" is available in the DVD's Software folder. If the user manually installs the software, please make sure that the user starts the application by clicking 'MET.exe'.

b. Your browser needs to be Java-enabled. If the user did not enable Java when installing your browser, the user may need to download some additional files from your browser manufacturer.

c. If your system does not support Autorun, then please explore the DVD contents, click on 'MET.exe' to start.

d. QuickTime version 6 or later must be installed in order to view the video clips. A version of QuickTime is available from www.apple.com/quicktime.

Acrobat Reader can be installed from the Software folder of the DVD.

Viewing Images
You can view images by chapter and export images to PowerPoint or an HTML presentation. Full details are available in the Help section of the DVD-Rom.

Technical Support
Technical support for this product is available between 7.30 a.m. and 7.00 p.m. CST, Monday through Friday.

Before calling, be sure that your computer meets the minimum system requirements to run this software.

Inside the United States and Canada, call 1-800-692-9010.
Inside the United Kingdom, call 00-800-692-90100.
Outside North America, call +1-314-872-8370.
You may also fax your questions to +1-314-997-5080, or contact Technical Support through e-mail:
technical.support@elsevier.com.